Promoting Integrated Healthcare Systems Through Team-Based Healthcare

Katsumi Fujitani
Bunkyo Gakuin University, Japan

Dawn Prentice
Brock University, Canada

IGI Global
Scientific Publishing
Publishing Tomorrow's Research Today

Vice President of Editorial	Melissa Wagner
Director of Acquisitions	Mikaela Felty
Director of Book Development	Jocelynn Hessler
Production Manager	Mike Brehm
Cover Design	Jose Rosado

Published in the United States of America by
IGI Global Scientific Publishing
701 East Chocolate Avenue
Hershey, PA, 17033, USA
Tel: 717-533-8845 | Fax: 717-533-7115
Website: https://www.igi-global.com E-mail: cust@igi-global.com

Library of Congress Cataloging-in-Publication Data

Names: Fujitani, Katsumi, 1959- editor http://id.loc.gov/rwo/agents/n2025016032 | Prentice, Dawn (Nurse), 1960- editor http://id.loc.gov/rwo/agents/n2025016033
Title: Promoting integrated healthcare systems through team-based healthcare / edited by Katsumi Fujitani, Dawn Prentice.
Description: Hershey, PA : IGI Global Scientific Publishing, [2026] | Includes bibliographical references and index. | Summary: "This book attempts to visualize the actual state of multi-professional collaboration in healthcare by making full use of existing indicators, established and proven metrics, and to clarify its specific content of interprofessional collaboration"-- Provided by publisher.
Identifiers: LCCN 2024057203 (print) | LCCN 2024057204 (ebook) | ISBN 9798369322307 hardcover | ISBN 9798369322314 ebook
Subjects: LCSH: Health care teams http://id.loc.gov/authorities/subjects/sh85059533 | Health services administration http://id.loc.gov/authorities/subjects/sh85059600
Classification: LCC R729.5.H4 P76 2025 (print) | LCC R729.5.H4 (ebook) | DDC 362.1068--dc23/eng/20250409
LC record available at https://lccn.loc.gov/2024057203
LC ebook record available at https://lccn.loc.gov/2024057204

British Cataloguing in Publication Data
A Cataloguing in Publication record for this book is available from the British Library.

Table of Contents

Detailed Table of Contents

The importance of team based healthcare and collaborative practice has globally received more attention since the release of the World Health Organization's (2010) Framework for action on Interprofessional education and collaborative practice. Studies reporting the many advantages to healthcare teams working collaboratively to promote patient-centered care and improve patient outcomes have also been published. In this introductory chapter the origins of teamwork will be discussed as well as the advantages of implementing team based health care and collaborative practice in clinical settings.

A theory is a system of reasoning based on clear facts, such as principles or laws, that describes, explains, elucidates, prescribes, or organizes a particular phenomenon (Walker & Avant, 2005). Theories also clarify various aspects of a phenomenon and provide a framework for understanding them. Furthermore, theories create complex and comprehensive understandings of phenomena that cannot be easily explained, such as how a particular culture works, how an organization functions, or why individuals interact in a certain way. Over the past few years, the use of theory in the interprofessional field has evolved and matured (Reeves & Hearn, 2013). This chapter reviews the foundational and related theories to better understand team-based healthcare.

This chapter provides an overview into collaborative leadership, its evolving impact on organizations and teams. A discussion is provided on defining collaborative

Addressing complex and systemic problems like health disparities require interdisciplinary, translational, and team-based approaches that take account of the social, cultural, economic, and environmental factors contributing to the persistence of such problems. By crossing disciplinary boundaries, researchers and stakeholders can integrate multiple perspectives into comprehensive solutions that can be translated into practice with a higher likelihood of reducing health disparities. Successful interdisciplinary collaboration hinges upon effective communication and leadership practices. In centering communication as a foundation for successful interdisciplinary and translational activities, this chapter considers the ways in which leadership—enacted through the design of strategies, processes, messages, and structures—may enable collaborative research efforts that productively address health disparities. The exploratory framework introduced in this chapter can help to inform the design of future initiatives for addressing health disparities across disciplines and with communities.

This study aims to identify factors that influence inter-professional collaboration (IPC) through text mining. While initial analysis using Co-occurrence networks captured the relevance of many words, it proved too complex to interpret. To address this issue, the researchers introduced coding rules to simplify the visualization of textual data and identified key concepts that support effective collaboration. In addition, correspondence analysis revealed significant differences in perceptions of collaboration based on professional roles and years of clinical experience. The finding underscores the importance of diverse perspectives within the healthcare team. While recognizing the limitations of text mining, our study recommends its use as a valuable complement to traditional quantitative approaches to understanding complex IPC structures.

Interprofessional collaboration includes relationships and decision making among health professionals, patients, families, and communities. Because its aim of high-quality care is consistent with acting in the best interest of patients, interprofessional collaboration is inherently ethical. Ethical knowledge is an important guidepost for interprofessional education, behaviors, and decision making. Interprofessional collaboration, however, also requires awareness of the impact of culture, context, emotion, disciplinary values and beliefs, and legal-centric views on the provision of ethical interprofessional, patient-centred care and on interprofessional relationships. This chapter discusses integration of ethics within interprofessional collaboration and decision making. Consideration is given to ethical theoretical frameworks and concepts and their application within interprofessional relationships and collaboration, as well as to the global predominance of traditional Western bioethics and informed consent and their limitations in selected cultural contexts.

The chapter studies how transformational leadership influences Human Resource Management practices within the organizational culture of Ethiopian healthcare. With data from 385 healthcare practitioners the research uses quantitative methods to analyze the connections between transformational leadership methods while studying human resource management and organizational culture. The Kaiser-Meyer-Olkin (KMO) test shows ideal data suitability for factor analysis. The research validates transformational leadership and organizational culture constructs through Confirmatory Factor Analysis to verify they produce reliable and valid results. Our SEM analysis with AMOS measures how transformational leadership affects HRM success paths mediated by organizational culture. Our analysis shows that when leaders embrace transformational behaviors they help HR practices with support cultures which create better employee work results and higher satisfaction. HRM systems in healthcare organizations and provides needed guidance for Ethiopian health care administrators.

The paper examines the adoption of Evidence-Based Management (EBM) as a fundamental model in healthcare management, emphasising evidence-based principles to address organisational strengths and weaknesses. EBM enables managers to navigate complex healthcare systems by systematically observing phenomena, formulating hypotheses and collecting data. It promotes effective multidisciplinary collaboration through mutual trust, psychological safety, clear objectives and meaningful work. By promoting social capital, organisational learning and collaborative leadership, EBM addresses systemic challenges, improves the quality of decision-making and aligns with sustainability principles, ensuring a dynamic and ethical response to the demands of the healthcare sector.

The rapid advancement of Artificial Intelligence (AI) and the increasing complexity of healthcare systems necessitate a shift from system-centric models to dynamic, team-based approaches for integrated healthcare. This chapter introduces a conceptual and theoretical framework that merges AI capabilities, team-based healthcare models, and dynamic capabilities to create sustainable, patient-centered healthcare systems. It explores the role of AI in enhancing collaboration, decision-making, and operational efficiency while addressing the challenges of siloed healthcare practices.

In this chapter, the researchers focus on the relationship between collaborative leadership and team-based healthcare implementation, while giving special attention to the role of Inter-professional education in the region of Horn of Africa. The research has a sample size of 390 respondents and employs KMO measure of

Preface

INTRODUCTION

In recent years, "team-based healthcare" has become a widely accepted concept—almost an assumed norm across healthcare systems worldwide. Yet, despite this consensus, a critical question remains largely unanswered: *What makes team-based healthcare effective?* And further, *how is such care actually delivered in real-world clinical settings?*

This book emerges from our shared effort to address those very questions. Our research team took on the challenge of examining the efficiency of interdisciplinary teamwork in healthcare and, importantly, of making its outcomes visible through empirical indicators and proven frameworks. Our aim is to contribute meaningful insights into how integrated care systems can thrive through genuine interprofessional collaboration (IPC).

Improving the quality and safety of care is a global imperative, and organizations such as the World Health Organization (WHO) emphasize the centrality of team collaboration in achieving that goal. This volume draws on both international theory and grounded data—most notably from Japan and Canada—to explore the structure, function, and impact of team-based practices in healthcare environments.

We began this research with several key assumptions about the nature of IPC. From there, we moved toward a more detailed articulation of how multidisciplinary collaboration can and should evolve. As healthcare professionals well know, the healthcare system is uniquely complex. Unlike many other industries, clinical environments are defined by frequent task interruptions, multiple simultaneous demands, unpredictable patient conditions, high-stakes decisions, immense informational loads, and time pressure—all occurring under conditions of constant tension and risk.

In such demanding contexts, four essential pillars sustain effective team-based care:

1. Mutual Trust – The foundation of open communication and error tolerance;
2. Psychological Safety – A climate where ideas and concerns can be freely shared;
3. Structure and Clear Goals – A framework that ensures every team member knows their role and objectives;
4. Meaningful Work and Impact – A shared sense that individual contributions matter to both the organization and the people it serves.

Our research included surveys conducted across approximately ten healthcare facilities in Japan and Canada, grounded in indices developed by Canadian researchers. A notable aspect of this project was the implementation of an interdisciplinary education program in Canada, built on the theoretical underpinnings explored in this book.

One recurring finding was the strong influence of psychological safety and workplace social capital on successful IPC. When team members feel safe to speak up and connect meaningfully with colleagues, collaborative leadership becomes more effective, and interprofessional relationships flourish. These findings highlight the vital role of workplace culture—not just in communication, but in shaping the very capacity for learning and adaptation within healthcare organizations.

This book is intended for a wide range of readers: healthcare researchers, clinical practitioners, and students across disciplines—doctors, nurses, dentists, pharmacists, caregivers, occupational and physical therapists, and more. It also serves as a resource for educators and healthcare administrators designing programs to foster effective team-based care.

A Japanese edition is also planned. With over two million healthcare professionals in Japan—including approximately 1.5 million nurses—we hope this work will support not only awareness of team-based healthcare but also the implementation of training programs that instill its core principles.

What makes this book distinctive is its integration of theoretical insight, practical application, and cross-national perspective. We believe it provides a comprehensive and useful resource for understanding the "why," "what," and "how" of team medicine, and the many forms it takes across real-world healthcare systems.

We are grateful to the many professionals and institutions that contributed to this effort, and we invite you—the reader—to explore how true interprofessional collaboration can transform not only teams, but the entire landscape of healthcare.

ORGANIZATION OF THE BOOK

This volume brings together a collection of interdisciplinary perspectives and empirical research aimed at advancing our understanding of team-based healthcare

(TBHC). The following chapters offer both theoretical grounding and practical insights for enhancing interprofessional collaboration (IPC) across diverse healthcare contexts.

We begin in Chapter 1 with an *Introduction to Team-Based Healthcare*. Here, the foundations and global relevance of collaborative practice are traced, particularly following the release of the WHO's 2010 framework on Interprofessional Education and Collaborative Practice. The chapter revisits the origins of teamwork in healthcare, highlighting the growing body of evidence supporting its benefits in improving patient-centered outcomes and overall care quality.

Chapter 2 deepens this conversation by examining the *Theoretical Foundations of Team-Based Healthcare*. Drawing from multiple disciplines, this chapter reviews essential theories that explain and contextualize how healthcare professionals interact, collaborate, and organize themselves within complex systems. It provides a necessary framework for understanding both the mechanics and the deeper implications of IPC.

Chapter 3 explores *Collaborative Leadership Within Team Learning*, focusing on leadership as a pivotal mechanism for team success. The chapter presents both theoretical and measurement-oriented perspectives on collaborative leadership, illustrating how it serves as a bridge between individual learning and team learning within clinical environments.

To support robust implementation of IPC, Chapter 4 addresses the critical issue of *Measuring and Evaluating Team Performance in Healthcare Practice*. This chapter presents the development and validation of two Japanese-language tools—AITCSII-J and AICLS-J—which reliably assess interprofessional collaboration and leadership. These tools represent a significant advancement for cross-cultural IPC research and practice evaluation.

In Chapter 5, the focus turns to *Interprofessional Education (IPE) and Collaborative Practice*. Recognizing that education is central to cultivating effective teams, the chapter reviews the evolution of IPE and its current challenges. It suggests pathways for future educational innovation that foster collaboration-ready healthcare professionals.

Chapter 6 shifts our attention to population health by addressing *Interprofessional Collaboration and Health Disparities in Public Health Interventions*. The chapter proposes a leadership framework for designing inclusive, cross-sectoral strategies aimed at reducing health disparities. It positions communication and leadership as essential tools in building equitable, community-engaged healthcare responses.

Implementation challenges take center stage in Chapter 7, which investigates the *Facilitators and Barriers of Team-Based Healthcare* using innovative text-mining and correspondence analysis methods. The chapter reveals how perceptions of collaboration vary by professional background and experience, offering new tools for navigating and strengthening IPC in diverse clinical settings.

Ethics are the focus of Chapter 8, titled *Interprofessional Collaboration: Ethical Knowing and Working Together*. This chapter explores the ethical dimensions of IPC, particularly the interplay between cultural values, professional norms, and patient-centered care. It also critically examines the dominance of Western bioethics and advocates for more inclusive, context-sensitive ethical frameworks.

Turning to leadership in emerging systems, Chapter 9 presents a case study on the *Transformational Leadership Effect on Human Resource Management in Ethiopia's Healthcare Sector*. The chapter offers valuable insights into how leadership styles can shape organizational culture and HR outcomes in resource-constrained settings.

In Chapter 10, the authors explore *Evidence-Based Management (EBM)* as a strategic model for multidisciplinary collaboration. This chapter highlights how EBM supports more ethical, data-driven, and psychologically safe environments where collaboration thrives and organizational learning is cultivated.

Chapter 11 pushes the boundaries of traditional system thinking in *Beyond Systems: Rethinking Integrated Healthcare with Team-Based Approaches, AI, and Dynamic Capabilities*. This conceptual chapter proposes a new model that integrates artificial intelligence and team-based care, arguing for a more adaptive, responsive, and patient-centered approach to complex healthcare systems.

Chapter 12 brings a regional focus to our discussion with an investigation into *Collaborative Leadership and Interprofessional Education in the Horn of Africa*. This empirical study uses structural equation modeling to show how leadership and education interact to enhance team-based healthcare implementation, particularly in low-resource environments.

Finally, Chapter 13 closes the volume by casting a forward-looking lens on *The Future of Interprofessional Collaboration*. The chapter addresses systemic enablers and barriers to IPC, underscores the importance of leadership commitment across both clinical and educational institutions, and speculates on the transformative role of artificial intelligence in shaping future care teams.

Together, these chapters provide a comprehensive, multi-layered understanding of what it takes to promote, implement, and sustain team-based healthcare across diverse contexts and cultures. We hope this collection will serve as a valuable resource for healthcare professionals, educators, researchers, and policy makers committed to advancing integrated healthcare systems through interprofessional collaboration.

CONCLUSION

As we bring this preface to a close, we wish to emphasize that *Promoting Integrated Healthcare Systems Through Team-Based Healthcare* is more than a compilation of academic chapters—it is a collective effort to reimagine how healthcare professionals learn, lead, and work together in increasingly complex and interdependent systems.

Each contribution in this volume reflects a shared commitment to improving healthcare outcomes by advancing interprofessional collaboration (IPC) at all levels—from education and leadership development to system design and front-line practice. Whether rooted in theory, empirical research, or practice-based reflection, these chapters reinforce the idea that collaboration is not incidental to high-quality care—it is fundamental to it.

The global nature of our contributors and case studies—from Japan and Canada to Ethiopia and the Horn of Africa—demonstrates that while healthcare systems differ in structure and resources, the core principles of trust, psychological safety, shared purpose, and meaningful work resonate universally. These pillars provide the scaffolding for effective team-based healthcare and the foundation for a culture of mutual respect, ongoing learning, and ethical accountability.

We hope this book serves not only as a resource for those already engaged in IPC but also as an invitation to those just beginning their journey. Whether you are a clinician, educator, researcher, or policymaker, we trust that the insights offered here will support your efforts to foster more collaborative, patient-centered, and resilient healthcare systems.

It is a great pleasure to be able to make the IPC content as up-to-date as possible in the complex and rapidly changing world of healthcare. We are greatly indebted to the contributors to this book, and we hope that they will be as pleased with the overall outcome of our collaboration as we are. We would like to thank the great Canadian researchers and colleagues, such as Dawn and Carole, and for encouraging our interprofessional research. We would especially like to thank our good friend and research colleague, Dr. Hironobu Matsushita. I am also indebted to the editors who have been so strict in ensuring that each chapter author and editor met their deadlines and delivered the book on time. Finally, I pray for peace and glory in heaven to my beloved my parents, Akira and Sachiko, who gave me life in this world and took their eternal journey to heaven several years ago.

In closing, we thank our contributors for their dedication and scholarship, and we thank you—the reader—for your interest in shaping the future of healthcare through the power of the team.

Chapter 1
Introduction to Team-Based Healthcare

Dawn Prentice
Brock University, Canada

ABSTRACT

The importance of team based healthcare and collaborative practice has globally received more attention since the release of the World Health Organization's (2010) Framework for action on Interprofessional education and collaborative practice. Studies reporting the many advantages to healthcare teams working collaboratively to promote patient-centered care and improve patient outcomes have also been published. In this introductory chapter the origins of teamwork will be discussed as well as the advantages of implementing team based health care and collaborative practice in clinical settings.

INTRODUCTION TO TEAM BASED HEALTHCARE

Throughout my 40-year career in nursing, I have worked with many teams in different healthcare settings in Canada ranging from critical care areas to rehabilitation and community settings. I have also had the opportunity to work in teams in the academic setting. Reflecting upon my experiences, I have worked with teams that functioned well and some teams that did function as well. For the teams that functioned well, there was excellent communication and collaboration among the members, respect for each team member's role and their area of expertise, and most importantly from my perspective, the shared, common goal of patient-centred care, whether taught, facilitated organizationally, or directly delivered.

The idea of team collaboration in the practice setting is not new; patients have been cared for by teams for many years. Forty years ago, Simms et al. (1984) ad-

DOI: 10.4018/979-8-3693-2230-7.ch001

dressed the need for making collaborative practice a reality in the clinical setting and the importance of collaboration to patient care. Furthermore, they discussed the need to focus on understanding the elements that make collaborative practice function well and recommended the need for further research to examine patient outcomes and healthcare provider outcomes resulting from collaborative practice (Simms et al., 1984).

For well over one hundred- and fifty-years physicians and nurses have worked together in hospitals (Helmstadter, 2002). Traditionally in the physician-nurse working relationship, there was a clear hierarchical structure with the physician being in charge and the nurse being in a subordinate role. The inequality in power between the two roles, without doubt, impacted on communication about patient care needs (Keddy et al., 1986) and was not seen as collaborative. Perceptions of power structures and hierarchy still exist in the workplace and can create barriers to interprofessional collaboration (Gergerich et al., 2019). This may may impact what healthcare workers communicate, as some individuals carefully consider what message would be appropriate to convey in a situation because of the continuing existence of power structures (Essex et al., 2023).

Since 2010, when the World Health Organization [WHO] released their initial paper on interprofessional education and practice, there has been increased emphasis on collaborative relationships not only between physicians and nurses but with the entire healthcare team. Many factors account for the need to have all healthcare professionals collaborate: the evolution of technology in patient care (Voyer, 2013), the complexity of patient care needs due to multiple patient co-morbidities (van Klaveren et al., 2024), and the escalating costs of health care (O'Rourke et al., 2018). These factors have necessitated that all healthcare providers work together to deliver safe and quality patient care, while bearing in mind the fiscal realities in healthcare. Moreover, with the emphasis on quality outcomes for patients (Wei et al., 2022), healthcare providers must focus on both system and patient outcomes such as decreasing length of stay in hospitals, increasing safety, preventing harm and error, and reducing infection rates (Musgrove et al., 2024; Srisatidnarakul et al., 2021;Walter et al., 2022), all of which has further underscored the need to have a collaborative practice environment where clear and timely communication among team members is paramount and the expertise of various team members is optimally and fully operationalized.

The structure of healthcare teams varies in hospital settings depending on the organization and model of care and this can contribute to initial difficulties with team formation, but these challenges are not insurmountable to collaborating well as a team. For example, in one rehabilitation healthcare setting, the structure is such that all healthcare providers (e.g., physiotherapists, occupational therapists) may be part of a core team situated on a unit with the foci of meeting the rehabilitation goals of the patient and on discharge planning (Dyer et al. 2020), whereas with other models of care team members (e.g., speech language pathologists, dietitians, social workers) may be responsible for patient care on more than one unit in the hospital and are therefore assigned to multiple units and need to collaborate with many teams across their organization. Despite the various team composition models and diverse healthcare settings that include hospital, homecare, community clinics, and long-term care, the importance of collaboration is not any different.

WHAT'S IN A NAME?

Generally, it is accepted that at least two people working together can be considered a team. In healthcare there are many names for team-based models of care including multidisciplinary, interdisciplinary, transdisciplinary, interprofessional and intraprofessional (Martin et al., 2022). With the many names for team-based models there can be confusion because the terminology may have different meanings for individuals and the structure of teams in the healthcare setting may also vary. Martin et al. (2022) suggest using standardized terms and definitions for each type of team to create a less ambiguous and clearer understanding of the different types of teams. However, until the nomenclature is standardized globally, for the purposes of this book all the above terms refer to types of healthcare teams.

TEAMWORK DEFINITION

Similar to the number of definitions for the term 'teams' in healthcare, there are many definitions of teamwork. The Canadian Interprofessional Health Collaborative (2024) uses the D'Amour et al., (2005) definition of teamwork in their glossary.

> *Describes an interdependent relationship that exists between members of a team. It is an application of collaboration. "Collaboration" deals with the type of relationships and interactions that take place between coworkers. Effective health care teamwork applies to caregivers who practice collaboration within their work settings (D'Amour, Ferrada-Videla & San Martin Rodriguez 2005).*

A later definition from The World Health Organization (2010) notes that "Collaborative practice happens when multiple health workers from different professional backgrounds work together with patients, families, carers and communities to deliver the highest quality of care across settings" (p. 7).

A concept analysis of 'team-based care' conducted by (Baik, 2016) reported three main attributes to team-based care including interprofessional collaboration, a patient-centred approach to care, and integrated processes, which means that teams need to understand each other's roles, be mutually respectful, and have organizational support for the teams to work together.

IMPORTANCE OF TEAMWORK AND QUALITY PATIENT OUTCOMES

Over the years there has been a plethora of reasons for promoting the need for teamwork and collaborative practice in healthcare documented in the literature. These include the need to ensure patient safety (Ma et al., 2017; Wei et al., 2022), high quality outcomes, patient satisfaction (Morgen et al., 2020; Will et al., 2019) staff satisfaction, (Espinoza et al., 2018), and effective teamwork, which in turn may contribute to retention of staff, (Kaiser et al., 2018).

Pomare et al (2020), conducted a systematic review of interprofessional collaboration in acute care hospitals and reported mostly positive outcomes in terms of patient and staff turnover, error rates, and organizational factors but still noted inconsistencies in the research findings due to differing patient cohorts and the complexity of the patient care. Pomare suggested further research using different methodological approaches needs to be conducted.

PATIENT SAFETY

Patient safety is a concern for every clinician working in healthcare. One in 10 patients are harmed by unsafe care and this can result in over 3 million deaths worldwide (Slawomirski & Klazinga, 2020). Canadian statistics from 2022-2023 show that 1 in 17 hospital stays involved at least one harmful event (Canadian Institutes for Health Information, 2024).

Patient safety indicators can include number of falls during hospitalization, incidence of hospital acquired pressure injury (Ma et al., 2018); infection rates, for example, in central line associated blood stream infections (CLABSIs) (Musgrove et al., 2024; Srisatidnarakul et al., 2021), or medication errors. There are many reasons that contribute to patient errors including communication breakdown on healthcare teams and teams that do not work effectively together (World Health Organization, September 11, 2023). Effective communication and good working relationships are key to interprofessional collaboration; individual team members who respect each other and are comfortable having open dialogue with other team members related to patient care issues (Gleeson et al., 2023) may assist in preventing errors. Patient care rounds are one example of a venue for interprofessional discussion about patients' care needs. Collaboration among healthcare teams is a suggested strategy for supporting patient safety outcomes (Ma et al., 2018).

PATIENT SATISFACTION

Patient satisfaction is an important quality indicator and can be measured in different ways depending on how a hospital or healthcare organization solicits patient satisfaction feedback. In a 2019 systematic review of different types of team composition in acute care hospitals, Willand and colleagues (2019) found that team-based care in hospital settings may affect patient satisfaction in a positive way. Yet Morgan et al. (2020), in their scoping review, reported that there was a paucity of literature on the patient's experience with interprofessional collaboration and suggested that future research should examine this outcome. Assessing patient satisfaction with interprofessional collaborative care is an example of an indicator that could benefit from further examination to understand the impact on patients.

STAFF SATISFACTION

Collaboration among team members can contribute to job satisfaction and potentially the retention of team members. Length of time working with a team, common goals and patient-centred care have been reported to increase staff satisfaction (Espinoza et al., 2018).

Nursing work environments can also be impacted positively in terms of job satisfaction and patient safety outcomes due to interprofessional collaboration (Labrague et al., 2022). Kaiser et al. (2018), in their systematic review of interprofessional work and employee outcomes, found the strongest positive relationship in participants' evaluation of the care they provided and interprofessional teamwork and another association was the positive relationship between interprofessional work and job satisfaction.

INTERPROFESSIONAL COLLABORATION

Since the release of the World Health Organization report on interprofessional education and collaboration in practice (2010), which provided a framework for moving forward in providing education on interprofessional collaboration, the importance of educating future practitioners together while they are still students has been increasingly highlighted. The goal of interprofessional education is that all new healthcare professional graduates will be ready to collaborate in the workplace upon graduation, which will result in improved patient outcomes and potentially contribute to a healthier workplace culture. As a guideline for learners, The Canadian Interprofessional Collaborative ([CIHC], 2024) published a National Competency Framework to assist healthcare students to learn about effective interprofessional collaborative care. Six competency domains were outlined in this framework that defined the skills, knowledge and values needed to promote successful interprofessional collaboration. The six competences include: interprofessional communication, patient/family-centred care, role clarification, team functioning, collaborative leadership and interprofessional conflict resolution (CIHC, 2010, p. 9). Ensuring all new healthcare provider graduates have achieved these six competencies should help with establishing the goal of interprofessional collaborative practice.

Despite the achievement of the six interprofessional competencies, how does interprofessional collaborative practice function in the real-world clinical settings? Given the complexity of many healthcare settings, staff shortages and time constraints, interprofessional collaborative practice may be difficult to achieve in the real-world setting. I contend that organizational leadership must promote interprofessional collaborative practice and provide the support for it to flourish. But what does this look like?

- Having time for teams to build and communicate and develop as a team.
- Ensuring a workplace where people are not afraid to speak up where all team members have an equal voice and are not afraid to speak up.
- Breaking down hierarchical barriers and having different channels of communication where individuals can express any concerns with team dynamics.

Furthermore, since conflict is inevitable in any workplace, organizations need to have clear policies that everyone is aware of and understands for addressing team conflict.

CONCLUSION

Given the known benefits of teams working together in collaborative practice both for patients and healthcare workers there is still a need for continued research in this area with the emphasis on linking patient and healthcare provider quality outcomes to interprofessional collaboration. The need for continued dialogue about interprofessional collaborative practice and the positive influences on patient care needs to occur and healthcare teams will still require organizational support to make interprofessional collaboration a reality in the workplace. Over the past forty years I have seen great strides in the implementation of interprofessional education in academia and interprofessional collaboration in the healthcare setting yet there is still work to be done to ensure interprofessional collaboration happens globally in all healthcare settings.

REFERENCES

Baik, D. (2016). Team-based care: A concept analysis. *Nursing Forum*, *52*(4), 313–322. DOI: 10.1111/nuf.12194 PMID: 27935047

Canadian Interprofessional Health Collaborative. (April 2024). CIHC competency framework for advancing collaboration. Retrieved June 20, 2024. https://cihc-cpis.com/wp-content/uploads/2024/06/CIHC-Competency-Framework.pdf

Canadian Interprofessional Health Collaborative. *Glossary*. Retrieved June 25, 2024. lhttps://cihc-cpis.com/resources/glossary/

D'Amour, D., Ferrada-Videla, M, San Martin Rodriguez, L., & Beaulieu, M.D. (2005). The conceptual basis for interprofessional collaboration: Core concepts and theoretical frameworks. *Journal of Interprofessional Care*, Supplement 1: 116 – 131DOI: DOI: 10.1080/13561820500082529

Dyer, S. M., Perracini, M. R., Smith, T., Fairhall, N. J., Cameron, I. D., Sherrington, C., & Crotty, M. (2020). Rehabilitation Following Hip Fracture. 2020 Aug 21. In: Falaschi P, Marsh D, editors. Orthogeriatrics: The Management of Older Patients with Fragility Fractures [Internet]. 2nd edition. Cham (CH): Springer; 2021. Chapter 12. Available from: https://www.ncbi.nlm.nih.gov/books/NBK565580/pdf/Bookshelf_NBK565580.pdf

Espinoza, P., Peduzzi, M., Agreli, H. F., & Sutherland, M. A. (2018). Interprofessional team member's satisfaction: A mixed methods study of a Chilean hospital. *Human Resources for Health*, *16*(30), 30. Advance online publication. DOI: 10.1186/s12960-018-0290-z PMID: 29996936

Essex, R., Kennedy, J., Miller, D., & Jameson, J. (2023). A scoping review exploring the impact and negotiation of hierarchy in healthcare organisations. *Nursing Inquiry*, *30*(4), e12571. DOI: 10.1111/nin.12571 PMID: 37338510

Gergerich, E., Boland, D., & Scott, M. A. (2019). Hierarchies in interprofessional training. *Journal of Interprofessional Care*, *33*(5), 528–535. DOI: 10.1080/13561820.2018.1538110 PMID: 30383437

Gleeson, L. A., O'Brien, G. L., O'Mahony, D., & Byre, S. (2023). Interprofessional communication in the hospital setting: A systematic review of the qualitative literature. *Journal of Interprofessional Care*, *37*(2), 203–213. DOI: 10.1080/13561820.2022.2028746 PMID: 35109753

Helmstadter, C. (2002). Early nursing reform in nineteenth-century London: A doctor-driven phenomenon. *Medical History, 46*(3), 325–350. https://www.cambridge.org/core/journals/medical-history/article/early-nursing-reform-in-nineteenthcentury-london-a-doctordriven-phenomenon/B78A155787D8643EFB9296ECC561B845. DOI: 10.1017/S0025727300069386 PMID: 12194424

Kaiser, S., Patras, J., & Martinussen, M. (2018). Linking interprofessional work to outcomes for employees. *Research in Nursing & Health, 41*(3), 265–280. DOI: 10.1002/nur.21858 PMID: 29906320

Keddy, B., Gillis Jones, M., Jacobs, P., Burton, H., & Rogers, M. (1986). The doctor-nurse relationship: An historical perspective. *Journal of Advanced Nursing, 11*(6), 745–753. DOI: 10.1111/j.1365-2648.1986.tb03393.x PMID: 3540064

Labrague, L. J., Al Subei, S., Al Rawajfah, O., AbuAlrub, R., & Burney, I. (2022). Interprofessional collaboration as a mediator in the relationship between nurse work environment, patient safety outcomes and job satisfaction among nurses. *Journal of Nursing Management, 30*(1), 268–278. DOI: 10.1111/jonm.13491 PMID: 34601772

Ma, C., Park, S. H., & Shang, J. (2018). Inter- and intra-disciplinary collaboration and patient safety outcomes in U.S. acute care hospitals: A cross sectional study. *International Journal of Nursing Studies, 85*, 1–6. DOI: 10.1016/j.ijnurstu.2018.05.001 PMID: 29783090

Martin, A. K., Green, T. L., McCarthy, A. L., Marcin Sowa, P., & Laakso, E. L. (2022). Healthcare teams: Terminology, confusion, and ramifications. *Journal of Multidisciplinary Healthcare, 15*, 765–772. DOI: 10.2147/JMDH.S342197 PMID: 35422626

Morgan, K. H., Barroso, C. S., Bateman, S., Dixson, M., & Conroy Brown, J. (2020). Patients' experiences of interprofessional collaborative practice in primary care: A scoping review of the literature. *Journal of Patient Experience, 7*(6), 1466–1475. DOI: 10.1177/2374373520925725 PMID: 33457603

Musgrove, H., Ruby, A., Chami, E., Pollak, E., Suleyman, G., & Gupta, A. (2024). Using interprofessional collaboration to reduce reported rates of central-line-associated bloodstream infection in an intensive care setting. *Infection Control and Hospital Epidemiology, 1-3*(5), 674–676. Advance online publication. DOI: 10.1017/ice.2023.279 PMID: 38163995

O'Rourke, B., Widenhoefer, T., Reimer, N., Vazquez, E., & Wolpert, C. (2018). Roles, Responsibilities, and implications of health care practitioners providing interprofessional collaborative practice to the geriatric population. *Topics in Geriatric Rehabilitation, 34*(3), 165–170. DOI: 10.1097/TGR.0000000000000189

Pomare, C., Long, J. C., Churruca, K., Ellis, L. A., & Braithwaite, J. (2020). Interprofessional collaboration in hospitals: A critical, broad-based review of the literature. *Journal of Interprofessional Care*, *34*(4), 509–519. DOI: 10.1080/13561820.2019.1702515 PMID: 31928245

Simms, L. W., Dalston, J. W., & Roberts, P. W. (1984). Collaborative practice: Myth or reality? *Hospital & Health Services Administration*, *29*(6), 36–48. PMID: 10268659

Slawomirski, L., & Klazinga, N. (2020). *The economics of patient safety: from analysis to action*. Organisation for Economic Co-operation and Development., https://www.oecd.org/health/health-systems/Economics-of-Patient-Safety-October-2020.pdf

Van Klaveren, L., Geukers, V., & de Vos, R. (2024). Care complexity, perceptions of complexity and preferences for interprofessional collaboration: An analysis of relationships and social networks in paediatrics. *BMC Medical Education*, *24*(1), 334. DOI: 10.1186/s12909-024-05304-6 PMID: 38528513

Voyer, B. (2013). Changes in the relations and roles of doctors and nurses. *British Journal of Health Care Management*, *19*(1), 16–21. DOI: 10.12968/bjhc.2013.19.1.16

Walter, C., Soni, T., Gavin, M. A., Kubes, J., & Paciullo, K. (2022). An interprofessional approach to reducing hospital-onset *Clostridioides difficile* infections. *American Journal of Infection Control*, *50*(12), 1346–1351. DOI: 10.1016/j.ajic.2022.02.017 PMID: 35569613

Wei, H., Horns, P., Sears, S. F., Huang, K., Smith, C. M., & Wei, T. H. (2022). A systematic meta-review of systematic reviews about interprofessional collaboration: Facilitators, barriers, and outcomes. *Journal of Interprofessional Care*, *36*(5), 735–749. DOI: 10.1080/13561820.2021.1973975 PMID: 35129041

Will, K. K., Johnson, M. L., & Lamb, G. (2019). Team-based care and patient satisfaction in the hospital setting: A systematic review. *Journal of Patient-Centered Research and Reviews*, *6*(2), 158–171. DOI: 10.17294/2330-0698.1695 PMID: 31414027

World Health Organization. (2010). Framework for action on interprofessional education and collaborative practice. Geneva, Switzerland: WHO https://www.who.int/publications/i/item/framework-for-action-on-interprofessional-education-collaborative-practice

World Health Organization. (September 11, 2023). *Patient safety*. Retrieved January 4, 2024. https://www.who.int/news-room/fact-sheets/detail/patient-safety

Chapter 2
Theoretical Foundations of Team-Based Healthcare

Yumi Tamura
https://orcid.org/0000-0003-0764-2383
Japanese Red Cross Hiroshima College of Nursing, Japan

Yuka Murata
Japanese Red Cross Hiroshima College of Nursing, Japan

ABSTRACT

A theory is a system of reasoning based on clear facts, such as principles or laws, that describes, explains, elucidates, prescribes, or organizes a particular phenomenon (Walker & Avant, 2005). Theories also clarify various aspects of a phenomenon and provide a framework for understanding them. Furthermore, theories create complex and comprehensive understandings of phenomena that cannot be easily explained, such as how a particular culture works, how an organization functions, or why individuals interact in a certain way. Over the past few years, the use of theory in the interprofessional field has evolved and matured (Reeves & Hearn, 2013). This chapter reviews the foundational and related theories to better understand team-based healthcare.

INTRODUCTION

"Health is everyone' s concern! "

Health care has changed enormously with more rapid pace in the last 20 years. With the complexity of modern health care, patients are rarely looked after by just

DOI: 10.4018/979-8-3693-2230-7.ch002

one health professional. In the context of a complex health care system, health care professionals need transit from being soloist to members of teams who work together. Since the WHO framework in 2010, the importance of team-based health care is now globally recognized as an essential approach for more effective and patient-centered health care delivery system.

However, the term "team-based health care" use interchangeable of other terms, such as interprofessional collaboration and its concept involve patient-centered care. For example, this term is used Japanese "team iryou" as same. And "team iryou" consists four concepts such as "professional specialty-oriented"; "team composition-oriented"; "patient-centered oriented" and "collaboration oriented" by Hosoda's sociological research (2021, p.95). The last two concepts are key components for team-based health care. At this point, those concepts are defined below:

Team-Based Health Care

Team-based care is defined as "the provision of health services to individuals, families, and/or communities by at least two health care providers who work collaboratively with patients and their caregivers – to the extent preferred by each patient – to accomplish shared goals within and across settings to achieve coordinated high-quality care" by the Institute of Medicine (IOM). The incorporation of sharing responsibilities with accountability between team members in health care systems offers great benefit.

Interprofessional Collaboration

Interprofessional collaboration (IPC) is one of the key concepts for team-based health care. IPC is interprofessional work that is the process whereby members of two or more different professions and/or agencies work together to provide integrated health and/or social care for the benefit of service users (Pollard et al, 2005, p.10). Barr et al. (2005) also mentioned that IPC involves different health and social care professions who regularly come together to negotiate and agree how to solve complex care problems or provide services. In other words, it differs from interprofessional teamwork as colleagues do not share a team identity and work together in a less integrated and interdependent manner based on their practice (Reeves et al., 2010).

Patient-Centered Care

Patient-centered care (PCC) and team-based and/or Interprofessional collaborative care (IPC) remain important goals for all health care systems. Patient-centered care is a model for providing health care that focuses not only on the patient's symptoms and medical history but also on the emotional, social, and financial factors that affect their life, as well as their values. It is often thought of as a partnership between a patient and a healthcare provider, in which the patient's perspective is as important as that of the doctor or nurse. In patient-centered care, the patient and the patient's family play an integral part in making decisions about the patient's care and treatment. This approach is very different from the traditional top-down doctor-patient model in which the healthcare provider makes all the decisions on the patient's behalf.

THEORETICAL FRAMEWORKS

Team-based healthcare has evolved significantly over the years, influenced by various theories and paradigms. This section presents various theoretical frameworks that underpin team-based healthcare. Those theories and paradigms have collectively shaped the development of team-based healthcare, leading to more effective, collaborative, and patient-centered care.

Systems Theory

Systems theory, also known as systems thinking, sees the world as a collection of interconnected systems. Instead of focusing only on individual components, it emphasizes the interdependencies and interactions between each part of the system. In systems theory, any change in one part of the system can have a ripple effect throughout the system. The fundamental aspects of systems theory are interconnections and interactions. These describe the relationships between system elements and how they interact with each other. Interconnections can take various forms such as communication channels, feedback groups, and dependencies. Also, interactions between elements can be direct or indirect. Systems theory has applications in various fields such as psychology, management, and sociology. Systems theory views health care as a complex system where each member's role and interactions affect the overall performance. It emphasizes the importance of understanding the interdependencies within the team and broader healthcare environment.

Social Identity Theory

Social identity theory is a theory that has significant influence on group processes and intergroup relations. Social identity is defined as "various aspects of a person's self-concept, emotions, evaluations, and other psychological correlates based on membership in a social group or social category" (Tuner, Hogg, Oakes, Reicher & Wetherell, 1987, p.29). Social identity theory explains the process of intergroup conflict and phenomena such as in-group bias and resulting out-group discrimination in intergroup cognition. It posits that social groups are motivated to distinguish themselves from other groups through social comparisons between in-groups and out-groups, in order to positively evaluate their own in-group. Tajfel and Turner (1979) explain social identity as the bias towards one's own in-group due to a sense of belonging and increased self-esteem associated with that group. Therefore, an individual's self-image within a social group can be attributed to the social category they belong to.

On the other hand, people tend to assume that out-groups are made up of people who are different from themselves, and they tend to discriminate and attack them, and the recognition of heterogeneity increases the likelihood of emotional conflicts between members (Yamaguchi, 2024). Heterogeneity includes the diversity of members. In order to utilize the cognitive stimuli leaked by member diversity as a variable that promotes team creativity and innovation, the culture and climate of the team, in which members accept and respect each other's thoughts and values, plays an important role (Yamaguchi, 2024). In this way, when individuals belonging to a group they are exposed to external and internal stimuli, influence each other, interact with each other, and demonstrate creativity, transforming into an innovative organization, this can be said to be an excellent performance of group dynamics.

Complexity Theory

Complexity Theory allows us to better understand systems as diverse as cells, human beings, forest ecosystems, and organizations, that are only partially understood by traditional scientific methods (Zimmerman et al., 2001). While it represents a relatively nascent field of study, it spans across a wide variety of disciplines in the physical, biological, and social sciences, and has profound implications for the way we think about and act within the world (Schneider & Somers, 2006).

This is especially important in the study of organizations, organizational change, and leadership, where complexity theory can offer insights into how organizations become more sustainable, adaptive, and innovative (Uhl-Bien et al., 2007).

Relational Coordination Theory

Relational coordination is an emerging theory for understanding the relational dynamics of coordinating work. According to the theory of relational coordination, coordination that occurs through frequent, high-quality communication supported by relationships of shared goals, shared knowledge and mutual respect enables organizations to better achieve their desired outcomes. Specifically, "relational co-ordination is a mutually reinforcing process of interaction between communication and relationships carried out for the purpose of task integration" (Gittell, 2011). According to this theory, three dimensions of relationships are integral to the process of coordination: shared knowledge, shared goals and mutual respect.

Transdisciplinary Model

A transdisciplinary model is an approach to curriculum integration that dissolves the boundaries between conventional disciplines and organizes teaching and learning around the construction of meaning in the context of real-world problems or themes. This approach includes a collaborative process where members offer their expertise to contribute to the larger ideas of the group. Transdisciplinary emphasizes collaboration across different healthcare disciplines to address complex patient needs.

KEY PRINCIPLES AND MODELS

This section outline of key principles that guide effective team-based healthcare.

Clear Roles and Responsibilities

There are clear expectations for each team member's functions, responsibilities, and accountabilities, which optimize the team's efficiency and often make it possible for the team to take advantage of division of labor, thereby accomplishing more than the sum of its parts.

Mutual Trust and Respect

Team members earn each other's trust, creating strong norms of reciprocity and greater opportunities for shared achievement. They respect and appreciate the role of each other. They also respect each other's talents and beliefs, in addition to their professional contributions. Effective teams also accept and encourage a diversity of opinions among members.

Effective Communication Strategies

This is crucial for the teamwork success. The team prioritizes and continuously refines its communication skills. It has consistent and accessible channels for complete communication, and used by all team members across all settings.

Shared Decision-Making Processes

According to a concept analysis on shared decision-making by Tsuji (2022), the attributes of shared decision making were found to be that "the patient is involved" and "it is a dynamic decision process where persons involved mutually influence one another". This process acts as an agency of communication and interaction. Through numerous two-way communications, persons involved share information gathered concerning choices available, the current situation, outlook, goals, values, preferences, and ideas.

Working together they move toward a desirable decision and come to agreement. The antecedents were 1) a change in health concept-variation in disease structure and response system characteristics, 2) medical uncertainties and advances in scientific technologies, 3) the certainty of a paradigm shift in the medical model, 4) characteristics of those involved, including the patient, and perception of authority.

The consequences were 1) maximizing people's health and QOL, 2) psychological changes and growth in the patient, 3) patient satisfaction with decisions, and 4) the practice of ethical clinical care, including the use of appropriate scientific technology. This concept analysis provides concrete support to person-centered care.

Continuous Learning and Improvement

A team is a group of members with a common purpose and goal, and it is only when members participate in team building that they can fulfill their role as a team. The purpose of promoting team medical care is to improve the quality of medical care and provide efficient medical services by actively utilizing specialized professions and promoting collaboration between multiple professions. In order to improve the quality of medical care, three perspectives are important: 1) communication, 2) information sharing, and 3) team management. In order to provide efficient medical services, 1) information sharing and 2) standardization of work are necessary. In order to improve the quality of the team approach, it is important for each profession to respect each other, evaluate each other from their own perspective toward a clear goal, and provide specialized skills efficiently. Furthermore, in order to practice a team approach, it is important to recognize that there are many tasks that are shared by multiple professions involved, rather than limiting the implementation of various tasks to a specific profession, and to respond flexibly according to the patient's condition and the medical care system (Ministry of Health, Labor and Welfare, 2010). In order to achieve these things, the team needs to continue to function continuously. Here, we first discuss the team development stage model and group rigidity, and then focus on team learning to outline the continuous learning and improvement of teams that can respond to today's rapidly changing society. To explain the stages of team development, we use the five-stage model of group development (Tuckman & Jensen, 1977). This model shows the process in which team members work together and develop and change over time. 1. The "formation stage" in which members understand each other, 2. The "tumultuous stage" in which members experience conflicts such as disagreements, 3. The "normative stage" in which roles and norms are established, 4. The "performance stage" in which members actively work on challenges, and 5. The "dissolution stage" for groups that have achieved their goals. However, not all groups reach the "performance stage," and some groups may reach the "dissolution stage" without achieving their goals (Figure 1).

Figure 1. Tuckman's team development model

Fig.1

Tuckman's Team Development Model

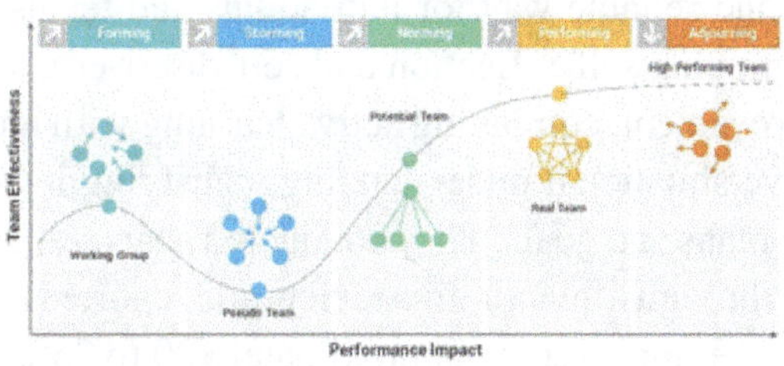

Source: https://www.test-correct.nl/blog/colearning-het-tuckman-model

Even if a group grows and improves its performance for a certain period of time, it may become dysfunctional along the way (Katz, 1982). Furukawa (1990) calls the phenomenon in which a group loses vitality after a long period of time in a stable state "rigidity." There are five reasons for this "rigidity": 1) The division of roles and the way members interact become fixed (excessive structuring), 2) The way members think and act becomes fixed (excessive standardization), 3) The communication channels become fixed and active discussions about work decrease (flattening of communication), 4) They lose interest in information outside the group (internalization and trivialization of interests and concerns), and 5) The leader is bound by past precedents and experiences and resists change (self-entrapment). To overcome this rigidity and prevent dysfunction, continuous change through team learning is important.

Team learning is defined as a cyclical team-level process that creates change or improvement for the team or its members (Decuyper et al., 2010). Argyris and Schön (1978) explain organizational learning as the addition or replacement of the existing knowledge and values of the organization by members of the organization with newly acquired knowledge and values, and list two types of learning: single-loop learning and double-loop learning. Single-loop learning refers to learning that modifies existing norms and frameworks acquired through past experiences. On the other hand, double-loop learning refers to learning that attempts to incorporate new ways of thinking and behavior that are performed when existing norms and frameworks are incompatible with the problem, and can be seen as transformative behavior. Senge (2006) also explains team learning as one of the five disciplines of the "learning organization," exploring complex problems through dialogue among members and narrowing down the best options through discussion among members.

Among team learning, team debriefing has been attracting attention in recent years. Tannenbaum and Christopher (2013) state that debriefing is designed to provide a systematic and reliable way for individuals and teams to improve their performance by encouraging self-reflection and self-discovery, targeting potential opportunities for improvement, combining active learning with multiple sources of information to improve situational understanding, clarifying lessons learned, and setting specific future plans and goals. They conducted a meta-analysis of the effectiveness of debriefing through a quantitative review and reported that individual and team performance can be improved by approximately 20 to 25% if team members engage in self-correction and improvement of teamwork by utilizing situations such as meetings and project closings.

FUTURE DIRECTIONS AND IMPLICATIONS ON TEAM-BASED HEALTH CARE

In this section, emerging trends and future directions in team-based healthcare will be explained, considering advances in technology, changing patient demographics, and evolving healthcare policies. And also, reflect on the implications of theoretical insights for healthcare practice, education, and policy development with leverage key points from Mitchell, P. et.al. (2012).

Embracing Digital Transformation

The integration of digital tools and technologies is set to revolutionize team-based health care. This includes the use of telemedicine, electronic health records (EHRs), and AI-driven diagnostic tools, which can enhance communication, streamline workflows, and improve patient outcomes.

Enhancing Adaptive Teamwork

Future research emphasizes the need for adaptive teamwork, where health care teams can dynamically adjust to changing conditions and patient needs. This involves studying the temporal and contextual aspects of teamwork to develop better strategies for coordination and flexibility.

Addressing Teamwork Challenges

Identifying and overcoming common challenges in teamwork, such as communication barriers, role clarity, and conflict resolution, is crucial. Evidence-based solutions and case studies can provide valuable insights into effective teamwork practices.

Interprofessional Education and Training

Ongoing education and training programs for health care professionals are essential to foster a culture of collaboration and mutual respect. This includes simulation-based training and interprofessional workshops to enhance team skills and competencies.

Policy and Organizational Support

Supportive policies and organizational structures are necessary to promote team-based care. This includes creating environments that encourage collaboration, providing resources for team development, and implementing policies that support team-based approaches.

Patient-Centered Care

Involving patients and their families as active members of the health care team can lead to better health outcomes. Future directions include developing strategies to effectively integrate patient perspectives and preferences into the care process.

These directions highlight the evolving nature of team-based health care and its potential to improve patient care through enhanced collaboration and innovation.

REFERENCES

Argyris, C., & Schön, D. A. (1978). *Organizational learning: A theory of action perspective.* Addison Wesley.

Barr, H., Koppel, I., Reeves, S., Hammick, M., & Freeth, D. (2005). *Effective interprofessional education: Argument, assumption, and evidence.* Blackwell. DOI: 10.1002/9780470776445

Decuyper, S., Dochy, F., & Van den Bossche, P. (2010). Grasping the dynamic -complexity of team learning: An integrative model for effective team learning in organizations. *Educational Research Review, 5*(2), 111–133. DOI: 10.1016/j.edurev.2010.02.002

Furukawa, H. (1990). Indispensable theoretical place to practice organizational transformation, a critical challenge for corporate organizations. "Ko-zo kowashi – soshiki henkaku no shinrigaku". In *Japapanese.* Seisin-Shobo.

Gittell, J. H. (2011). *Relational Coordination: Guidelines for Theory, Measurement and Analysis.* Relational Coordination Research Collaborative.

Hosoda, M. (2021). *"Team-iryo" towa nani-ka 2nd edi. Toward Patient/service user-centered approach.* Japanese Nursing Association Publishing Company. (in Japanese)

Katz, D. (1982). The effects of group longevity on project communication and performance. *Administrative Science Quarterly, 27*(1), 81–104. DOI: 10.2307/2392547

Mitchell, P., Wynia, M., Golden, R., McNellis, B., Okun, S., Webb, C. E., Rohrbach, V., & Kohorn, I. V. (2012) Discussion Paper: Core Principles & Values of Effective Team-Based Health Care - National Academy of Medicine (IOM).

Pollard, K., Sellman, D., & Senior, B. (2005). The need for interprofessional working. In Barret, G., Sellman, D., & Thomas, J. (Eds.), *Interprofessional Working in Health and Social Care: Professional Perspectives.* Palgrave Macmillan.

Reeves, S., & Hean, S. (2013). EDITORIAL Why we need theory to help us better understand the nature of interprofessional education, practice and care. *Journal of Interprofessional Care, 27*(1), 1–3. DOI: 10.3109/13561820.2013.751293 PMID: 23256880

Reeves, S., Lewin, S., Espin, S., & Zwarenstein, M. (2010). *Interprofessional teamwork for health and social care.* Blackwell- Wiley. DOI: 10.1002/9781444325027

Senge, P. M. (2006) *The fifth discipline: The art and practice of the learning organization.* Broadway.

Tannenbaum, S.I., Beard,R.L., & Cerasoli, C.P.(2013) Conducting team debriefings the work.

Tannenbaum, S. I., & Cerasoli, C. P. (2013) Do Team and Individual Debriefs Enhance Performance? A Meta-Analysis._https://journals.sagepub.com/doi/epub/10.1177/0018720812448394

Tuckman, B. W., & Jensen, M. A. (1977). Stages of Small-Group Development Revisited. *Group & Organization Studies*, *2*(4), 419–427. Advance online publication. DOI: 10.1177/105960117700200404

Walker, L., & Avant, K. C. (2005). *Strategies for theory construction in nursing* (4th ed.). Pearson Prentice Hall.

World Health Organization. Health Professions Network Nursing and Midwifery Office within the Department of Human Resources for Health (2010) Framework for action on interprofessional education and collaborative practice. Geneva Switzerland: World Health Organization. https://www.who.int/hrh/nursing-midwifery/en/

Chapter 3
Collaborative Leadership Within Team Learning

Carole A. Orchard
https://orcid.org/0000-0001-9942-7992
Western University, Canada

ABSTRACT

This chapter provides an overview into collaborative leadership, its evolving impact on organizations and teams. A discussion is provided on defining collaborative leadership over recent times. Next a focus on collaborative leadership perspectives at a theory and measurement level associated with health care teams is discussed. The chapter then focuses on how collaborative leadership fits into relationship-focused team practice and how it is related to organizational learning as a bridge between individual and team learning.

INTRODUCTION

This chapter will provide an overview into the significance of collaborative leadership and its development within health care teams to provide a means for transitions between individual health professionals' knowledge, skills, and expertise that can be integrated into inter-professional collaborative relationship-focused practices and in turn to evolving organizational learning within health organizations. Why is this important to explore?

One of the hallmark domains in health providers competence is to enact inter-professional relationship-focused collaborative practice within teams working together guided by their collaborative leadership. Collaborative leadership approaches provide a means to guide shared partnership, cooperation and coordination with the goal to improve outcomes of persons care. However, to date, health systems have

DOI: 10.4018/979-8-3693-2230-7.ch003

been reluctant to invest in this form of team-based care. An investment that requires continuing education training programs to develop such teams.

At the same time there is a great deal of rhetoric around the need for patients and their care partners (we will term persons in this chapter) being part of decision-making processes for their care. For example, recent additional federal funding to provincial health systems in Canada requires innovative approaches to improve delivery of health to the population. However, there is limited evidence of any significant innovative changes addressing development of such teams for more effective practice, a direction supported by the World Health Organization (WHO) and many countries (WHO, 2010). Furthermore, some provincial governments in Canada including Ontario, Saskatchewan and British Columbia have repeatedly discussed the need to move to patient-centred approaches to their care, with little evidence of wide-spread support for preparing their health provider teams in relationship-focused collaborative team care. Why might inter-professional team development be a potential solution to achieving the above?

BACKGROUND

While all provincial health systems in Canada are experiencing high burnout rates among primary care physicians, and registered and licenced practical nurses, impacts of burnout has included closures of Emergency Departments (ER) across smaller communities, delays in elective surgeries, closures of hospital beds, and the inability to fully deliver home care into communities. The outcome of burnout across many Canadian communities is the absence of sufficient primary care physicians to provide health care leading more persons to seek help with their health care issues in Emergency Departments. Even when nurse practitioners are being adopted into provision of primary care, there are limitations as to how provincial health systems are up-taking collaborative teams to deliver health services.

Various solutions are being put forward to address the impacts on health care services due to healthcare professional burnout and healthcare professional shortages. These solutions include privatization of health services, increasing salaries of key professionals in short supply, recruitment of health professionals from other low-income countries (depleting their health providers), and using paramedics to visit people in communities for those who are frequent users of ER services. All these examples seem to be ‘band-aided solutions’.

Solutions proposed focus on health providers, but not on how to meet the needs of persons. Why is this important? Current health systems were developed several decades ago to reflect a country’s populations of that time. Concomitantly, health providers were and continue to be prepared to meet population needs that do not fit with the realities of the current population.

What has changed in the population? Today, many previous diseases that caused decreased life expectancy are now treatable. Tuberculosis, lung cancers from smoking, treating heart and vascular diseases, cancers and renal failure are a few examples. At the same time, wars, climate changes, and economic situations have caused greater numbers of persons being displaced in their own countries who then seek refugee status in such countries as Canada, the United States of America and within European countries. The results are many persons with chronic conditions and other health and mental health issues seeking health care assistance.

As life expectancy has improved in populations, persons are now living much longer lives. Emphasizing the need for persons to become more able to deal with maintaining their own health. However, our health system is still providing its major funding on acute care interventions. The most expensive approach.

Occasionally we hear a political leader suggesting major re-thinking of health systems to address the 'real' issues. Several authors have pinpointed the situation, "the majority of work occurring in human service organizations (HSOs) today, is ameliorative in nature, leaving the original sources of problems in our communities or society unchanged" (Evan & Kivell, 2015, p. 760), "healthcare organizations have often been a decade or more behind other industries in the development and understanding of effective service and support ideologies" (Van Vactor, 2012, p. 556) and further "change becomes problematic for many health care leaders… [and] the tendency of many managers of healthcare is to await a perfect solution prior to moving ahead with new approaches and technology" (Van Vactor, 2012, p.556).

RENEWAL OF HEALTH SYSTEMS THROUGH COLLABORATIVE TEAMS

Why then might relationship-focused collaborative team care be one major solution? It offers a means for health providers and persons working together to develop a person agreed to plan of care to achieve an expressed goal for their health. It transforms the role of persons from passive recipients of directed care from health providers to one where there is a shared expertise brought together to enhance a fuller understanding of what might be achievable. Thus, it is the person who shares their situations (lived experience) and desires for their health with health providers responding with potential realistic means to create the plan. A collaborative approach then reflects adult education theory by Malcom Knowles that adults are problem focused (Jarvis, 2010) and persons are only willing to focus on their identified health issues. Often health providers provide directive care beyond the person's problem focus. The outcome is frustration among both persons and health providers. Hence, if health providers found out key goal(s) persons wish helped with through enhanced listening, and explored what the person's capacities, financial abilities, transportation access to meet the plan and willingness to act on the plan, will persons health improvement then be achieved. Therefore, how well persons participate in their ongoing plans of care are the true outcomes of health professional work. However, this is rarely a focus of measurement of outcomes and population health. Current approaches to care rarely provide persons with the opportunity to share their own expertise in working on their health and being effectively listened to by the health provider to gain the above information critical to the outcomes.

While there are excellent care and treatment options available today, the focus on limited time intervals available to provide this care based on government funding models, results in failures to often achieve possible improved health outcomes from lack of this critical communication interaction. One of the most valuable changes in health care delivery to decrease the use of hospitals, EDs, and visits to health providers is to provide sufficient timing at the initial interface with persons and their care partners with teams of health providers. These initial visits then provide for person, care partners and relevant health providers to collaboratively meet and create realistic and acceptable plans of care, guiding to implementation of the agreed upon plan. As part of the plan to consider the teaching/training needs for persons and or care partners to implement the care agreed to. Finally, to have a member of the team serve as a connector to the person to monitor implementation of the care plan with these persons and care partners to ensure movement towards their chosen goal(s). Will it take more time? Yes, but the time saved from dealing later with complications from a lack of ongoing interventions will save both health professionals time and also decrease the costs for the health system through decreased repeat ER visits and hospitalizations. Currently, our system prevents this intake approach and results in wasted treatments, lack of developed abilities and follow through by persons and their care partners from a lack of adequate education and training for their home care needs (Orchard et al., 2024). All these gaps then likely cost the health system more funds than if the system shifted to a focus on these initial team meetings with persons and their care partners.

While this chapter is about collaborative leadership it cannot be separated from how health care team members work collaboratively together. At the present time this form of team-based care is largely missing within delivery of care in most health services nationally and internationally.

What is proposed is not simple to change. Change can only occur if government funding models change to support such team care, and health organization administrations are willing to invest in the training required for this form of team-based care to be implemented as a norm of their organizations.

The post-secondary education system also has a responsibility to support their health professional programs integrating development of relationship-focused collaborative competencies within all their health program graduates. Current education that isolates health professional students learning across their programs within only their own discipline remains a block to their students and graduates leaving their programs with the skills and knowledge required to work collaboratively with persons, care partners and other health providers. Thus, faculty teaching in these programs also require in-service training to transform their thinking about health system practices to reflect a significant change in how they educate these students. Why is this a key to this transformation?

The means in which professionals' practice is set by that profession's signature pedagogy. This term was first coined by Shulman (2005) who used Law and Legal Education as an initial example and subsequently both medicine and nursing were studied in a similar way. Signature pedagogies comprise a *surface, deep, and implicit structure* for the learning required to enact each profession's roles. Surface structures include "concrete, operational acts of teaching and learning, of showing and demonstrating, of questioning and answering, of interacting and withholding, of approaching and withdrawing" (Shulman, p. 54-5). Deep structures include "a set of assumptions about how best to impact a certain body of knowledge and know-how" (p. 55). There is also an *implicit structure* comprised of "a moral dimension that comprises a set of beliefs about professional attitudes, values, and dispositions" (p. 55). These three professional components of their pedagogy are the means for, development of, and demonstration of the profession and are common around the world. Educators then determine within their settings, how development of each professional occurs across the three structures and evaluation of student capacities to graduate and be considered for their regulated/licensed practice. There are advantages to signature pedagogies, for example allowing the same professionals working together, even if they gained their preparation from different educational institutions. Their disadvantage is a rigidity in their practices when working across professions. Alterations can occur when there is uncertainty or other disruptions in their professional practice. For example, the current challenges to existing health care delivery models by professionals has a potential to open the 'door' to a rethinking of their professions' practice.

Over the past couple of decades there has been efforts to ensure that all health professionals within their post-secondary institutions learn about other health professionals related to their roles, knowledge and skills as health providers. But there remain limited cross-professional opportunities for these students to learn to work across health professions to develop relationship-focused collaborative practice and to enact collaborative leadership.

When these professionals move into their graduate practice this gap in team development is rarely resolved through in-service or continuing education by their employers and in primary care settings. The argument by health administrators is limited funding to both release health professionals from their delivery of care to participate in training programs due to lack of replacement staff is real. Such arguments often remove time for administrators and other health system leaders working on innovative changes to re-think their health care delivery.

Today all leaders function within complex adaptive systems, change is constant and unpredictable… "sense making is never exhaustive, decision making is never final and action taking needs constant course corrections" (Jiang, 2023, p. 4). Therefore, current health care delivery that seeks leaders who can function with complexities need to embrace different approaches to leading than in the past.

LEADERS AND LEADERSHIP

To begin this part of the chapter we will differentiate between leaders and leadership. Crevani et al (2009) suggested "…the leader is described as a member of a group, albeit with specific possibilities to influence the group, and leadership is… a series of interaction processes where leaders inspire followers by creating common meaningful images of the future" (p. 78). While Ahlquist and Levi (2011) suggested "leaders have power over others as a consequence of office, personal influence, persuasive capacity, charisma, or coercion, but all express power in interaction with followers" (p.3) they need to be chosen based on their capacities to "command the attention and respect of followers…" (p.5). Jiang (2023) then adds "leadership… [needs to be] distributed, collective, collaborative and shared across representatives" (p.2). Hsieh and Liou (2018) emphasized for collaborative leadership to be enacted it needs to evolve into "working with groups inside and outside the organization" (p. 84) and Van Vactor (2012) suggested then "every member of a team has a leadership role in the health care environment" (p. 559). Thus, leadership involves processes of social influence within teams (Kruse 2013, p. 3).

Strong proponents of collaborative leadership are Raelin (2014) and Pearce (2004), Boyle and Kochinka (2004) who termed this form as 'shared leadership' and Edmonstone (2009) in health care teams advocated exhibiting 'clinical leadership.' Raelin (2016) further isolated discussion to only the team and how teams envisioned what he termed leadership as practice that "emphasizes the patterns of connected action" (p. 25) and more recently as collaborative agency "mobilized through engaged social interaction" (p. 2). Raelin (2016) pushes his view of collaborative leadership to a point where organizations do not have any leaders only groups enacting collaborative leadership. Collaborative leadership is also called facilitative leadership, adaptive leadership, integral leadership, and catalytic leadership (Hsieh & Liou, 2018). In health care it is unlikely that leaders will not exist to ensure accountabilities for health services and assurances of safety and effectiveness of provisions of services.

Initially the focus of collaborative leadership was viewed as part of communities of practice (Frydman et al., 2000), it then expanded to situations where government and the public came together (Chrislip, 2002) and then on to organizations (Archer & Cameron, 2009). At the organizational level pundits of collaborative leadership focused on structural and financial aspects associated with mergers of businesses developing a new form of its management. As the term evolved collaborative leadership was viewed within groups across wide varieties of organizations and focused on behaviours of persons within teams and how their behaviours resulted in performance.

Researchers in the fields of social and behavioural science, management, business, and human resources and leadership have focused on teams and collaborative leadership over the past couple of decades. Jiang has suggested it contains cycles of sense making, decision-making and action taking. It is "distributed, collective, collaborative and shared across representatives" (Jiang, p. 02), Van Vactor suggested it is a "unique style of leadership… (p. 561) [that] evolves with change and embraces innovative thinking and the continual creation of new processes… (p. 556) for the future. Senge shared the value of collaborative learning as allowing for enhanced insights and thinking than can occur individually.

Collaborative leadership is a process ontology related to interactions that are embedded in a cultural context (Crevani et al.,2009). Ang'ana and Kilka (2022) suggested it requires (vertical) leaders to enable and provide an environment for their teams to develop the skills and behaviours necessary to collaborate successfully… (p. 54). When in place Hogan and Kariser (2005) suggested that leadership assessment must be focused on group performance over time with emphasis on intrapersonal skills, interpersonal skills, planning, budgeting, coordinating and monitoring. Ang'ana and Kilika (2022) suggested decentralization of collaborative leadership from the centrality of the (vertical) leader to enable an organization to understand why teams are needed to collaborate.

Pierce and Sims Jr. (2002) studied how there could be an interaction between those who hold formal leader roles they termed 'vertical leadership' and 'shared leadership' within practice teams. They then studied the interface with vertical and shared leadership amongst private sector organizations to determine what leadership styles could result in team effectiveness. They found that vertical and shared leadership is significantly related to team effectiveness, while shared leadership was a predictor to team effectiveness (Pierce & Sims Jr., 2002). They concluded that vertical leaders need to enact transformative, transactional, and empowering leadership practices to effect team effectiveness (2002). Pierce (2004) presented findings that when transformative, empowering forms of leadership are exercised by the vertical (formal) leader it can support collaborative/shared leadership within teams. However, this form of leadership is only recently being a focus within health care, with limited attention to how it can be developed within teams. One of a few studies focused on collaborative leadership and organizational performance was carried out by Hsieh and Liou (2018) who examined the relationship between collaborative leadership as comprised of activating resource assistance, framing work environment, mobilizing stakeholder support and synthesizing collaborative process, and organizational performance. They found collaborative leadership dimensions except for mobilizing stakeholder support were supported (Hsieh & Liou, 2018).

Theorizing Vertical & Collaborative Leadership. Orchard was interested in how health care interprofessional teams might be theorized and considered Pierce and Sims' concept of vertical and collaborative leadership. This resulted in Orchard and Rykhoff's (2015) theorized model of collaborative leadership. The model presents the vertical leader at the top of the model with collaborative teams at the bottom. The two dimensions are then connected through application of Gitell et al.'s (2013) relational coordination leading to team effectiveness and member empowerment enacted through application of Kouzes and Posner's leadership elements adapted to collaborative interactions (2012). These being:

Modelling the way: In teams this means: Knowing your own personal values and how these may enhance or interfere in working with others; Helping the team to stay focused on patient care

Inspire a shared vision -- In teams this means...Focusing on patient-specified goals and helping the team to consider how to get there, helping team members to bring their ideas together in an agreed upon plan with the patient

Challenge the process: In teams this means encouraging... On-going reflection on how the team is working together with each other and with the patient and based on feedback making needed changes; Members thinking about their professional roles within an interprofessional patient-centred context.

Enable Others to Act: In teams this means the collaborative leader...Helps to guide the team in promoting respect for all members, and in arriving at shared goals with patients and team members; Encouraging other team members to take on the leadership role and supporting patients in their decision making with the team.

Encourage the heart: In teams this means...the collaborative leader recognizes the positive work of all team members, including the patient, towards meeting patient-set goals for care; the team with the patient celebrate achievement of steps towards patient-set goals of care (Orchard, 2020) (see figure of model below).

Figure 1. Theorized model of combined vertical and collaborative leadership in teams (Orchard 2020)

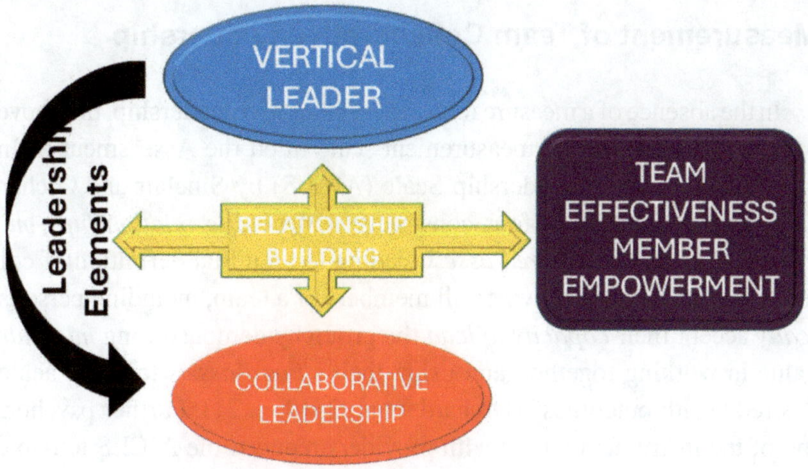

Vertical leaders then need to demonstrate strong person-focused leading (Klein et al (2010). Thus, for relationship-focused collaborative practice within teams "leadership [needs to be] replaced by less individualism and more humane constructs in social interactions," (Crevani, 2010, p. 84) it is about performance of teams (Hogan & Kariser, 2010). DiBello further asserts what is unique about collaborative leadership is that the role of the 'leader' may shift between team members, depending on varying circumstances (2019, p. 15). Yet this theorized model has not been empirically tested in healthcare organizations.

Defining Collaborative Leadership

A clear definition of collaborative leadership remains elusive. To arrive at such a definition a clearer understanding of collaborative leadership in teams was deemed needed by Rykhoff, Orchard and Wong (2015) who carried out a concept analysis of the phrase. The outcome was identification of its key attributes being (1) a situational interactive process that included mindfulness, complexity of care required, and facilitation of engagement; (2) collaborative interdependence that included symbiotic relationships, respect, trust for each other's expertise, (3) shared assets inclusive of information, mental models, decision making and power leading to collective action, and (4) capacity to lead inclusive of professional competence, knowledge, skills, experience, and creditability in the team. From the concept analysis, Sinclair and Orchard then considered how to develop a measure for collaborative leadership as none other was found in the literature.

Measurement of Team Collaborative Leadership

In the absence of a measure for team collaborative leadership, the above attributes were transformed into a measurement scale titled the Assessment of Interprofessional Collaborative Leadership Scale (AICLS) by Sinclair and Orchard, (2018). The scale comprised of four constructs -- *symbiotic relationships*, *mindfulness*, *capacity to lead* and *shared assets* leading to an initial definition of collaborative leadership as occurring "when all members of a team, including persons, *symbiotically* accept their *capacity to lead* the group by demonstrating *mindfulness* of the value in working together, and using their *shared assets* to reach achievable and desired health outcomes" (Orchard, et al. 2019, p. 21). Further psychometric testing of the instrument with health providers reduced the AICLS to two constructs, these being *valuing and supporting each other* comprises 6-items, focuses on "how team members show leadership through supporting and valuing of all inputs into shared decision making with and for their persons" (Orchard, 2022). The second construct as sharing of responsibilities also comprised of 6-items, focuses on how "all members show leadership by willingly ensuring there is an equitable sharing of their planning for, implementing of and evaluating for planned care goal achievement with all members" (Orchard, 2022). Collaborative leadership is then defined as persons, who value and support each other by sharing team responsibilities for working together and using their shared capacities to reach achievable and desired health outcomes" (Orchard, 2022).

Collaborative Leadership and Team Effectiveness

Collaborative leadership cannot exist in a vacuum of other competency domains associated with relationship-focused collaborative practice. Healthcare team members must also enact their capacity to partner with all team members (inclusive of persons and care partners) to work together to achieve a shared approach in planning of, implementation of, and evaluation of care. To work effectively in teams, all members need to participate in team building. Bard et al. (2014) stressed that "team formation is the first phase where individuals are socialized into the team through the creation of team norms, goals, and climate perceptions… [followed by acquiring] task knowledge and self-regulation skills in task compilation [and]… identify their roles and develop routines for task exchange" (p. 78). Kozlowski (2018) proposed a framework for teams comprised of inputs, processes, and outputs (IPO). Inputs focus on members' knowledge, skills, expertise, and attitudes that combine to create shared resources in the team. Processes relate to those actions needed to carry out the team's work. Outputs relate to the team's performance and its effectiveness. Studies of teams have been grouped by Kozlowski (2018) within the IPO framework summarizing the areas of research as focused on team design, team training and development, and team leadership. He further stresses that the area of team training is weak in research and how these "shape team processes and subsequent team effectiveness" (p. 209). There are also gaps in "new methodologies, measurement tools, and analytic systems" (Kozlowski, 2018, p. 210). Many reported studies of teams and their work are experimental in design and used subjects who are students in post-secondary institutions. The other area where there are further studies is related to project teams in both business and Information Technology sectors. However, there is limited research referring to health care team processes related to their collaborative leadership and its impact on team performance. Further intervention studies that focus on team training and the transfer of that learning into practice is needed (Yoon, 2010).

Integration of Collaborative Leadership into Teams

For teams to be effective in healthcare settings all members (inclusive of persons) need to be socialized into their working group. This socialized process needs to be reflective of Pettigrew's Intergroup Contact Theory Processes – *Learning about the outgroup*, *changing behaviour*, and *generating affective ties* (Pettigrew, 1998). These processes were uncovered in a study by Khalili and Orchard (2020) who focused on dual identity development in interprofessional students. Pettigrew and Tropp (2008) studied three mediators (decreased anxiety, valuing of enhanced empathy, and role clarity) and found all three as mediators that need to be presented in the above sequence for socialization processes to occur within teams. Thus, the initial step to team-based collaborative learning is to be socialized to work together using the ICT processes.

Once socialized, Jiang (2023) stressed that developing team collaborative leadership needs to comprise cycles of sense making, decision-making, and action taking. In a team, all members are expected to ensure they acquire clarity to arrive at shared meanings between members to ensure effectiveness of their collaborative planning, implementing and evaluating of performance effectiveness. Collaborative leadership in a team needs to ensure cycles of sense making that can lead to shared decision-making approaches for care needs of persons. This requires, team functioning, which is the ability to both listen and communicate with each other, and to explore what goals are for persons and treatments, advice, or other guidance that each provider could provide, then to allow persons to select those aspects that they are willing to engage in and work collaboratively with all team members. During such communicative interactions it is likely that disagreements will occur. Such disagreements are a healthy part of collaborative interchanges but do require all members being prepared to deal with disagreements using a process for addressing various viewpoints and then arriving at an acceptable agreement within the team. Therefore, collaborative leadership is the means to set a plan forward, agree to assignment of team members and participation in each aspect of the plan, and how evaluation of progress in reaching the goal(s) set is to be monitored. This will require participation in ongoing reviews of progress or needs to modify the plan as needed with all parties. It is these cycles and connections that are needed for healthcare teams to enact relationship-focused collaborative team practices. Thus, collaborative leadership is but one interactive component in this form of practice, albeit important as are all the other domains. In a recent survey conducted through the CIHC two domains were identified by participants that remain somewhat unclear – these being collaborative leadership and team differences/disagreement processes, please see Orchard et al. (2023) for more details on other domains.

The need for healthcare teams to provide effective care to persons is then associated with team functioning together and achieving innovative plans to address the complex needs of persons of today. Within the Canadian Interprofessional Health Collaborative's Relationship-focused Competency Framework are six competency domains shown below. The explanation of these domains and the framework are available at the Canadian Interprofessional Health Collaborative website https://cihc-cpis.com/.

Figure 2. CIHC competency framework for advancing collaborative practice

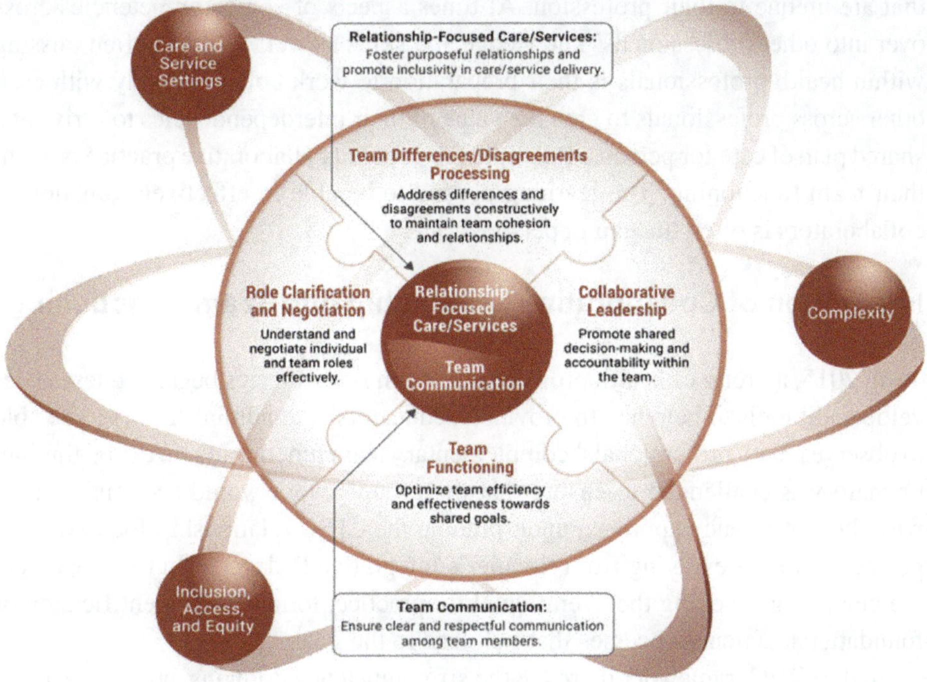

While collaborative leadership relates to a sharing of leading within teams, it is comprised of individuals bringing into the team's work intrapersonal and interpersonal skills, a capacity to plan, budget, coordinate and monitor towards a high-performance team (Hogan & Kariser, 2005). Jiang (2023) explored conceptual frameworks to consider how collaborative leadership enactment might enhance sense making, decision making and action taking processes. He concluded by bringing aspects of several together into what Miranda and Watts (2022) termed the RACI framework (responsible, accountable, consulted and informed) . However, in relationship-focused collaborative practice the person and care partners are integral team members. The remainder of the team will vary depending on the needs of the person. Unlike most team research, healthcare teams are cross-functional, time-limited by each patient with secondary members such as physiotherapists, social workers, dietitians, occupational therapist etc. who serve in teams only when needed for specific patient situations (Agbejule et al. 2021; Babnik et al. 2014). Most health care teams likely comprise registered nurses, physicians and pharmacists with persons and care providers varying with each situation. Teams in healthcare then are comprised of individuals who bring unique and shared assets into their work. Because of their assets then these team members have interdependencies needed to provide to the unique care of each person. Each health professional is licenced to provide a set of competencies that are unique to their profession. At times aspects of some competencies cross over into other professionals' knowledge and skills as well. What is often missing within health professionals is their preparation to work collaboratively with each other across professionals to gain the value of their interdependencies to arrive at a shared plan of care for persons. Relationship-focused collaborative practice is about their team functioning. The learning needed to be able to effectively function as collaborators is often the gap in persons' care.

Integration of Collaborative Leadership into Team Functioning

In 2015, a group of health professionals from six countries began a quest to develop audit tools to help health providers, educators, and administrators to be able to observe health professionals' complementary team functioning. In the beginning, Orchard was challenged to ensure that the group's work would accomplish a fit with the competency approach underpinning the CIHC relationship-focused competency domains evolving from Roegier's Integrative Pedagogy. In this approach, the beginning is setting the overall goal for practice, followed by identification of foundational actions/processes that will lead to the goal.

In the CIHC framework there are the six competency domains, previously mentioned. However, these domains or foundational actions do not stand alone, they interact with each other. For example, in collaborative leadership discussing what this is in practice is difficult without indicating how that domain interacts with the other five domains. Therefore, team functioning is underpinned by collaborative leadership and communication, and disagreement processing and the inclusion of all persons as well as clarity on roles and negotiating these as needed within the team to achieve relationship-focused collaborative practice.

To capture team processes there needed to be demonstrated steps for enactment of collaborative relationship-focused practice. Initially a set of ten steps needed to enact this form of practice were identified. The processes associated with each competency domain that were likely to be demonstrated to achieve each step were generated. These steps and processes were then shared with collaborators on the audit project, resulting in Anderson and Ford reducing the ten into four steps– *getting ready*, *working together to assess, diagnose, and plan care*, *delivering care*, and finally *reviewing care* (See figure below).

Figure 3. Collaborative Client-centred Practice Audit Framework

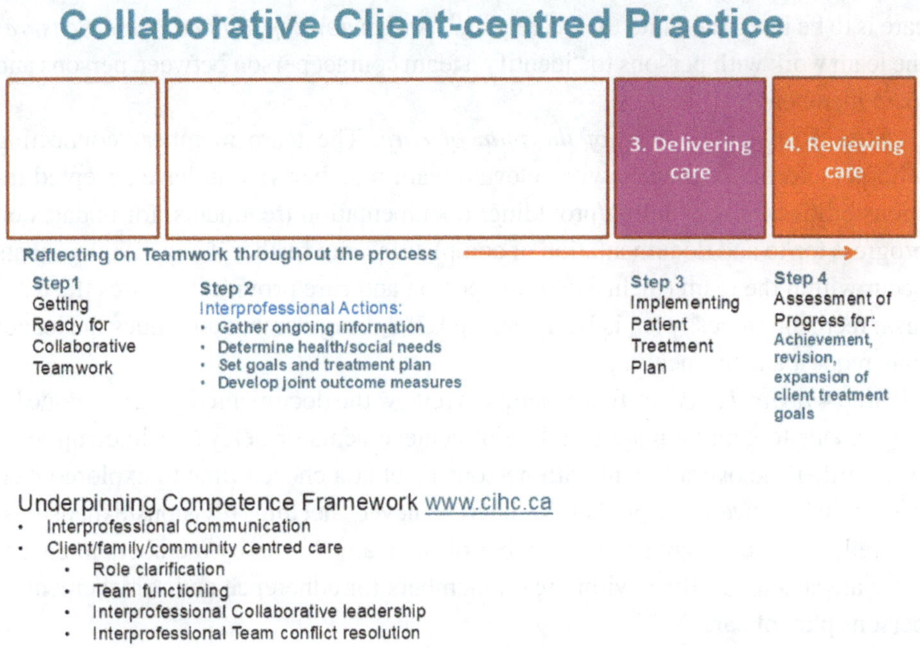

Since collaborative leadership is the means to achieve the team functioning outcome, the processes at each step are shared below as an example.

Step 1 *getting ready*. This step is about a team undergoing the learning to be able to enact relationship-focused collaborative practice. Each step is comprised of a set of criteria. The criteria are integrative of all the processes needed to enact each of the competency domains. There is a total of nine criteria in this step. Two examples are (1) team develops agreed processes for inclusion of all team members viewpoints and reflection on effectiveness of team, and (2) team develops processes for sharing leadership in the team.

Step 2 *working together to assess, goal set and plan care*. This step is the most complex of the steps as it involves the greatest change to current practice. Step 2 involves what are termed collaborative actions. There are 4 – (1) gather ongoing information; (2) determine required health/social needs; (3) set goals and treatment plans to address identified needs; and (4) develop joint outcome measures. An example of a criterion for each collaborative action will be provided. Within *gathering ongoing information*, "team members complete their individual assessments and share them with one another." Within *determine required health/social needs* the team "explores what the person is currently doing to address health issues and impact actions have had on overcoming problems." In *set goals and treatment plan to address identified needs* the "team members discuss with persons what suggested care is to be integrated into their care plan." And in *develop joint outcome measures* the team work with persons to "identify a team contact person between persons and team members"

Step 3 *implementation of the plan of care*. The team member "connecting with persons also connects with relevant team member(s) who have accepted responsibilities for scheduling/providing/ documentation treatments, for updates on progress for/to and documentation of completion" and further if any disagreements occur within the team (inclusive of the person and care provider) ensures the team disagreement process plan is being enacted. If a disagreement continues the leader may request a team meeting.

Step 4 *reviewing care*. Team members review the documented progress done by the persons to gain an understanding of achievements or delays /or interruptions. And further the overall team with persons meet at a chosen time to explore when their collaboratively set goals have been achieved, needing revisions/expansions. Overall, the leader may be any member of the team chosen by members to ensure there are accountabilities within team members for adherence and achievement of persons plan of care.

The Relationship-focused Collaborative Practice Audit Framework (Orchard et al., 2024) is now moving into testing of the audit tools. There likely will be some modifications as an outcome of this testing before it can be widely used to assist in determining when this form of practice in teams has been realized.

Collaborative Leadership and Team Learning

What then is the role of the person who chairs or leads the team? In collaborative leadership within this form of team-based care, team leadership requires all members to be responsible for the team's functioning. To select the lead for each persons' care may vary or be consistent. This is determined within the team. For organizations to support this form of team leadership, organizations need to establish an organizational learning culture. To achieve this culture, Sumeth and Li (2013) suggested there needs to be open-mindedness at the organizational leadership level "to question long held routine assumptions and beliefs" (p. 5). Then, to move towards a learning culture, defined as one that occurs at an individual, team and organizational level.

Individual learning "is a psychological change that takes place within the person… through acquisition of knowledge of facts… and linking application of facts to enabling consideration and... development of strategic knowledge that can be shared and exchanged… through informal social communication with experience develop strategic knowledge to guide prioritization and sharing" (Kozlowski & Bell,

2007, p.18). Team learning is defined as "the process of aligning and developing the capacity of a team to create the results its members truly desire" (Senge, 2006, p. 218). Organizational learning is limited to only "the sum of learning through the experiences and actions of their workers" (Stelmaszczyk, 2016, p. 110). Hence, it is individual learning among all members in an organization that when shared into any team facilitates its integration into broader thinking processes that can lead to innovative approaches to care and operations. When any changes are successful, they are more likely to be integrated at the organizational level. However, this tri-level of learning cannot occur unless there are opportunities for teams to be developed. Lack of attention within health care agencies to team development seems to be limited by both releasing professionals from care implementation, and funding for the cost of such programs.

SUMMARY

While there have been many studies of health care leader traits and behaviours, Ang'ana and Kilika (2022) suggested "many organizations today are struggling because they have not effectively transitioned from traditional management and leadership approaches to contemporary shared, collaborative leadership approaches" (p.49). For many organizations, a leader is an individual who leads. Those chosen to assume roles as leaders are often selected based on observed traits within them. These traits are believed to be needed to guide others. But these views are now obsolete.

Globalization of supply chains and the need to decrease costs of goods and services causing increasing pressures for employees 'to do more with less' have further pressured organizations towards newer thinking related to leaders and leadership within and across their businesses. These transitions in thinking have brought forward different ideas about this newer leading. Further changes have resulted from the COVID pandemic. The world was pushed from a communication age quickly into a digital age. This new age requires rapid thinking and evolution of ideas to address urgent issues. Time is no longer present for careful thinking and exploring potential options in addressing an issue. Rapidity of responses that provide for testing of directions is now the norm. Discounting those that prove not to work and up-taking those that do. This is no different in health systems.

Relationship-focused collaborative practice allows for this above movement to be enacted. This is a solution to the problems explored in this chapter.

Why can this team-based practice meet the above? The knowledge, skills and expertise of each health professional are complimentary to each other and needed to address the complex needs for care of persons today. The strength of the health provider's interdependencies can be captured in this form of teamwork to benefit persons and enhance the means used to provide effective care that improves the real outcomes of persons. Teams who exist to perform organizationally "relevant tasks, share one or more common goals, interact socially, exhibit task interdependencies (i.e. workflow, goals outcomes), maintain and manage boundaries, and are embedded in an organizational context that sets boundaries, constrains the team, and influences exchanged with outer units in the boarder entity" (Kozlowski & Bell, 2007, p. 16).

While we have focused in this chapter on single teams we are now in a time where intersectoral team development is also an essential reality. Intersectoral teams are defined as occurring "when all parties across a variety of agencies gather together to cooperatively plan coordinated support for a client who requires a variety of services to augment his/her capacity to manage activities of daily living within his/her own living environment leading towards enhanced their physical and mental health" (Orchard, 2021). This is an emerging new challenge needing attention. It is relevant within any health agency or organization as often there is a need to connect groups from different services to address key issues. We do not have the time to send an email and wait for responses from a variety of representatives of each group. We need to learn to bring them together and apply the learning from relationship-focused collaborative practice as well. The challenge is here, the need is for many persons who can practice using collaborative leading approaches to find innovative solutions within the constraints we all experience today. The need is for solutions for problems not being inundated with problems for which solutions are not explored.

REFERENCES

Agbejule, A., Rapo, J., & Saarikoski, L. (2021). Vertical and horizontal trust and team learning: The role of organizational climate. *International Journal of Managing Projects in Business*, *14*(8), 1425–1443. DOI: 10.1108/IJMPB-05-2020-0155

Ahlquist, J. S., & Levi, M. (2011). Leadership: What it means, what it does, and what we want to know about it. *Annual Review. Annual Review of Political Science*, *14*(1), 1–24. DOI: 10.1146/annurev-polisci-042409-152654

Ang'ana, G., & Kilika, J. M. (2022). Collaborative leadership in an organizational context: A research agenda. *Journal of Human Resource & Leadership*, *6*(1), 48–71. DOI: 10.53819/81018102t2050

Archer, D., & Cameron, A. (2009). *Collaborative leadership: How to succeed in an interconnected world.* Elsevier. DOI: 10.4324/9780080943008

Babnik, K., Sirca, N. T., & Dermol, V. (2014). Individuals learning in work teams: Support of knowledge management initiatives and an important source of organizational learning. *Procedia: Social and Behavioral Sciences*, *124*, 178–185. DOI: 10.1016/j.sbspro.2014.02.475

Bard, S. K., Rench, T. A., & Kozlowski, S. W. J. (2014). Performance adaptation: A theoretical integration and review. *Journal of Management*, *40*(1), 48–99. DOI: 10.1177/0149206313488210

Boyle, D. K., & Kochinda, C. (2004). Enhancing collaborative communication of nurses and physician leadership in two intensive care units. *The Journal of Nursing Administration*, *34*(2), 60–70. DOI: 10.1097/00005110-200402000-00003 PMID: 14770064

Chrislip, D. D. (2002). *The collaborative leadership fieldbook: A guide for citizens and civic leaders*. Jossey-Bass.

Crevani, L., Lindgfren, M., & Packendorff, J. (2009). Leadership, not leaders: On the study of leadership as practices and interactions. *Scandinavian Journal of Management*, *26*(1), 77–86. DOI: 10.1016/j.scaman.2009.12.003

DiBello, K. (2019). Collaborative leadership. *AAACN Viewpoint: Pitman*, *41*(4), 15–16.

Edmonstone, J. (2009). Clinical leadership: The elephant in the room. *The International Journal of Health Planning and Management*, *24*(4), 290–305. DOI: 10.1002/hpm.959 PMID: 18770874

Frydman, B., Wilson, I., & Wyer, J. A. (2000). *The power of collaborative leadership: Lessons for the learning organization*. Butterworth-Heinemann. HD58.82. F79 2000 658.4'063-dc21

Gitell, J. H., Godfrey, M., & Thistlethwaite, J. (2013). Interprofessional collaborative practice and relational coordination: Improving healthcare through relationships. *Journal of Interprofessional Care*, *27*(3), 210–213. DOI: 10.3109/13561820.2012.730564 PMID: 23082769

Hogan, R., & Kariser, R. B. (2005). What we know about leadership. *Review of General Psychology*, *9*(2), 169–180. DOI: 10.1037/1089-2680.9.2.169

Hsieh, J. Y., & Liou, K. T. (2018). Collaborative leadership and organizational performance: Assessing the structural relation in a public service agency. *Review of Public Personnel Administration*, *38*(1), 83–109. DOI: 10.1177/0734371X15623619

Jarvis, P. (2010). *Adult education & lifelong learning: Theory and practice* (4th ed.). Routledge.

Jiang, G. (2023). Collaborative leadership in team science: dynamics of sense making, decision making, and action taking. *Frontiers in Research Metrics and Analytics*, 01-06. DOI: 10.3389/frma.2023.1211407

Khalili, H., & Orchard, C. (2020). The effects of an IPS-based IPE program on interprofessional socialization and dual identity development. *Journal of Interprofessional Care*, ●●●, 1–11. DOI: 10.1080/13561820.2019.1709427 PMID: 32019374

Klein, K. J., Knight, A. P., Ziegert, J. C., Lim, B. C., & Slatz, J. L. (2010). When team members' values differ: The moderating role of team leadership. *Organizational Behavior and Human Decision Processes*, *114*(1), 25–36. DOI: 10.1016/j.obhdp.2010.08.004

Kouzes, J., & Posner, B. (2012). *The leadership challenge: How to make extraordinary things happen in organizations* (5th ed.). Jossey-Bass.

Kozlowski, S. W., & Bell, B. S. (2007). Team learning, development, and adaptation. In *Work group learning* (pp. 39–68). Psychology Press.

Kozlowski, S. W. J. (2018). Enhancing the effectiveness of work groups and teams: A reflection. *Perspectives on Psychological Science*, *13*(2), 205–212. DOI: 10.1177/1745691617697078 PMID: 29232536

Kruse, K. (2013). *What is leadership?* Forbes.com, April 9, 2013. 1-3

Miranda, D., & Watts, R. (2022). What is a RACI chart? How this project management tool can boost your productivity. www.forbes.com

Orchard, C., (2024). (in review). Health Care Transitions: A critical literature review. *The Journal of Continuing Education in the Health Professions.*

Orchard, C. (2020). The advanced practice nurse and interprofessional collaborative practice. In E. Staples, R. Pilon, & R.A. Hannon (Eds) *Canadian perspectives on advanced practice nursing (2nd. Ed.)* (pp. 406-432). Canadian Scholars. ISBN: 9781773382173

Orchard, C. (2022). *A further update of the Assessment of Interprofessional Collaborative Leadership Scale (AICLS*). Unpublished.

Orchard, C., King, G., Tryphonopoulos, P., Gorman, E., Ugirase, S., Lising, D., & Fung, K. (2023). Interprofessional team conflict resolution: A critical literature review. *The Journal of Continuing Education in the Health Professions*, *44*(3), 203–2010. DOI: 10.1097/CEH.0000000000000524 PMID: 37458607

Orchard, C., & Rykhoff, M. (2015). Collaborative leadership within interprofessional practice. In *Leadership and collaboration: Further developments for interprofessional education* (pp. 71-94). Palgrave Macmillan UK.

Orchard, C., Sinclair, E., & Rykhoff, M. (2019). The new leadership in health care teams: Progress report of development on a promising measure. *Archives of Healthcare*, *1*(1), 20–26.

Pearce, C. L. (2004). The future of leadership: Combining vertical and shared leadership to transform knowledge work. *The Academy of Management Perspectives*, *18*(1), 47–57. DOI: 10.5465/ame.2004.12690298

Pearce, C. L., & Sims, H. P.Jr. (2002). Vertical versus shared leadership as predictors of the effectiveness of change management teams: An examination of aversive, directive, transactional, transformational, and empowering leader behaviours. *Group Dynamics*, *6*(2), 172–197. DOI: 10.1037/1089-2699.6.2.172

Pettigrew, T. F. (1998). Intergroup contact theory. *Annual Review of Psychology*, *49*(1), 65–85. DOI: 10.1146/annurev.psych.49.1.65 PMID: 15012467

Pettigrew, T. F., & Tropp, L. R. (2008). How does intergroup contact reduce prejudice? Meta-analytic tests of three mediators. *European Journal of Social Psychology*, *38*(6), 122–134. DOI: 10.1002/ejsp.504

Raelin, J. A. (2016). Imagine there are no leaders: Reframing leadership as collaborative agency. *Leadership*, *12*(2), 131–158. DOI: 10.1177/1742715014558076

Raelin, J. A. (Ed.). (2016*). Leadership-as-practice: Theory and application*. Routledge Studies in Leadership Research, ISBN: 978-138-92485-7

Rykhoff, M., Orchard, C., & Wong, C. (2015). *Interprofessional Collaborative Leadership: a concept analysis*. Unpublished PhD work. University of Western Ontario.

Senge, P. M. (2006). *The fifth discipline: The art and practice of the learning organization*. Doubleday Publishing Group, Inc.

Shulman, L. S. (2005). Signature pedagogies in the professions. *Daedalus*, *134*(3), 52–59. DOI: 10.1162/0011526054622015

Sumeth, T., & Li, X. (2013). Is there a relationship between individual learning, team learning, and organizational learning? *The Alberta Journal of Educational Research*, *59*(1), 1–16. DOI: 10.55016/ojs/ajer.v59i1.55542

VanVactor, J. D. (2012). Collaborative leadership model in the management of health care. *Journal of Business Research*, *65*(4), 555–561. DOI: 10.1016/j.jbusres.2011.02.021

World Health Organization (WHO). (2010). *Framework for action on interprofessional education and collaborative practice. (WHO/HRH/HPN/10.3)*. WHO.

Yoon, S. W., Song, J. H., Lim, D. H., & Joo, B.-K. (2010). Structural determinants of team performance: The mutual influences of learning culture, creativity, and knowledge. *Human Resource Development International*, *13*(3), 249–264. DOI: 10.1080/13678868.2010.483815

Chapter 4
Measuring and Evaluating Team Performance in Healthcare Practice:
Two Major Scales

Katsumi Fujitani
Bunkyo Gakuin University, Japan

ABSTRACT

Background: The purpose of this study is to translate the AITCS (Assessment of Inter-professional Team Collaboration Scale), a measurement scale of IPC (Inter-Professional Collaboration), and the AICLS (Assessment of Interprofessional Leadership Scale), a measurement scale of leadership in IPC, into Japanese and to examine their reliability and construct validity. Methods: AITCS and AICLS were translated from English into Japanese, AITCSII-J and AICLS-J were created, and their reliability and construct validity were examined. Results: The Cronbach'sα coefficient for AITCSII-J was 0.9, indicating excellent internal consistency. For AICLS-J, Cronbach'sα, which indicates good reliability of the data, was 0.987, indicating good internal consistency of the questions. The original AICLS scale consists of 28 questions, but was refined to 10 questions after verification. Conclusion: AITCSII-J and AICLS-J show acceptable evidence of validity and reliability, suggesting that these scales are useful for measuring IPC in Japanese healthcare settings.

INTRODUCTION

Collaborative leadership, a new form of leadership style, is essential for effective multidisciplinary collaboration. Collaborative leadership is a concept based on or-

DOI: 10.4018/979-8-3693-2230-7.ch004

ganizational learning, and is applied in the context of action learning, where leaders appropriately guide teams toward goals to promote strategies in which teams work collaboratively to solve problems. This term, collaborative leadership, is understood to better fit within healthcare to reflect the ever-changing strategies that need to be implemented with each patient. The AICLS (Assessment of Inter-professional Collaborative Leadership Scale) was developed by a team at Western University in Canada (Sinclair & Orchard, 2019). The original questionnaire consisted of 28 items and four subscales (Symbiotic relationships, Mindfulness, Shared assets, Capacity to lead). In this paper, we will describe? a survey using the Japanese version of the Collaborative Leadership Scale at medical facilities in Japan and will report on the results that verified the reliability and validity of the Japanese version of the scale. Collaborative leadership is generally considered to be a current need to cultivate and strengthen leadership in the management of welfare and medical facilities and integrated community care systems (Matsushita, 2010). On the other hand, regarding leadership, various discourses have been proposed, from servant leadership (Greenleaf, 1977) to humble leadership (Schein, 2018). In recent years, collaborative leadership has been attracting attention as a leadership theory that leads to multidisciplinary collaboration in healthcare and contributes to improving the quality and safety level of healthcare. According to Orchard et al., in multidisciplinary collaboration and patient-centered healthcare practice, team leadership has a significant impact on providing better quality care and safety to patients and healthcare users (Orchard & Rykhoff, 2015). In previous research, multiple pieces of evidence have shown that Inter-professional Collaboration Education (IPE), which contributes to inter-professional collaboration, has a high learning effect and influences healthcare outcomes (Hammick et al., 2007; Reeves et al., 2007). There are also reports that link inter-professional collaboration and the need for organizational learning in healthcare settings to share member's mental morel, (Matsuo 2009; Yamamoto 2014; Yamaguchi 2017). However, research that quantitatively examines multi-disciplinary collaboration from a leadership perspective is rare.

METHOD

Reliability of the AICLS was calculated using Cronbach's αcoefficient, and exploratory factor analysis and confirmatory factor analysis were used for validity. In accordance with the previous studies of AITCS, Cronbach's alpha was chosen to evaluate the reliability of this psychometric construct. The internal consistency of a scale is to measure the degree to which different statements intend to measure the same characteristic. Statements that are supposed to measure the identical characteristic should be highly correlated with each other. Consequently, Cronbach's alpha coefficient is used to investigate the internal consistency; when it is above 0.70, it is considered acceptable (Tavakol & Dennick, 2011). A robust cloud environment was built to implement the survey using the Internet. All the respondents read the study description on a poster, and those who wanted to participate accessed the survey site through the Internet from devices such as mobile phones, tablets, and personal computers, through predetermined quick response codes and addresses from their respective workplaces. The survey on the AITCS was implemented from April 15 to May 17, 2019. The responses were limited to only on per person. The results were encrypted using Secure Socket Layer technology, then stored in the cloud and managed by the primary researcher. First, we confirmed the equivalence of the Japanese version of the questionnaire. We conducted interviews with multiple medical professionals, including doctors, nurses, and medical safety department managers, to ask if they understood each item that had been translated from the original version, and confirmed whether the content of the questions was as intended in the original version. We then conducted a back-translation and asked a Canadian researcher to review it again to check for any differences from the original version, thereby confirming the equivalence of the Japanese version of the questionnaire. Next, based on the translated questionnaire, we requested cooperation from Hospital A, an acute care medical facility located near Tokyo, and asked all medical and administrative staff employed at Hospital A to complete a survey using the cloud-based AITCSII-J (Assessment of Inter-professional Team Collaboration Scale II-J), a scale for measuring the actual state of inter-professional collaboration, and the AICLS-J (Assessment of Inter-professional Collaborative Leader Scale-J), a scale for measuring leadership. To request cooperation, with the permission of the hospital administrator, a poster clearly stating the survey contents was posted in the healthcare settings, and each staff member was asked to voluntarily access the questionnaire form on the website using the displayed QR code and submit the data. The system was set up so that participants could proceed to the input form only if they read the research explanation in the questionnaire form, agreed to cooperate in the research, and clicked the consent button on the web. The survey on AICLS was conducted from November 1, 2021 to January 31, 2022. Approval was obtained from the ethics committee of A Hospital and the ethics committee of Bunkyo Gakuin University Faculty of Health and Medical Technology (No. 2021-0006) to conduct the survey. To verify reliability and validity, factor analysis (exploratory factor analysis and confirmatory factor analysis) was performed using structural equation modeling (SEM). First, an exploratory factor analysis was performed to verify reliability (internal consistency), and then a confirmatory factor analysis was performed using maximum likelihood estimation. The model fit was verified using the chi-square value, Goodness of fit index (GFI), Adjusted goodness of fit index (AGFI), Comparative fit index (CFI), and Root mean square error of approximation (RMSEA). Canadian researchers had already completed exploratory and confirmatory factor analysis of the AITCS, so we adopted those results and only conducted exploratory factor analysis in order to confirm the number of factors in the Japanese version. IBM SPSS Statistics (Version 26) was used to verify reliability (internal consistency), and IBM SPSS Amos Version 27) was used for confirmatory factor analysis, with a p value of less than 0.05 considered statistically significant. In addition, to verify criterion-related validity, the correlation between the AITCSII-J and AICLS-J scales was evaluated as an external criterion.

RESULTS

In our research, we conducted the IPC survey first and the collaborative leadership survey later, so we conducted the AITCS and AICLS surveys on different occasions and at different institutions.

① AITCSII-J

The AITCS was developed by Canadian researchers and revised from the original 37 questions to 23 questions (AITCS II), which has already obtained high reliability and internal validity (Orchard et al., 2018). Therefore, in this study, we conducted a two-stage validation. In the first stage, we evaluated the methodological translation and cultural adaptation of AITCS II from English to Japanese and created the first version of AITCS II-J. In the second stage, we examined the reliability and content validity of AICTS II-J. In our main survey, the number of participants was 364. Based on the above criteria, six were judged as invalid responses; consequently, 358 were finally regarded valid responses. Of these, 82.1% were female, 15.4% were male and 0.6% were unknown or unwilling to be identified. Since this study was an empirical study on IPC practices, it targeted all professionals employed by the hospital, both full-time and part-time, and in all departments. Cronbach's α for the three subscales and the original AITCS (37 questions) total sum score varied from 0.917 to 0.962. As shown in Table 1, Cronbach's α for the three subscales of AITCSII-J were: partnership 0.912, cooperation 0.940, and coordination 0.917. Exploratory factor analysis used an unweighted least square method with vari-max rotation.

Table 1. Factor loadings of AITCSII-J

	Factor		
	Partnership	2 Cooperation	3 Coordination
Item 11	**.821**	.239	.082
Item 12	**.760**	.207	.316
Item 4)	**.757**	.178	.107
Item 1)	**.740**	.142	.232
Item 16	**.727**	.198	.348
Item 2	**.726**	.203	.121
Item 2)	**.714**	.195	.133
Item 5)	**.714**	.155	.292
Item 18	**.656**	.339	.188
Item 3)	**.655**	.128	.274
Item 15	**.627**	.144	.421
Item 1	**.591**	.230	.146
Item 8	**.489**	.144	.244
Item 6	**.467**	.136	.429
Item 21	.214	**.860**	.142
Item 7)	.211	**.854**	.128
Item 6)	.238	**.829**	.130
Item 8)	.138	**.822**	.117
Item 13)	.187	**.806**	.193
Item 12)	.217	**.793**	.283
Item 11)	.214	**.780**	.239
Item 10)	.228	**.771**	.301
Item 9)	.229	**.748**	.279
Item 29	.383	**.651**	.322
Item 28	.376	**.603**	.304
Item 17)	.271	.408	**.671**
Item 19)	.209	.283	**.666**
Item 20)	.310	.174	**.661**
Item 16)	.353	.279	**.653**
Item 15)	.207	.466	**.603**
Item 18)	.394	.490	**.566**
Item 14)	.262	.351	**.455**

② AICLS-J

Valid responses were obtained from 729 out of a total of 1,221 employees (response rate: 60.0%). In order to perform factor analysis using IBM AMOS, data with missing values were removed, leaving 675 valid data (valid response rate: 55.28%). The reliability statistic (Cronbach's α), which indicates the reliability of the data, was 0.987, indicating that the internal consistency of the questions was ensured.

Furthermore, after confirming that there were no ceiling or floor effects in the items of the original AICLS Japanese version scale, factor analysis was performed for each item. First, an exploratory factor analysis was performed on the 28 AICLS questions (four factors), and the results converged the questions down to 10 items (three factors). Furthermore, a confirmatory factor analysis was performed on the 10 questions, and the goodness-of-fit indices for the factor structure were high, GFI = 0.963, AGFI = 0.936, and CFI = 0.986, respectively, with an RMSEA = 0.07 ($\chi 2$ = 136.887, DF = 32, $p < 0.00$) (Table 2). Therefore, the model showed a moderate fit. Based on these results, the AICLS-J was selected as the formal measurement scale. Below is a path analysis diagram showing the factor loadings for each question item (Figure 1). In addition, the correlation between the AICLS and the AITCSII-J was r = 0.809 (Table 3), which was significantly high ($p < 0.01$).

Figure 1. Path analysis diagram showing the factor loadings for each of the 10 questions

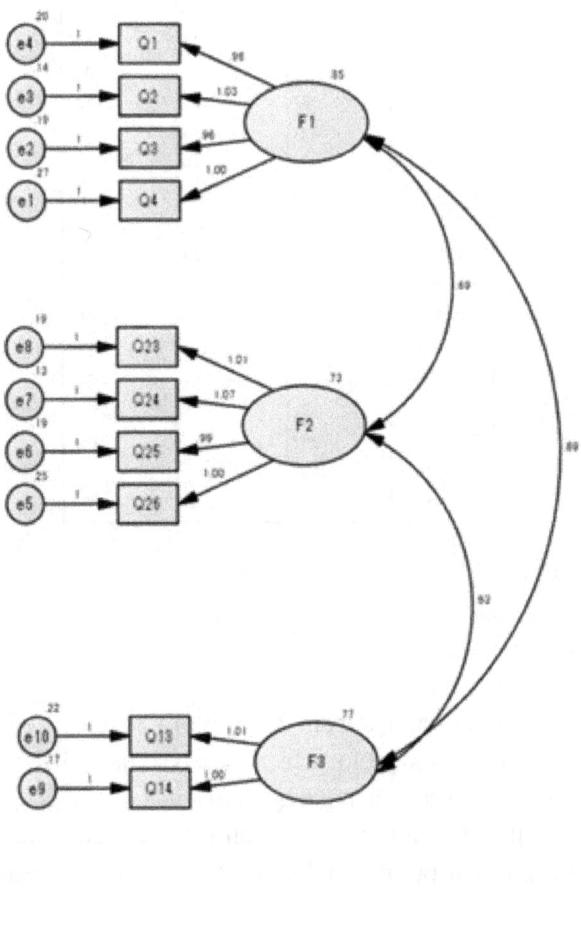

Table 2. Factor description and model fit

F1	Factor 1	Mutual understanding and cooperation
F2	Factor 2	Psychological safety and innovation
F3	Factor 3	Empowerment among members
Model fit:GFI=.963, AGFI=.936, RMSEA=.070, CFI=.986		

Table 3. Correlation between AICLS and AITCSII-J

Speraman		AITCS II -J	AICLS-J
AITCS II -J	Correlation coefficient	1.00	.809**
	Significance probability		0.00
	frequency	729.00	729.00
AICLS-J	Correlation coefficient	.809**	1.00
	Significance probability	0.00	
	frequency	729.00	729.00
**The correlation coefficient is significant at the 1% level (two-tailed).			

DISCUSSION

The fit indices used in this study are considered to be appropriate when the CFI is ≥ .90 and the RMSEA is ≤ .06 (.07 or .08) (Hu & Bentler 1999). The results of this study showed high fit indices of GFI = 0.963, AGFI = 0.936, and CFI = 0.986, and the factor structure was confirmed with RMSEA = 0.07. The values of GFI, AGFI, CFI, and RMSEA were also generally within the standard range, so it can be said that the construct validity of this scale was confirmed. Furthermore, in order to verify criterion-related validity, the correlation with the AITCSII-J, a scale for measuring the actual state of inter-professional collaboration, was examined, and a significant correlation of r = 0.809 was observed, indicating the concurrent validity of the two concepts of inter-professional collaboration and collaborative leadership. The AITCSII-J is a scale that measures the perception of the actual state of inter-professional collaboration, and since it correlated well with the AICLS-J evaluation scale, criterion-related validity was confirmed. Furthermore, in the verification of internal consistency, the Cronbach alpha, which indicates reliability, exceeded the generally accepted standard of 0.70 (Bland & Altman 1997, Devellis, 2003, Nunnaly & Bernstein 1994), and it was determined that sufficient internal consistency was obtained. The AICLS-J created in this study is evaluated as having a certain degree of reliability and validity.

CONCLUSION

We developed a 10-question Japanese version of the Collaborative Leadership Scale (AICLS-J) and verified its reliability and validity. In this study, we conducted a factor analysis on the 28 original questions of the AICLS. This resulted in further refinement, and a certain degree of validity and reliability was confirmed, so it is judged that it can be used in Japanese environments in the future. In this study, the results of exploratory factor analysis and confirmatory factor analysis of the data confirmed the reliability and validity of the Japanese version of the AICLS as an evaluation index. In the future, we would like to verify the relationship between the confirmation of collaborative leadership and indicators of other elements such as organizational learning and psychological safety in relation to leadership functions and multi-professional collaboration, and further consider the possibility of applied use.

REFERENCES

Bland, J. M., & Altman, D. G. (1997). Cronbach's Alpha. *British Medical Journal, 314*(7080), 572. DOI: 10.1136/bmj.314.7080.572 PMID: 9055718

DeVellis, R. F. (2003). *Scale Development: Theory and Applications* (2nd ed.). Sage.

Greenleaf, R. K. (1977). *Servant Leadership: A Journey into the Nature of Legitimate Power and Greatness*. Paulist Press.

Hammick, M., Freeth, D., Koppel, I., Reeves, S., & Barr, H. (2007). A best evidence systematic review of inter-professional education: BEME Guide no.9. *Medical Teacher, 29*(8), 735–751. DOI: 10.1080/01421590701682576 PMID: 18236271

Hu, L. T., & Bentler, P. M. (1999). Cutoff Criteria for Fit Indexes in Covariance Structure Analysis: Conventional Criteria versus New Alternatives. *Structural Equation Modeling, 6*(1), 1–55. DOI: 10.1080/10705519909540118

Matsushita, H. (2010). *Creative Leadership and Team Medical Care*. Japan Medical Planning.

Orchard, C., & Rykhoff, M. (2015). Collaborative leadership within inter-professional practice. In Forman, D., Jones, M., & Thistlethwaite, J. (Eds.), *Leadership and collaboration: Further developments for inter-professional education* (pp. 71–94). Palgrave Macmillan. DOI: 10.1057/9781137432094_5

Orchard, C., Sinclair, E., & Rykhoff, M. (2019). The new leadership in health care teams: Progress report of development on a promising measure. *Archives of Healthcare, 1*(1), 20–26.

Orchard, C., Sonibare, O., Morse, A., Collins, J., & Al-Hamad, A. (2017). Collaborative leadership, part 1: The nurse leader's role within inter-professional teams. *Nursing Leadership, 30*(2), 14–25. DOI: 10.12927/cjnl.2017.25258 PMID: 29083290

Orchard, C. A., King, G. A., Khalili, H. L., & Bezzina, M. B. (2012). Assessment of inter-professional team collaboration scale (AITCS): Development and testing of the instrument. *The Journal of Continuing Education in the Health Professions, 32*(1), 58–67. DOI: 10.1002/chp.21123 PMID: 22447712

Reeves S, Perrier L, Goldman J et al (2007). Inter-professional education: effects on professional practice and healthcare outcomes, Cochrane Database of systematic reviews 3,h t t p s: / / w w w. c o c h r a n e l i b r a r y. c o m / c d s r / d o i /, accessed on Jul 3, 2021DOI: 10.1002/14651858.CD002213.pub3/full

Schein, E. H., & Schein, P. A. (2018). *Humble Leadership: The Power of Relationships, Openness and Trust*. Berrett-Koehler Publishers.

Tavakol, M., & Dennick, R. (2011). Making sense of Cronbach's alpha. *International Journal of Medical Education*, *2*, 53–55. DOI: 10.5116/ijme.4dfb.8dfd PMID: 28029643

Yamaguchi, E. (2017). Cultivating a learning hospital organization: striving for better quality and safety in medical care (Japanese) *System/Control/Information*, Vol. 61, No. 6, pp. 233–239.

Yamamoto, T. (2014). Empirical research on organizational change in hospitals through team medical care (Japanese). *Kawasaki Medical Welfare Journal*, *23*(2), 255–267.

Chapter 5
Interprofessional Education (IPE) and Collaborative Practice

Jenn Salfi
Brock University, Canada

ABSTRACT

Interprofessional Education (IPE) is not a new concept but how it is defined, what it encompasses, modes of delivery, and how it is evaluated are constantly evolving as research evidence emerges and work environments change. This chapter will (1) revisit some of the history of IPE, including common facilitators and barriers that still present challenges today; (2) review recent research literature to better understand the current perspectives on the effectiveness of IPE; and (3) propose and share ideas for future IPE that take into consideration the existing barriers and challenges, while acknowledging what is required to successfully develop collaborative professionals in today's taxing healthcare environment.

INTERPROFESSIONAL EDUCATION

Interprofessional education remains a popular strategy for educating students and professionals about teamwork and collaboration and can be described in the literature as education taking on many different shapes and forms, and in a variety of settings. A review of the literature on IPE reveals differences in definitions and approaches to delivery, among a variety of stakeholders such as healthcare providers, professional associations, and post-secondary institutions. To some, IPE as an occasional activity or workshop is viewed as sufficient to encourage a collaborative mindset and behaviors, while others argue that IPE can only be effective if embed-

DOI: 10.4018/979-8-3693-2230-7.ch005

ded in health and social care curriculum, mandated by professional programs, and included in accreditation processes of all health professions (Grymonpre et al., 2021). Other differences in perspective in how IPE should be delivered include delivery right from the beginning of a student's pre-licensure studies, as opposed to a delayed exposure to allow for students to gain adequate knowledge on their own professional roles and scope of practice; and IPE delivered as a single method of teaching and learning versus IPE as a repertoire of experiences and methods upon which teachers can employ the most appropriate approach to learning.

Whatever the format or delivery, a few key points should always be upheld when designing and implementing IPE experiences for learners. First, interprofessional education should expose and foster role clarity, which includes learning about one's own scope of professional practice and how to articulate it to others, as well as includes an awareness of where one's role fits within a variety of health and social care teams. This role clarity is further enhanced by "learning with, from and about others" present in any given interprofessional learning environment, which includes exposure to the skills, language, values and distinctive experiences and expertise that all participating professionals bring to the healthcare team from their respective backgrounds (CAIPE, 2021).

Second, IPE should provide opportunities for the development and improvement of both basic and more complex skills required for effective team functioning. Communication, mutual goal-setting, and shared-decision-making are essential for successful collaborative experiences and are skills that are only developed with repeated exposure and practice. Competence in these areas depends on one's ability to trust and respect others, listen attentively and be open-minded, flexible, and accountable. Possession of all these team functioning skills is required as the building blocks for more advanced skills in collaboration such as in collaborative leadership and conflict management.

One final key principle of effective IPE is that it should not be viewed in isolation but rather as a continuum over a pre-licensure curriculum, that is revisited and reinforced on an ongoing basis as the student develops as a professional. Ideally, interprofessional education experiences should be thoughtfully embedded within existing professional programs and planned with intentional and shifting goals for each level of the learner, using a variety of pedagogical methodologies. When IPE is threaded throughout the content and the processes of an entire prelicensure curriculum, there is a recontextualization of the traditional uni–professional knowledge, into a knowledge of one's unique and valuable professional role within an interprofessional practice. In turn, these interprofessional experiences afford students the opportunity to accumulate essential knowledge, skills, attitudes, and confidence necessary to be an effective member of a health care team upon graduation (Grice et al., 2018; Salfi et al., 2012).

IPE COMPETENCIES AND FRAMEWORKS

Embedded within these key principles of effective IPE are several competencies (knowledge, skills, values, and behaviors) that are required for interprofessional collaborative practice. IPE competency frameworks are instrumental in fostering a collaborative-ready workforce as they aim to provide a common lens through which a variety of professionals can understand, implement, and assess team-based practices. Although the number and specificity of interprofessional competencies varies across countries and academic institutions, the overall content is similar.

On an international level, the World Health Organization (WHO) revealed its commitment to IPE to the world audience with the release of their publication, *Framework for Action on Interprofessional Education and Collaborative Practice* (2010). Their framework identified six key interprofessional learning domains required for collaborative practice: teamwork, roles and responsibilities, communication, learning and critical reflection, relationships with the patient, and ethical practice. Similar in content, yet differing in categorization, are the six core competencies of the Canadian *Competency Framework for Advancing Collaboration* (Canadian Interprofessional Health Collaborative (CIHC) (2024), which include team functioning, role clarification and negotiation, team communication, collaborative leadership, team differences/disagreements processing, and relationship-focused care/services. The two domains that ground the framework and support the other areas of competence are team communication and relationship-focused care/services, with the four remaining domains providing support and completing the whole integrated structure: role clarification, team functioning, team differences/disagreements processing and collaborative leadership. This updated framework also acknowledges the importance of inclusion, access and diversity in collaborative care, as well as advancements in technology and communication tools (CIHC, 2024).

Similar to the Canadian framework (CIHC, 2024), the interprofessional competency framework for Japanese healthcare professionals also includes two core domains and four peripheral domains. *Patient/client/family/community-centered* and *interprofessional communication* are the two core domains upon which the entire framework is built around, with four supporting "peripheral" domains including competence in *role contribution, facilitation of relationships, reflection and understanding of others* (Haruta et al., 2018).

Some IPE frameworks have condensed the number of primary competencies into four broader areas, for example, the Interprofessional Education Collaborative (IPEC). First adopted in 2011, then updated in 2016, and recently revised in 2023, four key competencies currently guide American professional curriculum and accreditation standards. The IPEC identifies these core domains for collaborative practice as: *Values and Ethics, Roles and Responsibilities, Communication and Teams and*

Teamwork. Included within these four key areas of competence are thirty-three additional sub-competencies, which provide more detail and specificity to help guide curricular decisions in interprofessional education (IPEC, 2023).

IS IPE EFFECTIVE?

An established competency framework that is grounded in best available evidence, inclusive of diverse stakeholder perspectives, and reflective of socio-cultural norms and values, is a significant facilitator for the development, implementation and evaluation of effective IPE. Regardless of the variation in competencies and viewpoints across these collaborative practice frameworks, one stance that seems to be universally agreed upon is the notion that there is a lack of research evidence establishing the overall effectiveness of IPE and the development of these competencies within interprofessional education. Are these competency frameworks effective in informing IPE aimed at cultivating a collaborative workforce? Does IPE promote a collaborative mind and skill set? How long do the "effects" of IPE last after an experience is over, and what is the most effective length/form of delivery of interprofessional educational?

According to a situational analysis on global IPE, involvement in IPE-related scholarship or research was revealed as being extremely low (less than one tenth), as the result of multiple challenges such as lack of funding and administrative support, and limited time for research. These challenges have led to poor attitudes and little motivation to pursue any research or scholarly work in this pedagogical area (Khalili et al., 2022), contributing to an already limited amount of credible published research measuring the impact of IPE.

Although the quest to produce rigorous research evidence supporting the connection between effective IPE - interprofessional collaborative practice - improved patient outcomes remains, some research has surfaced in the meantime that demonstrates little correlation. In a mixed method study that aimed to compare the outcomes of IPE and single professional education (SPE) during a simulation training course, no significant difference between groups was noted. The simulation education experience, overall, was determined to be effective for enabling the development of critical medical management and team behavior performance in all students – but outcome differences *between IPE and SPE groups* was insignificant. The study concluded that SPE-simulation could be an acceptable alternative to IPE-simulation, in the development of team performance outcomes (Chen et al., 2022).

In addition, there is a desire to determine whether IPE experiences in pre-licensure curriculum has long-lasting effects on collaborative behaviours, post-graduate. Most studies evaluating IPE strategies show significant improvements in the skills and attitudes of health and social care professional students *immediately following* the IPE experience, but there is a noticeable lack of research assessing the lasting effects, if any, of IPE and the long-term influences of IPE experiences. This is a critical area to explore, as it is possible that a discrepancy exists between short-term and long-term effects of IPE on interprofessional collaborative practice. To highlight this point, a sequential explanatory mixed-methods study design was conducted to assess what students learned about interprofessional collaboration and teamwork, after an intensive 10-week interprofessional gross anatomy dissection course (data collected from class cohorts spanning from 2011 to 2014 (n = 97)). Immediately following this interprofessional course, quantitative data revealed statistically significant positive change ($P < 0.05$) in areas of teamwork and collaboration, positive professional identity, and roles and responsibilities. Qualitative findings reinforced these results, highlighting key themes of learning about self and others, experiencing the benefits of a long-duration IPE initiative (developing pride and faith), and going forward (commitment to future interprofessional practice) (Fernandes et al., 2015).

To assess the long-term effects of this same 10-week interprofessional gross anatomy dissection course, a follow-up study was also conducted collecting data from the same cohort of students, years after completing this IPE experience. Quantitative analysis revealed a significant decrease in teamwork and collaboration subscales, despite qualitative analysis revealing

that even after several years, graduates greatly appreciated this IPE opportunity and were still able to recall what they had learned and gained from this interprofessional experience. The overall conclusion after this research had been completed was that exposure to current clinical environments may have eroded some of the gains made from the safe, somewhat controlled, IPE experience offered in undergraduate curriculum. Exposure to the hierarchy and stereotypes that still exist in clinical practice are realities that have been identified to have a negative impact on a professional's collaborative attitude, creating an internal conflict between how one wishes to practice, and what results in a fast-paced clinical world (Zheng et al., 2017).

Despite the ongoing challenges and limited available research establishing a strong connection between IPE and the development of a collaborative workforce and improved health outcomes, there is still widespread consensus on the importance of developing competence in interprofessional collaboration. As such, the development and delivery of IPE has continued to evolve over the years and has expanded beyond typical short duration interprofessional activities. IPE-relevant accreditation standards for health and social care academic programs have been viewed as a significant driver of the implementation and ongoing evaluation of IPE curriculum (Azzam at al., 2022), as well as investing in IPE initiatives that are intentional, experiential, longer in duration, and sustainable (ie. in-person, hybrid or online courses) (Grice et al., 2018).

THE FUTURE OF IPE: NAVIGATING, NEGOTIATING AND NORMALIZING

It is well documented what knowledge, skills, attitudes and values need to be gained and reinforced in interprofessional education to become a collaborative professional and an effective team member. Key principles and a variety of IPE frameworks have been developed and updated over time to inform and help guide educators and practitioners in the development of effective IPE, however more evaluation and research is required to establish what interprofessional educational practices truly influence and help create a collaborative workforce. Learning from the past and taking into consideration existing curriculum-related challenges, limited human and financial resources, and an apparent disconnect between education and everyday health care environments, suggestions for future IPE strategies are proposed. Navigating barriers, negotiating importance, and normalizing behaviors are key to advancing IPE in an already strained and ever-changing health care environment.

Navigating Barriers

For IPE to continue to advance as an effective pedagogical practice in preparing health and social care professionals to work together, educators must learn to navigate and plan around the well-known barriers that have presented great challenges in the past (ie. curriculum scheduling conflicts across professional groups, limited human and financial resources, lack of support for faculty champions leading to lack of motivation and drive in IPE). Capitalizing on existing experiences and opportunities that are already well-resourced prevents the hurdles and challenges commonly associated with the creation of new IPE events.

One strategy is to embed a variety of IPE opportunities within the content and processes of undergraduate, prelicensure curriculums. When embedded throughout a professional program, there is a recontextualization of the traditional uni–professional knowledge, into a knowledge of one's unique and valuable professional role within an interprofessional practice. When a conscious effort is made to incorporate a variety of interprofessional experiences throughout a curriculum, students gain opportunities to accumulate the essential knowledge, skills, attitudes, and confidence necessary to be an effective member of a health care team upon graduation (Salfi et al., 2012). Behavioural change takes time, and therefore repetition and reinforcement of key interprofessional competencies over the course of one's prelicensure education is essential in fostering collaborative professionals.

One mechanism for ensuring the integration of IPE strategies throughout a professional curriculum is through accreditation. Accreditation of health profession programs help provide system-level support for interprofessional education and interprofessional collaborative practice - if the concepts of interprofessional education and interprofessional practice are clearly defined, and accountability is evident in identified outcome measures. A recent Canadian study concluded that a standardized approach to IPE accreditation is viewed by many across the country, as a significant driver of IPE and its continuous improvement (Azzam et al., 2022).

All health professional programs include clinical practicum components which are ideal opportunities for students to acquire and build competence in collaborative practice. IPE that is integrated into professional practice courses is already well-resourced with a variety of professionals present, bypassing a common barrier to IPE. To maximize the strengths of the clinical setting in preparing students to be effective collaborative practitioners, it is critical for educators of professional programs to be strategic and intentionally plan the integration and scaffolding of interprofessional competencies within each course, becoming more advanced and refined as students progress through the program. In doing so, and by the time the students have completed their professional program, they will have been provided with ample and consistent opportunities to learn with, from and about other professionals, which is essential for building a foundation for becoming an effective collaborative professional.

Negotiating Priorities

Waning support from management, government and leaders in both academic and health care settings as the result of financial constraints and other priorities, presents another great challenge for the advancement of IPE efforts. These challenges in turn lead to poor attitudes and little motivation in the academic sector to pursue any further activities, research or scholarly work in this pedagogical area (Khalili et al., 2022).

Negotiating priorities within and between academic and clinical centers is more critical than ever before, due to added pressures and strain placed on professionals in these environments. Due to the nature of IPE and the requirement of at least two different professional groups represented within the interprofessional learning experience, priorities and interests of all involved parties must align to achieve the desired outcome and sustainability. One such example highlighting the importance of negotiating priorities across the education and clinical sector was the planning and development of an Interprofessional Education Clinical Teaching Unit (IPE-CTU) in a Canadian community hospital. A steering committee comprised of three academic partners and multiple hospital stakeholders met for several months to plan an innovative clinical teaching unit. The negotiated priorities of the IPE-CTU included the intent to integrate IPE into core training for the pre-licensure students, as well as for the professionals on the clinical unit, for the purpose of developing competence in interprofessional collaborative practice, while simultaneously providing high quality, patient-centered care in the hospital setting (Prentice & Salfi, 2021).

The IPE CTU provided multiple opportunities for interprofessional engagement between both students and practitioners, such as daily rounds (team meetings) and case presentations and role discussions. A study that examined staffs' perception of IPE reported that everyone respected each other, but felt they needed more organizational support from the top to further develop their team skills and make adjustments to team processes (Prentice et al., 2016). Key themes generated from another study that collected data via open-ended survey questions from students participating on the IPE CTU described the importance of communication and respect, the importance of mentors and role modelling in IPE, and the importance of setting aside dedicated time and opportunities for IPE within their full professional curriculums (Salfi et al., 2019). Both studies revealed the importance of negotiating priorities to sustain the effectiveness of such an initiative as an IPE CTU: the staff requesting more support from management in order to develop their team skills, and the students requesting dedicated time for IPE within their already full, professional curriculums in order to continue with their development as collaborative professionals. When management and educators lose sight of these priorities, it is impossible for effective IPE initiatives such as an IPE CTU to continue and move forward.

Normalizing Behaviours

Based on the scholarly work and research evidence that does exist to date, it is apparent that there is a disconnect between the safe, somewhat controlled, typical IPE experience that occurs in the academic setting, with current realities that exist within the fast-paced clinical world (Zheng et al., 2017). There is a possibility that the focus of past and some current IPE activities may be too narrow and may need to extend beyond simply "learning with, from and about" one another, to also include individual preparation with key competencies and experiences to enable new graduates to recognize and manage the complexities and reality of interprofessional collaboration in health settings (Thistlethwaite, & Xyrichis, 2022).

One strategy to assist with preparing students with the transition to the reality of collaboration in health settings is to foster and solidify behaviours that are anchored by required competencies in collaboration, in conjunction with the development of one's soft skills set. In 2016, a large survey was administered to managers and new graduates to better understand what skills they were missing upon entering the workforce. Results clearly revealed "soft skills" (communication/listening, teamwork, conflict management, shared decision-making etc.) accounted for the largest skills gap in new graduates (PayScale, Inc. 2016).

To combat this deficiency, an interprofessional course on collaboration and teamwork was created and made its debut in 2020. The goal of the course is to develop and enhance the soft skills of current (graduate level) and soon-to-be professionals (undergraduate level), through a variety of intentional interprofessional experiential experiences. The layout of the course is guided by a national competency framework (Canadian Competency Framework for Advancing Collaboration (CIHC, 2024) and has two main components. The first half of the course exposes the students to foundational concepts and best evidence on collaboration, which is reinforced by multiple small group challenges and activities, completed face-to-face, within the safety of the classroom and with the faculty facilitator present to role model and assist, if required. The second half of the course focuses on remote teaming, completing a project with a different interprofessional group of students, independent of direct faculty assistance (only support as required); and culminating in a team product and presentation on the final day of the course. The course also includes a before/after video analysis of their team's performance, including their role as a team member; the opportunity to give and receive verbal feedback from their peers regarding their contributions to the team; and a personal reflection at the finale to connect the importance of the various interprofessional experiences throughout the course with their current (or desired) professional role.

The benefits of IPE in course form include (a) sustainability (if mandated by or within a professional program); (b) multiple opportunities to collaborate, manage conflict, and learn to work with different people/personalities; and (c) a stronger likelihood of acquiring some level of competence in "effective" collaborative behaviour as the result of repetitive group/team experiences throughout the course. Many common barriers to IPE are minimized when integrated into existing courses or as a stand-alone course while benefits of IPE are maximized, staying true to the goal of developing competent, confident, collaborative professionals.

The perpetual shortage of healthcare providers and ongoing financial constraints are just a few of the harsh realities currently impacting the care of individuals across a variety of health care sectors. Although IPE has shown the potential to produce graduates capable of working with other professionals in a climate of mutual respect and trust, it is no secret that traditional IPE experiences that were created at a time of ample funding and overwhelming support, were not sustainable, and their effectiveness has been called into question given the disconnect between what is learned in the academic setting and what occurs in the current clinical setting. Navigating barriers, negotiating priorities and normalizing behaviours are just a few ideas for future IPE that take into consideration the existing barriers and challenges, while acknowledging what is required to successfully develop collaborative professionals in today's complex healthcare environment.

REFERENCES

Azzam, M. B., Girard, M. A., Andrews, C., Bilinski, H., Connelly, D. M., Gilbert, J. H. V., Newton, C., & Grymonpre, R. E. (2022). RE. Correction: Accreditation as a driver of interprofessional education: the Canadian experience. *Human Resources for Health*, *20*(1), 77. DOI: 10.1186/s12960-022-00775-4 PMID: 36333726

Canadian Interprofessional Health Collaborative (CIHC). (2024) CIHC Competency Framework for Advancing Collaboration. Retrieved from: https://cihc-cpis.com/wp-content/uploads/2024/06/CIHC-Competency-Framework.pdf

Chen HW, O'Donnell JM, Chiu YJ, Chen YC, Kang YN, Tuan YT, Kuo SY, Wu JC. (2022). Comparison of learning outcomes of interprofessional education simulation with traditional single-profession education simulation: A mixed-methods study. *BMC Med Educ 30*, 22(1):651. . PMID: 36042449; PMCID: PMC9429663.DOI: 10.1186/s12909-022-03640-z

Fernandes, A. Palombella, J. Salfi, & B. Wainman. (2015). Dissecting through barriers: A mixed-methods study on the effect of interprofessional education in a dissection course with health care professional students. *Anatomic Science Education (ASE). Journal*, *8*, 305–316. PMID: 25641912

Grice, G., Thomason, A., Meny, L., Pinelli, N., Martello, J., & Zorek, J. (2018). Intentional interprofessional experiential education. *American Journal of Pharmaceutical Education*, *82*(3), 6502. https://www.ncbi.nlm.nih.gov/pmc/articles/PMC5909877/pdf/ajpe6502.pdf. DOI: 10.5688/ajpe6502 PMID: 29692445

Grymonpre, R. E., Bainbridge, L., Nasmith, L., & Baker, C. (2021). Development of accreditation standards for interprofessional education: A Canadian Case Study. *Human Resources for Health*, *19*(1), 12. DOI: 10.1186/s12960-020-00551-2 PMID: 33472633

Haruta, J., Yoshida, K., Goto, M., Yoshimoto, H., Ichikawa, S., Mori, Y., Yoshimi, K., & Otsuka, M. (2018). Development of an interprofessional competency framework for collaborative practice in Japan. *Journal of Interprofessional Care*, *32*(4), 436–443. https://doi-org.proxy.library.brocku.ca/10.1080/13561820.2018.1426559. DOI: 10.1080/13561820.2018.1426559 PMID: 29381091

Interprofessional Education Collaborative (IPEC). (2023). *IPEC Core Competencies Revision: Version 3 (2021-2023)*. Retrieved from: https://www.ipecollaborative.org/assets/core-competencies/IPEC_Core_Competencies_Version_3_2023.pdf

Khalili, H., Lackie, K., Langlois, S., Wetzlmair, L. C., & the Working Group. (2022). Global IPE Situational Analysis Result Final Report. InterprofessionalResearch. Global Publication (ISBN: 978-1-7366963-2-3). Available at: https://interprofessionalresearch.global/wp-content/uploads/2022/10/Global-IPE-Situational-Analysis-Final-Report-October-2022-1.pdf

Payscale (2016). *2016 Workforce-Skills Preparedness Report.* Retrieved June 28, 2024 from https://www.payscale.com/data-packages/job-skills

Prentice, D., & Salfi, J. (2021). Translating evidence into practice: An experience with interprofessional education (IPE). In Matsushita, H. (Ed.), *Health Informatics. Translational Systems Sciences, 24.* Springer., DOI: 10.1007/978-981-15-3781-3_7

Salfi, J., Prentice, D., Podwinski, K., Triemstra, C., & Hildebrand, L. (2019). The Impact of an Interprofessional Education (IPE) Clinical Teaching Unit on Developing Collaborative Skills and Behaviors: A Pilot Case Study. Unpublished manuscript.

Salfi, J., Solomon, P., Allen, D., Mohaupt, J., & Patterson, C. (2012). Overcoming all obstacles: A framework for embedding interprofessional education (IPE) into a large, multi-site BScN program. *The Journal of Nursing Education*, *51*, 106–110. DOI: 10.3928/01484834-20111230-05 PMID: 22201276

Thistlethwaite, J., & Xyrichis, A. (2022). Forecasting interprofessional education and collaborative practice: Towards a dystopian or utopian future? *Journal of Interprofessional Care*, *36*(2), 165–167. DOI: 10.1080/13561820.2022.2056696 PMID: 35484900

World Health Organization (WHO). (2010) *Framework for action on IPE & collaborative practice.* WHO, Geneva, Switzerland. Retrieved from: https://iris.who.int/bitstream/handle/10665/70185/WHO_HRH_HPN_10.3_eng.pdf

Zheng, Y., Palombella, A., Salfi, J., & Wainman, B. (2018). Dissecting through barriers: A follow-up study on the long-term effects of interprofessional education in a dissection course with healthcare professional students. *Anatomic Science Education (ASE). Anatomical Sciences Education*, *12*(1), 52–60. DOI: 10.1002/ase.1791 PMID: 29659188

Chapter 6
Interprofessional Collaboration and Health Disparities in Public Health Interventions:
An Exploratory Leadership Framework

Ralph A. Gigliotti
https://orcid.org/0000-0001-6060-9270
Rutgers University, USA

Sara E. Spear
Yale University, USA

Christine Goldthwaite
Yale University, USA

ABSTRACT

Addressing complex and systemic problems like health disparities require interdisciplinary, translational, and team-based approaches that take account of the social, cultural, economic, and environmental factors contributing to the persistence of such problems. By crossing disciplinary boundaries, researchers and stakeholders can integrate multiple perspectives into comprehensive solutions that can be translated into practice with a higher likelihood of reducing health disparities. Successful interdisciplinary collaboration hinges upon effective communication and leadership practices. In centering communication as a foundation for successful interdisciplinary and translational activities, this chapter considers the ways in

DOI: 10.4018/979-8-3693-2230-7.ch006

which leadership—enacted through the design of strategies, processes, messages, and structures—may enable collaborative research efforts that productively address health disparities. The exploratory framework introduced in this chapter can help to inform the design of future initiatives for addressing health disparities across disciplines and with communities.

INTRODUCTION

Addressing intractable problems, such as health disparities, requires interdisciplinary and translational approaches that take account of the social, cultural, economic, and environmental factors contributing to the existence and persistence of such challenges. The interplay of these factors contributes to complex problems that must be explored through meaningful engagement with diverse stakeholders and the crossing of disciplinary boundaries in pursuit of applied research. These efforts require collaboration among individuals from different disciplines, the integration of different methods or propositions from various areas of study, or even the creation of new hybrid interdisciplinary fields (Klein, 2017). More broadly, translating scientific and operational observations from laboratories and clinics to effective healthcare and public health interventions requires working with the communities who ultimately receive the care (Gilliland et al., 2019; Smith et al., 2017). Given the need to integrate contributions from numerous constituencies, higher education institutions and academic health centers are uniquely situated to design, implement, and lead such efforts (Karpf, 2019).

The growing research on interdisciplinary and translational science continues to highlight communication as a critical ingredient for successful collaboration—and this emphasis on communication has become especially pronounced in response to the investigation of recent public health challenges, including the COVID-19 pandemic. Leading a diverse network of collaborators and stakeholders is more effective and strengthened by the thoughtful design of engagement strategies, structures, processes, and messages that are grounded in communication theory and that reflect the underlying assumptions associated with effective communicative practice (Aakhus, 2007; Aakhus & Bzdak, 2015). Despite the many opportunities for interdisciplinary research and collaboration, the barriers are abundant, and failure to consider individual and collective communication practices can negatively impact efforts to address healthcare disparities. This paper explores how leadership, which we view as "the design and implementation of messages, strategies, processes, and structures to facilitate social influence" (Ruben & Gigliotti, 2019, 2021), enables interdisciplinary and translational activities for addressing health disparities.

RESEARCH QUESTIONS

Given the ongoing presence of health disparities and the need for broader interdisciplinary and transdisciplinary interventions to respond to these disparities, we engaged in a comprehensive review of the scholarly literature to explore relevant linkages to leadership and communication theory and practice that could be used by scholars and practitioners engaged in this work. The following research questions served as a guide for this exploratory project:

RQ1) What are the relevant concepts in the literature that could inform the development, study, and practice of collaborative efforts for addressing health disparities?

RQ2) In what ways can leaders of these collaborative engagements focus upon messages, strategies, processes, and structures to influence the success of these comprehensive interventions?

This qualitative inquiry led to the design of an exploratory framework—grounded in communication and leadership theory and practice—that could be used to guide the development, study, and practice of collaborative efforts for addressing health disparities. Future research and practice might further refine the conceptual framework proposed in this paper.

LITERATURE REVIEW

Situating the Study of Health Disparities

Health disparities can be described as differences in health outcomes between groups of people, reflecting inequalities where disadvantaged groups "systematically experience worse health or greater health risks than more advantaged groups" (Braveman, 2006, p. 180). In 2003, the Institute of Medicine issued its landmark report, *Unequal Treatment: Confronting Racial and Ethnic Disparities in Health,* documenting the extent of health disparities and their contributing factors, along with recommended strategies for reducing such disparities (Smedley et al., 2003). This report brought national awareness to the issue of health disparities, acknowledging the need to view health disparities from multiple levels. Ten years later, in 2013, the U.S. Department of Health and Human Services concluded that no significant progress had yet been made in lessening disparities, and "health care quality and access [remain] suboptimal, especially for minority and low-income groups" (Gold, 2014). Since then, significant research has been conducted on health outcomes across groups in the United States, with overwhelming evidence to confirm the prevalence of health disparities including morbidity (e.g., HIV and diabetes) and mortality rates (e.g., infant deaths), behavioral risk factors, access to healthcare, and exposure to environmental hazards (Harrington, 2013). These disparities reflect social inequalities and have an adverse impact on individuals, community wellbeing, and economic prosperity (Cameron, 2013). There is a moral imperative in addressing health disparities, with some advocating for a shift in language to *health inequality* or *inequity* to underscore these differences as both unnecessary and avoidable (Harrington, 2013; Koh et al., 2010). The goal of reaching health equity is one where "everyone has the opportunity to attain full health potential and no one is disadvantaged from achieving this potential because of social position or any other socially defined circumstance" (Weinstein et al., 2017, p. 32).

The topic of health disparities remains one of widespread interest for scientists, agencies, and individuals with community health and public health responsibilities. For example, the COVID-19 pandemic brought health disparities to the forefront given the disproportionate impact of the virus on people of color (CDC, 2020). Furthermore, given the increased emphasis on team science and recent efforts to analyze and understand the competencies associated with leading interprofessional and interdisciplinary teams (Gigliotti et al., 2024), the subject of this paper is one of timely importance. The realization of health equity requires well-coordinated thinking and the design of interventions across system levels and domains, and ultimately, a commitment to effective communication and leadership in guiding the work of interprofessional and interdisciplinary teams dedicated to this work.

The Role of Multilevel Interventions

Despite growing awareness of systemic inequities, healthcare is still frequently discussed on a micro level, focused narrowly on interactions between physicians and patients, where poor health is attributed to individual genetic or behavioral factors. Additionally, research examining the political, organizational, and cognitive dynamics that impede patient-physician medical collaborations is limited (Touati et al., 2018). However, a broadened focus on population health at a macro level considers the impact of environmental factors, psychosocial variables, political and economic determinants, and the healthcare system more broadly. Since the *Unequal Treatment* report, numerous research initiatives have examined the structural drivers of health disparities (Brown et al., 2019) that put certain groups at a systemic disadvantage in the United States, such as race and ethnicity, socioeconomic status, gender or gender identity, sexual orientation, geographical location, and disability status (Weinstein et al., 2017). For example, the recommendation for women to start receiving annual mammograms at age 40 is widely advertised and closely followed by insurance companies. This recommendation, however, is based on research of breast cancer among white women, disregarding data that shows breast cancer emerges earlier among Black and Hispanic women (Gehlert et al., 2010). When such benchmarks and policies are based on white populations, individuals of other races are put at risk, all the while reinforcing existing health disparities.

Social determinants of health are the conditions that both reflect and reinforce inequalities. The U.S. Department of Health and Human Services categorizes these determinants into five domains: economic stability, education access and quality, health care access and quality, neighborhood and built environment, and social and community context (U.S. Department of Health & Human Services, n.d.). These five domains and their structural drivers are often interconnected and overlapping where the systemic determinants of racism or poverty span multiple domains and create a deeply embedded system of "complicated roots" that disproportionately impact specific populations and are difficult to disentangle (Koh et al., 2010, p. S72). For example, socioeconomic status is correlated with chronic stress (Agurs-Collins et al., 2019) and people of color are significantly less likely to have health insurance, a critical factor for access to high-quality care (Cameron, 2013). When such factors are combined, as in the case of people with intersectional identities, the likelihood of experiencing health disparities significantly increases (Weinstein et al., 2017).

Since healthcare has traditionally been viewed as a collection of individual patient and doctor interactions, interventions have typically focused on the individual level. Considering the complex and inextricable web of factors, one-level interventions are not as adequate in eliminating the health disparities that exist within populations (Agurs-Collins et al., 2019; Gehlert et al., 2010). In response, various frameworks and models have emerged to systematically consider the multiple levels and factors involved in addressing health disparities. For example, the CDC's Social-Ecological Model considers the interplay of individual, relational, community, and societal factors (CDC, 2021) and a framework utilized by the National Institute of Minority Health and Health Disparities (NIMHD), spans individual, interpersonal, community, and societal levels of influence across the five domains of biological, behavioral, physical environment, sociocultural environment, and health system (NIMHD, 2017). These models can guide the design of interventions that span the micro-macro continuum. For example, the quest to reduce obesity includes the promotion of a healthy diet and exercise, but must also acknowledge the role of safe recreational spaces and free or reduced meal programs (Brown et al., 2019). Similarly, individual smoking cessation programs are more likely to be effective when paired with family programs, antismoking work policies, and tobacco taxes (Agurs-Collins et al., 2019). Strategic multilevel interventions are more comprehensive and therefore, more likely to have wide-reaching and significant implications across social groups.

Crossing Disciplinary Boundaries

In 1990, the National Institutes of Health (NIH) established the Office of Minority Programs (OMP), and as a result of the Minority Health and Health Disparities Research and Education Act in 2000, the National Center for Minority Health and Health Disparities (NCMHD) was established (Gehlert et al., 2008). Another initiative was the creation of the Federal Collaboration on Health Disparities Research (FCHDR), an organization that works with a wide variety of federal and nonfederal partners to support and disseminate research that aims to reduce or eliminate disparities in health and health care (Rashid et al., 2006). Over the years, numerous summits have been convened by what is now named the National Institute on Minority Health and Health Disparities (NIMHD), with the most recent event focusing on health disparities resulting from the COVID-19 pandemic (NIH, 2020).

These interdisciplinary efforts consist of teams who possess diverse expertise and who share a goal in determining the multilevel, evidence-based interventions that can help to reduce health disparities. In fact, the landmark *Unequal Treatment* report specifically recommended the use of multidisciplinary teams consisting of individuals from different professions (Smedley et al., 2003), recognizing that to address some of the most complex health issues—such as AIDS, climate change, or opioid addiction—a diversity of fields and disciplines, like the behavioral and social sciences, must be embraced (Mabry et al., 2008).

With a recognition that "the tangled roots of health disparities" (Arnst, 2018, n.p.) are grounded in culture, racism, environmental settings, and policies that disproportionately affect racial, ethnic, or gender group health outcomes, interdisciplinary and transdisciplinary activities can maximize the diverse expertise needed to address these interconnected challenges (Brown et al., 2019). Multiple disciplines, including medicine, psychology, epidemiology, economics, social and political sciences, health services research, humanities, geography, and legal science, can help to drive the development of solutions that are informed by the collective body of expertise (Kivits et al., 2019). Such efforts serve as an important "nexus for developing research, strategies, interventions, measures, tools, policies, and institutional shifts that will directly change health care outcomes among vulnerable populations" (Dankwa-Mullan et al., 2010). That is, when experts work across disciplines, collective interdisciplinary efforts have the potential to create comprehensive and sustainable change in pursuit of health equity (Gehlert et al., 2010).

Despite the value of interdisciplinary and transdisciplinary research efforts, the barriers for engaging in this collaborative work are formidable (Gehlert et al., 2010, p. 420). For example, tensions often arise based on the "ontological and epistemological differences and power inequalities between the disciplines" (Thorpe et al., 2020, p. 19). Many factors contribute to the failure of interdisciplinary efforts including organizational limitations, leadership deficits, mismatched skill sets, and team dynamic dysfunctions (Brown et al., 2019; Gehlert et al., 2010; Klein & Porter, 1990; Siedlok & Hibbert, 2014). Limited by existing institutional and organizational structures, interdisciplinary and translational collaborations require a reimagined organization that can motivate and support such initiatives (Feller, 2002; Rhoten, 2004; Sá, 2007; Whitmer et al., 2010). A review of the literature on interdisciplinarity offered by Siedlok et al. (2015) notes, "a gap exists in our knowledge of how such collaborations are accomplished and the kinds of emergent organizational forms in which it occurs" (p. 96). Facing many potential obstacles, an integrated focus on leadership and communication can be useful in supporting teams that are dedicated to interdisciplinary pursuits.

SYNTHESIS OF KEY CONCEPTS

A Communicative View of Interdisciplinary and Transdisciplinary Collaborations

In response to RQ1, the concepts detailed in the literature review point to the complexity and urgency associated with addressing health disparities through multilevel interventions. Furthermore, these concepts emphasize the importance of addressing such issues in ways that leverage expertise across disciplines. Furthermore, as detailed in this section, leadership and communication become critical to the success of these interdisciplinary and transdisciplinary efforts. The synthesis of this existing scholarship will contribute to the development of a preliminary framework to follow.

As Keyton, Ford, and Smith (2008) note, communication is not merely a component of collaboration, rather communication is "the essence of collaboration" (p. 376). Likewise, communication lies at the "heart" of interdisciplinarity and transdisciplinary activities where it is through communication that the collaborative process unfolds. Therefore, leading a diverse network of collaborators and stakeholders requires the thoughtful design of engagement strategies, structures, and processes that consider the unique disciplinary and community stakeholder perspectives about communication (Aakhus, 2007; Aakhus & Bzdak, 2015; Ruben & Gigliotti, 2019).

A prominent idea in the scholarly literature centers on the importance of interaction and integration across disciplinary boundaries (Jensen & Lund, 2014; Klein, 2017; Paxson, 1996). Fundamentally, interdisciplinary and translational collaborations are constituted through a range of discursive practices including dialogue, questioning, negotiation, and even humor. Dialogue that is structured around building a shared understanding of an issue can enable interdisciplinary groups with members who have "different frames of reference" to productively engage in divergent and/or convergent thinking together (Barge, 2002; Ellinor & Gerald, 1998; Garmston & Wellman, 1999). Questioning is particularly critical for facilitating the development of shared understanding. Critical questions can examine assumptions, raise potential challenges, and reveal tensions that derail interdisciplinary activities including important dialogue about the nature and validity of knowledge or perceptions of quality and credibility across disciplines (Monteiro & Keating, 2009; Ôberg, 2009). Additionally, questioning in the form of appreciative inquiry (Cooperrider & Srivastva, 1987), which calls attention to what is working well, can also surface potential solutions and new directions. Negotiation practices can bring clarity to partial or erroneous understandings, helping team members to translate and interpret concepts and ideas across the unique representational systems of different disciplines (Monteiro & Keating, 2009). The behaviors of group members contribute to the collective communication competence of the team. For example, members can demonstrate attentiveness to others through active listening, using humor and a positive tone when challenging ideas, reserving time for informal conversation and reflection, using shared language, and maintaining a commitment to ongoing learning. While not surprising, sarcasm, inattentiveness, judging others, challenging the expertise of others, and some non-verbal cues such as displays of boredom, all have a detrimental effect (Thompson, 2009). Since communication is a key factor associated with the success or failure of any collaboration, leaders must approach the subject with intentionality, recognizing the value of negotiating and clarifying communication norms at the start of interdisciplinary inquiries and initiatives.

Leading Interdisciplinary and Translational Collaborations

Scholars and practitioners of interdisciplinary and translational science have emphasized the essential role of leadership in supporting the success of such collaborations (Gehlert, et al., 2010; Lengwiler, 2006). However, the expansive literature highlights a range of potential styles, such as transformational, servant, and empowering, along with a wide range of competencies associated with management and leadership, including disciplinary knowledge, problem solving skills, managing schedules and core tasks, budgeting, performance monitoring, and communication and public relations (Benoliel & Somech, 2014; Klein & Porter, 1990; Porter et al., 2006). As conveners and coordinators of interdisciplinary activities, leaders must also engage in the work of project management, including guiding, monitoring, and supporting research output, clarifying goals, melding objectives, providing direction, and managing deadlines (König et al., 2013).

Perhaps most importantly, productive collaborations require leadership practices that are attuned to the fundamentals of communication and relationship-building.

Leaders are typically responsible for facilitating knowledge exchange, requiring skills that enable them to integrate diverse intellectual contributions and encourage their translation (König et al., 2013; Porter et al., 2006). They must attend to interpersonal and team dynamics in order to balance the need for broad participation against the potential for "information overflow and chaos" (König et al., 2013, p. 266), encourage inclusive decision making, balance formal and informal sources of authority, and effectively manage conflict (Jehn, 1997; Vasconcellos, 1990), while also engaging in ongoing coordination and communication with key external stakeholders (Benoliel & Somech, 2014). Finally, germane to the focus on leading interdisciplinary and transdisciplinary teams, leaders play a key role in "establishing and maintaining a balance among disciplines" through building consensus, encouraging cooperation, focusing teams on the big picture, minimizing competition and defensiveness, and creating a context for the free exchange of ideas (Gehlert et al., 2010, p. 413).

By facilitating a productive communication climate, ensuring equal participation, encouraging shared decision making, and nurturing interpersonal relationships within the group and beyond (Boix Mansilla et al., 2015), leaders can influence communication dynamics in creating an environment that is conducive to interdisciplinary and translational collaborations. Providing opportunities for both formal and informal interaction are critical for reducing uncertainty and complexity and building cohesive groups for interdisciplinary initiatives. In addition to ensuring the operational success of the collaboration, leaders can positively impact the collective identity of a unified group. Activities such as building trust and nurturing well-being, framing and focusing the group's attention on objectives and common interests, and managing dynamic group membership can help to maintain and strengthen a shared identity (Boix Mansilla et al., 2015).

Finally, the development and cultivation of an inclusive culture that supports interdisciplinarity is a key leadership activity that can help to support the success of these efforts (Dean, Gill, & Barbour, 2016; Gigliotti & Goldthwaite, 2021). Intercultural awareness and communication competence are needed to support a range of diverse stakeholder groups and create an inclusive environment that welcomes their participation in the process. Leaders must play an active role in shaping communication processes by encouraging open and transparent discussion and decision making, supporting a climate of fairness, and upholding professional ethical standards (König et al., 2013).

AN EXPLORATORY FRAMEWORK FOR LEADING INTERDISCIPLINARY AND TRANSLATIONAL COLLABORATIONS

As supported by the existing literature, leading interdisciplinary and transdisciplinary collaborations is a complex endeavor that is most effective when guided by a thoughtful and systematic approach that recognizes the linkages to communication and leadership behaviors. Using Ruben and Gigliotti's (2019) definition of leadership, "the design and implementation of messages, strategies, processes, and structures to facilitate social influence" (p. 57), we present a concrete way to operationalize the key activities involved in facilitating and supporting interdisciplinary collaboration. This multi-dimensional approach can guide individuals and teams to consider their internal and external stakeholders, immediate and long-term goals, potential sources of resistance, and the impact of collaborative efforts.

Building upon the existing literature summarized in this article, coupled with our experience of engaging with units and teams at our institution, we propose an exploratory four-by-four matrix (Table 1) that delineates the four stages of team development (Tuckman, 1965) and explicates relevant cross-cutting leadership design practices to consider for each stage. While the matrix is presented in a linear fashion, groups are more likely to cycle in and out of these stages. For example, groups may return to the convening phase if new stakeholders join the effort or they may move to the clarifying stage when competing ideas lead to conflict. The stages and corresponding leadership design practices are discussed below.

Table 1. Framework for leading interdisciplinary research teams

Leadership	STAGES			
	Convening	**Clarifying**	**Committing**	**Collaborating**
Message Design	Establish a welcoming and safe context defined by mutual respect and trust	Identify shared purposes that prioritize community stakeholder concerns and advance a culture-centered approach	Build a sense of urgency and create buy-in among all stakeholder groups	Question, critique, and celebrate shared activities
Strategy Design	Initiate opportunities for inclusive engagement	Define clear and achievable measures for success	Develop action plans, clarifying tasks, responsibilities, and deliverables	Encourage learning and continuous improvement
Process Design	Establish open, participatory, and collaborative processes for participation	Identify gaps in understanding and barriers to participation	Review established participation approaches for potential refinement	Monitor and evaluate progress
Structure Design	Create inclusive frameworks to foster diverse networks for participation	Identify the necessary human, technological, organizational, and financial resources	Reinforce expectations for relationships, partnerships, and other areas for collaboration	Coordinate resource needs and availability for ongoing support

Message Design

When leading interdisciplinary research teams, the messages used to build support and awareness of the research discoveries are essential. Ideally, during the convening stage, the messages one uses to encourage a welcoming and safe environment for team members can provide a strong foundation for the initiative. Importantly, leaders should recognize and attend to the different cultural norms and communication practices represented within the group. Negotiating and clarifying communication norms early in the engagement can also contribute to greater long-term success. Regarding the second stage, one may find it useful to integrate community stakeholder concerns in the design and delivery of messages focused on the shared purpose of the team. The third stage focuses on building commitment, creating a sense of urgency, and encouraging buy-in from all stakeholders. In order to do this successfully, leaders will want to understand each individuals' unique values and motivation for participating. The fourth stage of collaborating is likely the most complex and requires the design and delivery of messages that help to create a psychologically safe communication climate (Edmondson,1999; Gibson & Gibbs, 2006) where the questioning or critiquing of ideas and contributions is encouraged (Monteiro & Keating, 2009; Ôberg, 2009). As part of this stage, the team will want to recognize and celebrate their progress internally, as well as communicate their ongoing success to and engagement with external constituents (Benoliel & Somech, 2014; Defila & di Giulio, 2017).

Throughout the research engagement, leadership messages should provide consistent and logical reasons for the problems to be addressed, along with guidance concerning the multiple constituencies and desired activities, the expected results and deliverables, and a timeline for achieving these results. Additionally, the importance of keeping stakeholders informed throughout the process cannot be overstated, especially when coordinating with community members. The repeated use of multiple messages through a variety of channels is also recommended, noting that what might seem repetitive and common sense to the leader may be new for various audiences, and that repetition purposefully builds awareness and commitment (Ruben et al., 2021). Thus, failure to craft intentional messages that support the ongoing progress of the project can derail even the most well-meaning goals.

Strategy Design

Leaders play a fundamental role in the development and dissemination of a strategic vision. Neglecting the development of a well-conceived strategy is an all-too common mistake, as is the hasty implementation of a poorly defined strategy. Shortcomings in either regard can result in unanticipated problems, such as limited commitment on the part of community members or an inability to understand the ways in which one's contributions align with the broader purpose of the research. Questions to consider when developing a strategy for interdisciplinary or transdisciplinary research teams might include the following:

- Why is it important to address this problem via interdisciplinary research?
- Who are the key stakeholders and how might they be best served?
- Who holds power and influence in the community, on the team, and in key institutions, agencies, and organizations that rely on and influence this research?
- Which of our combined strengths could be viewed as assets in the initiative and which weaknesses could be liabilities?
- What are the intended outcomes and what resources are needed to accomplish these?

Beginning with the convening stage, engaging the group in the development of a strategy can result in more meaningful involvement of all collaborators and community stakeholders through a process that allows for a high degree of input, engagement, and commitment. In the clarifying stage, the focus should be on articulating the purpose of the initiative, its intended (and potentially unintended) impact, and the inclusion of clear and achievable measures for success. In the third stage, strategy design should expand into the development of action plans with realistic timeframes, clear task assignments, manageable implementation procedures, and substantive deliverables. To create a realistic plan, the team must consider potential areas of resistance or opportunities to secure broadened support. The final stage might include a focus on refining the team's strategy to encourage ongoing learning and continuous improvement. The strategy needs to be reassessed to ensure the interdisciplinary team is operating in ways that will allow it to achieve its goals.

Process Design

Designing and implementing processes that enable researchers and stakeholders to engage with the initiative is a critical component for the productive integration of ideas and potential solutions. As Hirokawa (1988) notes, "Effective decision making demands that the group base its choice on an accurate (i.e., valid or reasonable) understanding of (a) the nature of the problem, (b) the extent and seriousness of the problem, (c) the possible cause(s) of the problem, and (d) the possible consequences of the not dealing effectively with the problem" (p. 489). Beginning with the first stage, the focus lies on identifying and establishing processes that are open, participatory, and collaborative. Within the clarifying stage, it is critical to implement processes that allow members of a team to identify gaps in understanding and potential barriers for effective participation. To mitigate potential resistance, stakeholders should be involved in decision-making and idea generation in a manner that encourages individuals to express feelings and receive validation and reassurance for doing so. Recognizing that resistance can serve a vital role in the success of the initiative, creating the opportunity for meaningful dialogue can heighten support while also surfacing unforeseen barriers (Reichers et al., 1997). During the commitment stage, leaders may adopt processes that enable each participant to discover what aspects of this work are personally and professionally meaningful. Guiding participants through a series of questions or activities that allow everyone to explore their own motivations for engaging in the effort can help to clarify one's reason for involvement. Additionally, processes that allow for a discussion of each person's passions, values, and skills, talents, and expertise can help to build a committed team where respect for the individual contributions of each member is valued. For the fourth stage, processes that enable the continuous monitoring and evaluation of progress are critical to the ultimate success of the initiative.

Structure Design

In order to achieve the goals of an interdisciplinary collaboration, a leader ought to consider ways of designing structures to organize the direction and management of core activities, including leadership and administrative structures, social structures and communication patterns, and information and communication technology structures. Siloed structures, a common feature of decentralized institutions of higher education, can present challenges for wide-scale interdisciplinary collaborations across distinct academic departments. Cross-cutting arrangements like matrix structures, networks, or ad hoc teams and working groups can provide greater opportunities for the integration of ideas across disciplinary boundaries. Matrix structures can be effective for managing interdisciplinary research given that they combine both hierarchy and project organization and thus "can facilitate a balance of power and increase intrateam communication and decision making, through lateral channels" (Klein & Porter, 1990, p. 15). Such structural dimensions include clear reporting arrangements that identify the critical roles and responsibilities needed to support processes, financial resources to reinforce and reward behaviors, and information and communication technologies to manage the flow of information throughout the process.

For the first stage, creating inclusive frameworks with low barriers for entry in order to foster diverse networks for participation is paramount. For example, on the surface, convening a meeting using virtual technologies might appear to be widely accessible and inclusive, however the use of such technologies might in fact create a barrier for participants with limited technology capabilities. For the clarifying stage, engaging all members in a discussion to determine the optimal human, technological, organizational, and financial structures that will be necessary to do the work in productive ways is key. For the third stage, one might consider reinforcing expectations for relationships, partnerships, and other areas for collaboration while addressing potential challenges or areas of resistance. Finally, the focus of the collaborating stage centers on structuring intra-team communication and decision making, balancing the need for formal authority and responsibility with flexibility and informal processes, integrating various contributions, and managing interpersonal relations or conflict (König et al., 2013).

APPLICATIONS TO HEALTH DISPARITIES

The existing scholarly literature across disciplines points to the existence of health disparities and the social determinants that underlie and contribute to these inequities. While most of this research tends to focus on health disparities and the outcomes of targeted community health initiatives, several studies have examined the factors that help or hinder the success of these efforts. These studies illuminate the various leadership practices that might be useful at each stage of a team research project and they can be mapped onto the strategies detailed in our proposed framework.

With communication at the core of any interdisciplinary team research, effective message design is a fundamental element that cuts across all of the stages. When bringing people from different backgrounds together, language differences can be difficult to overcome. In one study of the Community Child Health Network Study Los Angeles (CCHN-LA), researchers found that academic members used terminology that was unfamiliar to the community members involved in the project (Wright et al., 2011). This mismatch in communication led to a perceived division where academics continued use of inaccessible language, resulted in community members feeling devalued on the team. Developing a shared language is an important way to establish a cohesive team where people understand and respect one another. In addition to mutual respect, establishing trust is a key determinant of successful interdisciplinary research. Community members may be skeptical or cynical in working with academic researchers, especially if past experiences had little impact, or worse, a negative impact on their community (Wright et al., 2011). In a study of longitudinal academic-community collaborations, trust emerged as a primary precondition, mechanism, and outcome of sustainable partnerships (Jagosh et al., 2015). One participant of the study noted how a healthy level of skepticism allows members to ask critical questions and forge a stronger partnership over time (Jagosh et al., 2015). Feelings of distrust, however, can permeate team dynamics and can ultimately sink a project if not handled with care.

In the study of CCHN-LA, researchers found that team members possessed different definitions for project success. Academic partners described success as meeting the intended goals of the project as established in the grant submission, while community partners viewed success as one involving shared leadership and trusting communication (Wright et al., 2011). When they convened team meetings, academic partners often arrived with an agenda driven by their goals, which ultimately led to a breakdown in trust because community partners did not feel like shared partners in the leadership of the project (Wright et al., 2011). In a different study of a community-based participatory health research partnership with the Latinos Unidos por la Salud (LU-Salud) intervention project, academic scholars and Latinx immigrants worked together collaboratively to promote health and health equity in the community (Vaughn et al., 2018). All members were engaged in decision-making regarding recruitment, data collection, and measurement, and the co-researchers described an experience of *convivencia*, or a coexistence where team members valued the time they spent together, showing and perceiving a mutual respect for the expertise and ideas that other team members brought (Vaughn et al., 2018). Brush, et al (2020) provide additional examples of partnership success, along with the introduction of a tool to measure factors contributing to success in long-standing partnerships. As detailed across each of these examples, it is important for teams to establish trust in their messaging, creating an environment where all members feel comfortable to voice their concerns.

In a review of previously published studies covering hundreds of collaborative partnerships on issues related to public health, Roussos and Fawcett (2000) emphasize the criticality of having a clear mission and vision for the project. Those projects that had a broad or unfocused mission demonstrated lower rates of effectiveness in enacting community change. As the authors note, mission and vision clarity generate support for the initiative, reduce conflicting goals among those involved, help identify additional allies, and minimize distractions that can absorb time and resources (Roussos & Fawcett, 2000). In addition, they argue that successful collaborative projects treat the process of creating the vision and mission as important as the product itself. Collaborative teams that involved all constituents in the development of the project mission and vision were able to create shared commitment and ownership of the project's progress and success, and by periodically returning to these, teams were able to continuously monitor their progress and adapt accordingly (Roussos & Fawcett, 2000). The vision is likely what connects everyone on the team to a common cause (Carlton et al., 2009) and a shared motivation that propels the project in a forward direction (Vaughn et al., 2018).

A strategic vision should drive the process, serving as a guidepost where decision-making and actions are tied back to the shared vision of the project (Carlton et al., 2009). Therefore, successful team research projects need to be able to operationalize the vision into a foundational structure and action plan for the project (Carlton et al., 2009; Roussos et al., 2000). While creating a robust action plan can be time-intensive, research teams that invest time and effort to the systematic development of such a plan may be more likely to enact sustainable change in communities and systems (Roussos et al., 2000). When these action plans are complemented with careful documentation and ongoing feedback, project leaders can continuously evaluate and make modifications to ensure progress (Roussos et al., 2000). Through documentation, Roussos et al. (2000) found that research teams were able to map their progress which allowed them to celebrate their accomplishments, identify barriers, and redirect their efforts to the most effective activities along the way, as well as communicate these efforts to their stakeholders.

Lastly, creating a structure that fosters diverse participation is an important leadership practice for effective team research. Leadership requires the cultural competency to work with people of all different backgrounds and perspectives. Roussos et al. (2000) argued that homogenous teams can limit the level of change and that the variety of perspectives on a diverse team are better for enacting system-level change. Embracing such diversity and creating an inclusive environment that is conscientious of inherent power dynamics is important in communicating how each person is a valued member of the team (Wright et al., 2011). In the CCHN-LA study, community members recognized that the academic researchers had more education and may come from higher socioeconomic backgrounds, but they brought expertise from their lived experiences in those communities (Wright et al., 2011). Leaders must recognize and appreciate the different skills team members possess and model their commitment to the rest of the team, helping each person understand everyone's role in the collaborative partnership. In addition, projects supported by technical assistance and financial resources are more likely to succeed and be found sustainable over time (Roussos et al., 2000). When such resources are paired together with strong trusting partnerships, teams may be able to create spin-off projects where the partnerships are sustained through additional collaborative initiatives (Jagosh et al., 2015).

LIMITATIONS AND FUTURE RESEARCH

As an exploratory qualitative study, the conceptual model proposed in this paper has yet to be empirically tested. The framework is informed by the key concepts introduced in the relevant streams of literature; however, as a limitation, this preliminary model could benefit from additional application to collaborative research initiatives. We invite future research that could apply and build upon the strategies detailed in this article. Additionally, the research on interdisciplinary collaborations designed to address health disparities extends across academic disciplines including communication, leadership, medicine, and public health. As a result, another limitation involves the inability to adequately scan and integrate the findings from this extensive body of interdisciplinary scholarship. However, as we engage in future research involving this framework, we aim to incorporate additional perspectives that reflect the extensive and evolving literature on this subject.

CONCLUSION

In summary, the exploratory framework introduced in this article offers a systematic approach for designing and leading interdisciplinary and transdisciplinary teams. With an emphasis on leadership and communication theory and practice, we outline key considerations for leaders of interdisciplinary research efforts regarding messages, strategies, processes, and structures across the critical phases of team development. As a result of effective leadership and communication, interdisciplinary teams will be better enabled and empowered to translate reach into actionable steps that are informed by theory and evidence with a focus on implementing sustainable solutions that ultimately reduce health disparities and improve the health of our communities. It is our hope that this proposed framework and synthesis of relevant literature will contribute to future research and application regarding this area of focused attention.

REFERENCES

Aakhus, M. (2007). Communication as design. *Communication Monographs*, *74*(1), 112–117. DOI: 10.1080/03637750701196383

Aakhus, M., & Bzdak, M. (2015). Stakeholder engagement as communication design practice. *Journal of Public Affairs*, *15*(2), 188–200. DOI: 10.1002/pa.1569

Agurs-Collins, T., Persky, S., Paskett, E. D., Barkin, S. L., Meissner, H. I., Nansel, T. R., Arteaga, S. S., Zhang, X., Das, R., & Farhat, T. (2019). Designing and assessing multilevel interventions to improve minority health and reduce health disparities. *American Journal of Public Health*, *109*(S1), S86–S93. DOI: 10.2105/AJPH.2018.304730 PMID: 30699029

Arnst, J. (2018, February 1). Addressing the tangled roots of health disparities. *ASBMB Today*. https://www.asbmb.org/asbmb-today/science/020118/addressing-the-tangled-roots-of-health-disparities

Barge, J. K. (2002). Enlarging the meaning of group deliberation: From discussion to dialogue. (2002). In *New Directions in Group Communication* (p. 159). SAGE Publications, Inc., DOI: 10.4135/9781412990042.n9

Benoliel, P., & Somech, A. (2014). The role of leader boundary activities in enhancing interdisciplinary team effectiveness. *Small Group Research*, *46*(1), 83–124. DOI: 10.1177/1046496414560028

Boix Mansilla, V., Lamont, M., & Sato, K. (2015). Shared cognitive–emotional–interactional platforms. *Science, Technology & Human Values*, *41*(4), 571–612. DOI: 10.1177/0162243915614103

Braveman, P. (2006). Health disparities and health equity: Concepts and measurement. *Annual Review of Public Health*, *27*(1), 167–194. DOI: 10.1146/annurev.publhealth.27.021405.102103 PMID: 16533114

Brown, A. F., Ma, G. X., Miranda, J., Eng, E., Castille, D., Brockie, T., Jones, P., Airhihenbuwa, C. O., Farhat, T., Zhu, L., & Trinh-Shevrin, C. (2019). Structural Interventions to Reduce and Eliminate Health Disparities. *American Journal of Public Health (1971)*, *109*(S1), S72–S78. https://doi.org/DOI: 10.2105/AJPH.2018.304844

Brush, B. L., Mentz, G., Jensen, M., Jacobs, B., Saylor, K. M., Rowe, Z., Israel, B. A., & Lachance, L. (2020). Success in long-standing community-based participatory research (CBPR) partnerships: A scoping literature review. *Health Education & Behavior*, *47*(4), 556–568. DOI: 10.1177/1090198119882989 PMID: 31619072

Cameron, K. A. (2013). Advancing equity in clinical preventive services: The role of health communication. *Journal of Communication*, *63*(1), 31–50. DOI: 10.1111/jcom.12005

Carlton, E. L., Whiting, J. B., Bradford, K., Dyk, P. H., & Vail, A. (2009). Defining factors of successful university-community collaborations: An exploration of one healthy marriage project. *Family Relations*, *58*(1), 28–40. DOI: 10.1111/j.1741-3729.2008.00532.x

Centers for Disease Control and Prevention (CDC). (2020, December 10). Risk of severe illness or death from COVID-19. https://www.cdc.gov/coronavirus/2019-ncov/community/health-equity/racial-ethnic-disparities/disparities-illness.html

Centers for Disease Control and Prevention (CDC). (2021, January 28). The Social-Ecological Model: A framework for prevention. https://www.cdc.gov/violenceprevention/about/social-ecologicalmodel.html

Cooperrider, D. L., & Srivastva, S. (1987). Appreciative inquiry in organizational life. In Woodman, R. W., & Pasmore, W. A. (Eds.), *Research in organizational change and development* (Vol. 1, pp. 129–169). JAI Press., DOI: 10.1108/S1475-9152(2013)0000004001

Dankwa-Mullan, I., Rhee, K. B., Williams, K., Sanchez, I., Sy, F. S., Stinson, N.Jr, & Ruffin, J. (2010). The science of eliminating health disparities: Summary and analysis of the NIH summit recommendations. *American Journal of Public Health*, *100*(S1), S12–S18. DOI: 10.2105/AJPH.2010.191619 PMID: 20147660

Dean, M., Gill, R., & Barbour, J. B. (2016). "Let's sit forward": Investigating interprofessional communication, collaboration, professional roles, and physical space at EmergiCare. *Health Communication*, *31*(12), 1506–1516. DOI: 10.1080/10410236.2015.1089457 PMID: 27093130

Defila, R., & di Giulio, A. (2017). Managing Consensus in Inter- and Transdisciplinary Teams: Tasks and Expertise. In *The Oxford Handbook of Interdisciplinarity* (2nd ed.). Oxford University Press. https://doi.org/DOI: 10.1093/oxfordhb/9780198733522.013.27

Edmondson, A. (1999). Psychological safety and learning behavior in work teams. *Administrative Science Quarterly*, *44*(2), 350–383. DOI: 10.2307/2666999

Ellinor, L., & Gerard, G. (1998). *Dialogue: Rediscover the transforming power of conversation*. John Wiley.

Feller, I. (2002). New organizations, old cultures: Strategy and implementation of interdisciplinary programs. *Research Evaluation, 11*(2), 109–116. DOI: 10.3152/147154402781776862

Garmston, R. J., & Wellman, B. M. (1999). *The adaptive school: A sourcebook for developing collaborative groups*. Christopher-Gordon.

Gehlert, S., Murray, A., Sohmer, D., McClintock, M., Conzen, S., & Olopade, O. (2010). The importance of transdisciplinary collaborations for understanding and resolving health disparities. *Social Work in Public Health, 25*(3-4), 408–422. DOI: 10.1080/19371910903241124 PMID: 20446184

Gehlert, S., Sohmer, D., Sacks, T., Mininger, C., McClintock, M., & Olopade, O. (2008). Targeting health disparities: A model linking upstream determinants to downstream interventions. *Health Affairs, 27*(2), 339–349. DOI: 10.1377/hlthaff.27.2.339 PMID: 18332488

Gigliotti, R. A., Weidner, M., Jansen, M., Greenberg, P., Bachmann, G., Dominguez-Bello, M. G., Parmar, V., Panettieri, R. A., Reilly, N., Ayers, C. A., Cohen, B., Denzin, L. K., Feldman-Zohn, C., Fiedler, N., Jimenez, M. E., Laumbach, R. J., Malin, S. K., Mazzaferro, N., Pai, S., & Horton, D. B. (2024). Assessments of working group effectiveness in the planning of the New Jersey Kids Study: An applied mixed-methods study on the science of team science. *Journal of Clinical and Translational Science, 8*(1), e163.

Gibson, C. B., & Gibbs, J. (2006). Unpacking the concept of virtuality: The effects of geographic dispersion, electronic dependence, dynamic structure, and national diversity on team innovation. *Administrative Science Quarterly, 51*(3), 451–495. DOI: 10.2189/asqu.51.3.451

Gigliotti, R. A., & Goldthwaite, C. (2021). *Leadership in academic health centers: Core concepts and critical cases*. Kendall Hunt.

Gilliland, C. T., White, J., Gee, B., Kreeftmeijer-Vegter, R., Bietrix, F., Ussi, A. E., Hajduch, M., Kocis, P., Chiba, N., Hirasawa, R., Suematsu, M., Bryans, J., Newman, S., Hall, M. D., & Austin, C. P. (2019). The fundamental characteristics of a translational scientist. *ACS Pharmacology & Translational Science, 2*(3), 213–216. DOI: 10.1021/acsptsci.9b00022 PMID: 32259057

Gold, M. (2014). Reducing health care disparities: Where are we now? *Mathematica Policy Research.* Robert Wood Johnson Foundation. https://www.mathematica.org/our-publications-and-findings/publications/reducing-health-care-disparities-where-are-we-now

Harrington, N. G. (2013). Introduction to the special issue: Communication strategies to reduce health disparities. *Journal of Communication*, *63*(1), 1–7. DOI: 10.1111/jcom.12004

Hirokawa, R. Y. (1988). Group communication and decision-making performance: A continued test of the functional perspective. *Human Communication Research*, *14*(4), 487–515. DOI: 10.1111/j.1468-2958.1988.tb00165.x

Jagosh, J., Bush, P. L., Salsberg, J., Macaulay, A. C., Greenhalgh, T., Wong, G., Cargo, M., Green, L. W., Herbert, C. P., & Pluye, P. (2015). A realist evaluation of community-based participatory research: Partnership synergy, trust building and related ripple effects. *BMC Public Health*, *15*(725), 1–11. DOI: 10.1186/s12889-015-1949-1 PMID: 26223523

Jehn, K. A. (1997). A qualitative analysis of conflict types and dimensions in organizational groups. *Administrative Science Quarterly*, *42*(3), 530–557. DOI: 10.2307/2393737

Jensen, R., & Lund, A. (2014). Horizontal dynamics in an inter-professional school improvement team. *International Journal of Leadership in Education*, *17*(3), 286–303. DOI: 10.1080/13603124.2013.794302

Karpf, M. (2019). The role of academic health centers in addressing health equity and social determinants of health. *Academic Medicine*, *94*(9), 1273–1275. DOI: 10.1097/ACM.0000000000002834 PMID: 31460914

Keyton, J., Ford, D. J., & Smith, F. I. (2008). A mesolevel communicative model of collaboration. *Communication Theory*, *18*(3), 376–406. DOI: 10.1111/j.1468-2885.2008.00327.x

Kivits, J., Ricci, L., & Minary, L. (2019). Interdisciplinary research in public health: the "why" and the "how." *Journal of Epidemiology and Community Health (1979)*, *73*(12), 1061–1062. https://doi.org/DOI: 10.1136/jech-2019-212511

Klein, J. T. (2017). Typologies of interdisciplinarity: The boundary work of definition. In *The Oxford Handbook of Interdisciplinarity* (2nd ed.). Oxford University Press., DOI: 10.1093/oxfordhb/9780198733522.013.3

Klein, J. T., & Porter, A. L. (1990). Preconditions for interdisciplinary research. In *International Research Management*. Oxford University Press., DOI: 10.1093/acprof:oso/9780195062526.003.0002

Koh, H. K., Oppenheimer, S. C., Massin-Short, S. B., Emmons, K. M., Geller, A. C., & Viswanath, K. (2010). Translating research evidence into practice to reduce health disparities: A social determinants approach. *American Journal of Public Health*, *10*(1), S72–S80. DOI: 10.2105/AJPH.2009.167353 PMID: 20147686

König, B., Diehl, K., Tscherning, K., & Helming, K. (2013). A framework for structuring interdisciplinary research management. *Research Policy*, *42*(1), 261–272. DOI: 10.1016/j.respol.2012.05.006

Lengwiler, M. (2006). Between charisma and heuristics: Four styles of interdisciplinarity. *Science & Public Policy*, *33*(6), 423–434. DOI: 10.3152/147154306781778821

Mabry, P. L., Olster, D. H., Morgan, G. D., & Abrams, D. B. (2008). Interdisciplinarity and systems science to improve population health. *American Journal of Preventive Medicine*, *35*(2), S211–S224. DOI: 10.1016/j.amepre.2008.05.018 PMID: 18619402

Monteiro, M., & Keating, E. (2009). Managing misunderstandings: The role of language in interdisciplinary scientific collaboration. *Science Communication*, *31*(1), 6–28. DOI: 10.1177/1075547008330922

National Institute on Minority Health and Health Disparities (NIMHD). (2017). *NIMHD research framework*. https://www.nimhd.nih.gov/about/overview/research-framework.html

National Institutes of Health (NIH). (2020, December 4). *The NIH almanac: National Institute on Minority Health and Health Disparities (NIMHD)*. https://www.nih.gov/about-nih/what-we-do/nih-almanac/national-institute-minority-health-health-disparities-nimhd

Paxson, T. D.Jr. (1996). Modes of interaction between disciplines. *The Journal of General Education*, *45*(2), 79–94.

Porter, A. L., Roessner, J. D., Cohen, A. S., & Perreault, M. (2006). Interdisciplinary research: Meaning, metrics and nurture. *Research Evaluation*, *15*(3), 187–195. DOI: 10.3152/147154406781775841

Rashid, A. M., Ling, K., Tassone, R. D., Resnick, P., Kraut, R., & Riedl, J. (2006). Motivating participation by displaying the value of contribution. *Proceedings of the SIGCHI Conference on Human Factors in Computing Systems, 2*, 955–958. DOI: 10.1145/1124772.1124915

Reichers, A. E., Wanous, J. P., & Austin, J. T. (1997). Understanding and managing cynicism about organizational change. *The Academy of Management Perspectives*, *11*(1), 48–59. DOI: 10.5465/ame.1997.9707100659

Rhoten, D. (2004). Interdisciplinary research: Trend or transition. *Items & Issues*, *5*(1-2), 6–11. https://items.ssrc.org/from-our-archives/interdisciplinary-research-trend-or-transition/

Roussos, S. T., & Fawcett, S. B. (2000). A review of collaborative partnerships as a strategy for improving community health. *Annual Review of Public Health*, *21*(1), 369–402. DOI: 10.1146/annurev.publhealth.21.1.369 PMID: 10884958

Ruben, B. D., De Lisi, R., & Gigliotti, R. A. (2021). *A guide for leaders in higher education: Core concepts, competencies, and tools* (2nd ed.). Stylus.

Sá, C. M. (2007). 'Interdisciplinary strategies' in U.S. research universities. *Higher Education*, *55*(5), 537–552. DOI: 10.1007/s10734-007-9073-5

Siedlok, F., & Hibbert, P. (2014). The organization of interdisciplinary research: Modes, drivers and barriers. *International Journal of Management Reviews*, *16*(2), 194–210. DOI: 10.1111/ijmr.12016

Siedlok, F., Hibbert, P., & Sillince, J. (2015). From practice to collaborative community in interdisciplinary research contexts. *Research Policy*, *44*(1), 96–107. DOI: 10.1016/j.respol.2014.07.018

Smedley, B. D., Stith, A. Y., & Nelson, A. R. (Eds.). (2003). Unequal treatment: Confronting racial and ethnics disparities in health care. In *Journal of the National Medical Association*: Vol. 94. *Issue 8* (pp. 666–668). National Academies Press., DOI: 10.17226/12875

Smith, C., Baveja, R., Grieb, T., & Mashour, G. A. (2017). Toward a science of translational science. *Journal of Clinical and Translational Science*, *1*(4), 253–255. DOI: 10.1017/cts.2017.14 PMID: 29657860

Thompson, J. L. (2009). Building collective communication competence in interdisciplinary research teams. *Journal of Applied Communication Research*, *37*(3), 278–297. DOI: 10.1080/00909880903025911

Thorpe, H., Clark, M., Brice, J., & Sims, S. (2020). The transdisciplinary health research apparatus: A Baradian account of knowledge boundaries and beyond. *Health*. Advance online publication. DOI: 10.1177/1363459320961429 PMID: 33012195

Touati, N., Rodríguez, C., Paquette, M.-A., & Denis, J.-L. (2018). Understanding the emergence and development of medical collaboration across organizational boundaries: A longitudinal case study. *Health*, *22*(6), 580–602. DOI: 10.1177/1363459317724852 PMID: 28795577

Tuckman, B. W. (1965). Developmental sequence in small groups. *Psychological Bulletin, 63*(6), 384–399. DOI: 10.1037/h0022100 PMID: 14314073

U.S. Department of Health & Human Services (HHS). (n.d.). Healthy people 2030. https://health.gov/healthypeople/objectives-and-data/social-determinants-health

Vasconcellos, E. (1990). Organization design for interdisciplinary research: Conflicts and performance. In Birnbaum-More, P. H., Rossini, F. A., & Baldwin, D. R. (Eds.), *International Research Management*. Oxford University Press., DOI: 10.1093/acprof:oso/9780195062526.003.0013

Vaughn, L. M., Jacquez, F., & Zhen-Duan, J. (2018). Perspectives of community co-researchers about group dynamics and equitable partnership within a community-academic research team. *Health Education & Behavior, 45*(5), 682–689. DOI: 10.1177/1090198118769374 PMID: 29618239

Weinstein, J. N., Geller, A., Negussie, Y., & Baciu, A. (Eds.). (2017). *Communities in action: Pathways to health equity*. The National Academies Press. DOI: 10.17226/24624

Whitmer, A., Ogden, L., Lawton, J., Sturner, P., Groffman, P. M., Schneider, L., Hart, D., Halpern, B., Schlesinger, W., Raciti, S., Bettez, N., Ortega, S., Rustad, L., Pickett, S. T., & Killilea, M. (2010). The engaged university: Providing a platform for research that transforms society. *Frontiers in Ecology and the Environment, 8*(6), 314–321. DOI: 10.1890/090241

Wright, K. N., Williams, P., Wright, S., Lieber, E., Carrasco, S. R., & Gedjeyan, H. (2011). Ties that bind: Creating and sustaining community-academic partnerships. *Gateways : International Journal of Community Research & Engagement, 4*, 83–99. DOI: 10.5130/ijcre.v4i0.1784

Chapter 7
Implementing Team-Based Healthcare:
Facilitators and Barriers

Risa Suzuki
https://orcid.org/0000-0002-8448-1475
Waseda University, Japan

ABSTRACT

This study aims to identify factors that influence inter-professional collaboration (IPC) through text mining. While initial analysis using Co-occurrence networks captured the relevance of many words, it proved too complex to interpret. To address this issue, the researchers introduced coding rules to simplify the visualization of textual data and identified key concepts that support effective collaboration. In addition, correspondence analysis revealed significant differences in perceptions of collaboration based on professional roles and years of clinical experience. The finding underscores the importance of diverse perspectives within the healthcare team. While recognizing the limitations of text mining, our study recommends its use as a valuable complement to traditional quantitative approaches to understanding complex IPC structures.

INTRODUCTION

Many research reports on inter-professional collaboration (IPC) have shown positive results for healthcare in general. For example, in a systematic review, Reeves et al. (2008) reported the impact of interprofessional collaboration on healthcare processes and patient outcomes. Similarly, in a systematic review of IPC, Tsakitzidis et al. (2016) reported on the effects of interprofessional collaboration in elderly care.

DOI: 10.4018/979-8-3693-2230-7.ch007

Esperat and colleagues (2023) reported on the effect of IPC in chronic disease and showed that when different professionals work together to care for patients, improved health outcomes and follow-up rates are seen, indicating that ongoing IPC allows for patient oversight, patient education, and implementation of treatment plans. These studies show that IPC is essential in improving the quality and effectiveness of health care.

It has been reported that when various professionals work together to provide integrated care, they can improve patient health outcomes and treatment effectiveness, decrease hospitalization rates, and reduce health care costs. For example, according to Tsakitzidis et al. (2016), interprofessional collaboration (IPC) has generally had a positive impact on elderly care. In particular, significant improvements were reported in areas such as communication within the team, satisfaction among professionals and patients, and the quality of care. At the patient level, outcomes included reduced pain, fewer falls, improved quality of life, increased independence, shorter hospital stays, and lower mortality rates. However, the impact on costs was not consistently reported. However, these systematic reviews (Esperat et al., 2023; Reeves et al., 2008; Tsakitzidis et al., 2016) state that it takes time and effort to obtain significant results on the effectiveness of IPC and that it is difficult to conduct uniform research on the effects of IPC. Therefore, it is essential to understand the behaviors and attitudes of individual team members in order to implement IPC. Zwarenstein et al. (2009) report that it is difficult to generalize how IPC affects healthcare and to what extent improved collaboration contributes to patient outcomes and suggests the need for qualitative research. It is difficult to generalize because the organizational climate and culture of health care institutions are diverse. Therefore, causes need to be investigated individually to guide them in a more positive direction. Lindqvist et al. (2005) studied the attitudes of team members when healthcare professionals from different professions collaborate to provide care and found that the team members' attitudes toward mutual respect, mutual understanding, and participation in joint decision-making were significantly higher than those of the team members who were not involved in the collaboration. Mutual understanding and participation in joint decision-making indicate positive team member attitudes are associated with effective IPC.

There are various ways to investigate an organization's attitudes toward IPC. For example, the Assessment of Inter-professional Team Collaboration Scale (AITCS) (Orchard et al., 2012) which serves as an evaluation index for IPC, can be used to investigate the actual state of IPC. However, most IPC survey methods are based on Likert scales or two-choice questionnaires. Rosenman et al. (2015) studied tools used to assess team leadership in healthcare activity teams and reported that most were global rating scales. Since these methods are in the form of responses to questions prepared by the researcher, the findings are within the framework assumed by the researcher. In order to supplement the findings from these global rating scales, another method is needed to understand how team members think about collaboration in the form of interviews or free-response statements (Korner, 2010). The interview format has the disadvantages of taking a long time to conduct interviews, making it difficult to obtain the cooperation of busy healthcare professionals and challenging to hear from many people. In the accessible text format, in which many people can be interviewed at once, the methodology of analyzing the descriptions becomes essential.

This chapter deals with text mining using KHcoder3.beta.04a© (Higuchi, 2017), a method for analyzing accessible text description formats, to qualitatively investigate what each member thinks about IPC. The methodology, results, advantages, and limitations of this text mining will be described, along with the results of an actual study that was conducted using text mining. The research discussed in this chapter is a text-mining study on IPC in the clinical setting, in which we conducted text mining of free-answer statements from staff representing multiple professions who had a wide range of years of clinical experience and ideas about what they consider to be the things that promote or hinder IPC, to visualize how team members view IPC, and to examine the effects of IPC on the quality of care. This paper visualizes how team members perceive IPC and identifies the elements necessary for IPC.

MATERIALS & METHODS

The study period was from October 26, 2021, to January 31, 2022. The survey was conducted with the cooperation of Hospital X, an acute care hospital. To obtain data, recruitment posters inviting employees to participate in the survey on multidisciplinary cooperation were displayed in the participating hospital and distributed to all employees. A QR code leading to the survey site on the Internet was placed on the recruitment posters. Participants were asked to access the survey site from their smartphones, review the explanation of the study, and respond "I agree" to a check box asking whether or not they agreed to participate in the study. Two open-ended questions were also asked. Question 1 was "What do you think is needed to further promote IPC?" (hereafter referred to as "Facilitators") and Question 2 was "What are the obstacles to multidisciplinary cooperation? (hereafter referred to as "Barriers"). Demographic questions included age, gender, job title, and years of clinical experience. The survey was anonymous to maintain privacy and confidentiality.

This study used a text mining tool to create and visualize a co-occurrence network diagram or correspondence analysis diagram based on freely written opinions about the factors that promote and inhibit multidisciplinary collaborative care. The software used was KHcoder3.Beta.04a© (Free software, Higuchi, Japan).

In the first analysis, the aggregated descriptive data was tabulated by part of speech for each word that appeared to determine the number of times the word appeared in the sentence. When a noun appeared consecutively, it was extracted as a compound word. Next, to analyze the staff's awareness of the Facilitators and Barriers of IPC, a co-occurrence network analysis was conducted after analyzing the frequently occurring words, compound words, and frequently occurring words obtained from the morphological analysis results. A co-occurrence network is a network in which words used in a text are considered nodes (extracted words), and the co-occurrence between words is considered links (Morita et al., 2012). The distance between the links (the co-occurrence relationship) is represented by the Jaccard coefficient, expressed from 0 to 1 (Morita et al., 2012). The Jaccard coefficient is a coefficient that indicates the degree of similarity between two sets, and the higher the co-occurrence, the larger the value of the Jaccard coefficient (Higuchi, 2017). In the case of this study, two sets are the number of occurrences of two words in a sentence. Words with low Jaccard coefficients were also indicated if the frequency of occurrence was 60 times or more, referring to a previous study (Fukui et al., 2013). Although most of the Jaccard coefficients report 0.2 or more as a threshold value, the Jaccard coefficient was calculated from a Jaccard coefficient of 0.15 to a node's co-occurrence, referring to previous studies (Morita et al., 2012; Yasuda et al., 2021). The study focused on the co-occurrence of nodes based on the Jaccard coefficient of 0.15 (Morita et al., 2012; Yasuda et al., 2021).

In addition, as a secondary analysis, coding rules for extracting conceptual domain categories were created for two factors, Facilitators and inhibiting factors, to establish categories indicating conceptual domains related to IPC regarding the factors extracted in the primary analysis. Then, based on the classification by coding rules, a co-occurrence network diagram was created for each conceptual domain category, and the Jaccard coefficients were confirmed. In addition, we analyzed the correspondence between these domain categories, years of clinical experience, and the department to which the respondents belonged.

This research was supported by the Bunkyo Gakuin University Joint Research Grant for the fiscal years 2022 and 2023. In addition, approval was obtained from the Ethics Review Committee of the School of Health and Medical Technology of Bunkyo Gakuin University (2021-0006) to conduct the study.

RESULTS

During the survey, Hospital X had 765 beds and 1,295 employees (196 physicians, 181 medical technologists, 742 nurses, 56 other nursing personnel, 42 administrative staff, and five other staff). The number of survey responses was 729 (response rate:56.3%). Of these, 377 (29.1%) responded to the descriptive questionnaire, which was the respondents of this study (Figure 1). The gender breakdown of the respondents was 90 males (23.9%), 281 females (74.5%), four others (1.1%), and two no answers (0.5%)(Figure 1). The age breakdown of the respondents was as follows: 12 (3.2%) were in their teens, 70 (18.6%) were in their 20s, 75 (19.9%) were in their 30s, 96 (25.5%) were in their 40s, 106 (28.1%) were in their 50s, and 18 (4.8%) were in their 60s. The composition by occupation is shown in Table 1. The years of professional clinical experience composition is shown in Table 2. There were 11 blank responses in Question 1, resulting in 366 valid responses (response rate: 28.2%). There were 28 blank responses in Question 2, resulting in 349 valid responses (response rate: 26.9%).

Table 1. The composition of occupations

Occupation	Abbreviation	Number	(%)
Clinical engineer	CE	6	1.59%
Clinical psychologist	CP	2	0.53%
Clinical research coordinator	CRC	1	0.27%
Dental hygienist	DH	4	1.06%
Doctor	Dr	52	13.79%
General secretary	GS	10	2.65%
Medical radiology technician	RT	9	2.39%
Medical social worker	MSW	1	0.27%
Medical technologist	MT	14	3.71%
Midwife	MW	22	5.84%
Nurse	Ns	221	58.62%
Nurse assistant	NsA	2	0.53%
Occupational therapist	OT	4	1.06%
Pharmacist	Ph	6	1.59%
Physiotherapist	PT	7	1.86%
Registered dietician	RD	6	1.59%
Resident	Resident	2	0.53%
Speech therapist	ST	1	0.27%
Welfare technologist	WT	1	0.27%
Others	Others	5	1.33%
anonymous		1	0.27%
Total		**377**	

Note. The following table shows the job titles and abbreviations of the respondents and the number of those who fall into each category.

Table 2. The composition of years of clinical experience

Clinical experience(years)	Number	(%)
0-5years	59	15.60%
5-10years	54	14.30%
10-15years	39	10.30%
15-20years	38	10.10%
20-25years	44	1.70%
25-30years	41	10.90%
30-35years	64	17.00%
over 35years	25	0.07%
anonymous	13	0.03%
Total	**377**	

Note. This table shows the number of years of professional clinical experience of the respondents and the corresponding number of those who fall into each category.

The primary analysis revealed that the number of different words for Facilitators was 480 (words), and the average number of occurrences was 2.88 ± 5.68 (times). The number of different words for the inhibiting factors (Barriers) was 5.68 (times), and the average number of occurrences was 2.88 ± 5.68 (times). For the inhibitory factors, the number of different words was 530(words), and the mean number of occurrences was 2.52±5.12(times) (Figures 2 and 3). The list of words that appeared more than five times among the extracted frequent words is shown in Tables 3 and 4.

Figure 1. Flow diagram of the study

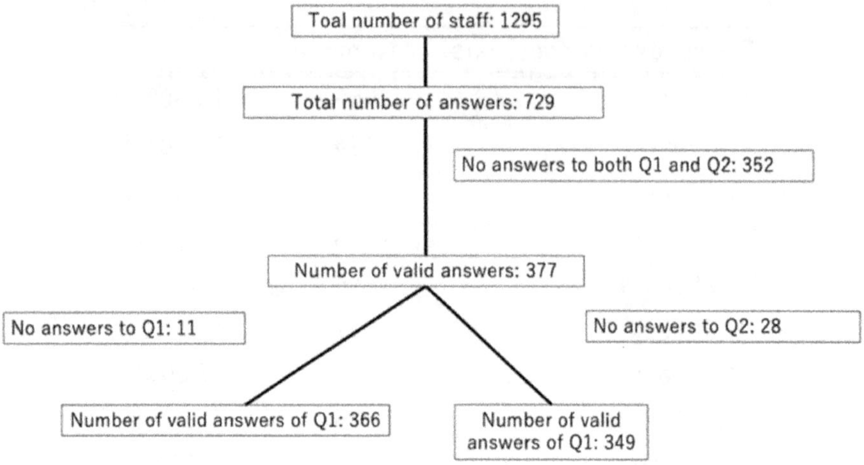

Note. A diagram of the procedures and number of respondents for this study is presented.

Figure 2. Term frequency of facilitators

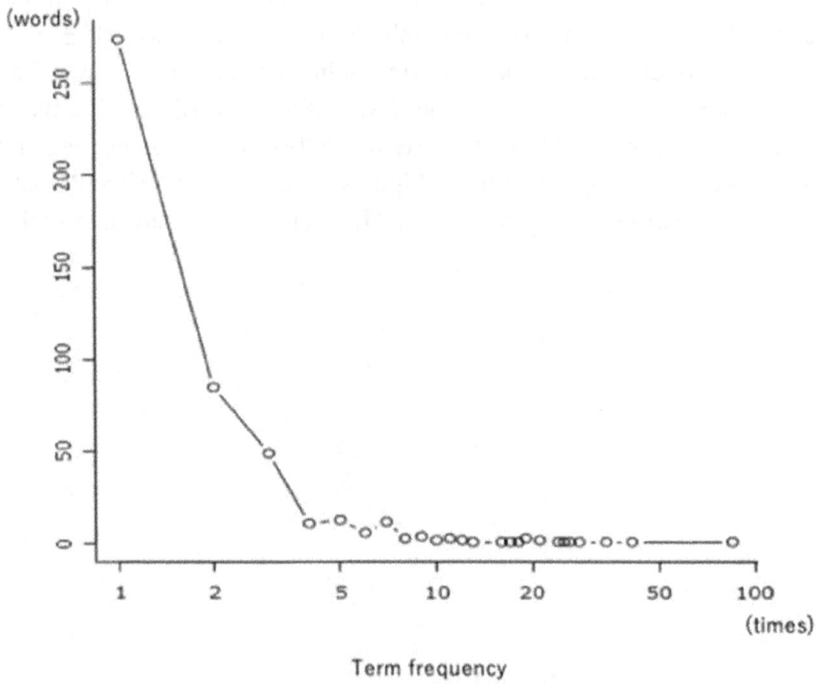

Note. This figure shows the number of occurrences of the word and its frequency in Facilitators.

Figure 3. Term frequency of Barriers

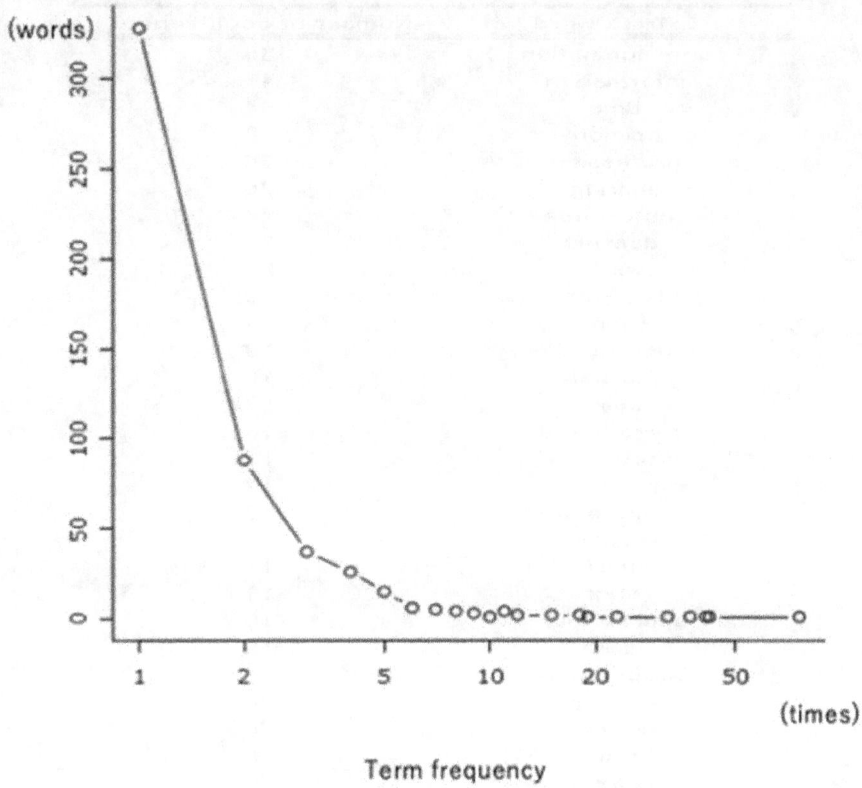

Note. This figure shows the number of occurrences of the word and its frequency in Barriers.

Table 3. The list of words with more than five occurrences (facilitators)

Extract word	Number of occurrences
communication	85
information	41
time	34
opinion	28
profession	26
sharing	25
conference	24
doctor	21
work	21
respect	19
team	19
understanding	19
mutual	18
easy	17
environment	16
discussion	13
atmosphere	12
cooperation	12
regular	11
share	11
staff	11
opportunity	10
talk	10
Cooperation	9
exchange	9
know	9
need	9
express	8
situation	8
skill	8
allow	7
collaboration	7
create	7
Environment	7
good	7
medicine	7
multidisciplinary	7
relationship	7
speak	7
trust	7
understand	7
what	7
communicate	6
consultation	6
Exchange	6
get	6
patient	6
person	6

Note. This table lists words that appeared more than five times in Facilitators.

Table 4. The list of words with more than five occurrences (barriers)

Extract word	Number of occurrences
lack	76
time	42
communication	41
opinion	37
doctor	32
busy	23
attitude	19
information	18
profession	18
understanding	15
work	15
busyness	12
listen	12
difference	11
inability	11
insufficient	11
staff	11
mutual	10
cooperation	9
department	9
due	9
difficult	8
discuss	8
sharing	8
team	8
own	7
position	7
Pride	7
think	7
workload	7
atmosphere	6
different	6
job	6
make	6
people	6
uncooperative	6

Note. This table lists words that appeared more than five times in Barriers.

After words extraction, a co-occurrence network was drawn to visualize the relationships in which words co-occur. The number of sentences used in the co-occurrence network for the Facilitators was 386(sentences), while the number used for the inhibiting factors (Barriers) was 361(sentences).

A method for detecting nodes that play the role of betweenness centrality in a co-occurrence network was implemented in this study. As Miyoshi et al. (2024) stated, betweenness centrality measures the degree to which a node mediates the set of nodes to which its links are strongly connected. We were able to classify six significant groups in terms of facilitators (Figure 4) and eight major groups in terms of Barriers (Figure 5).

Figure 4. The result of the co-occurrence network analysis in facilitators

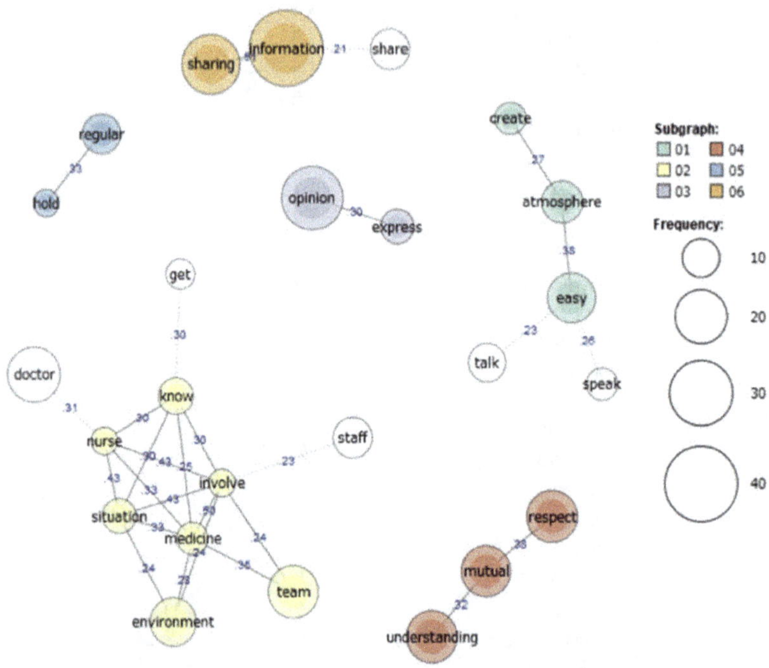

Note. This figure shows the results of the co-occurrence network for the respondents with Facilitators.

Figure 5. The result of the co-occurrence network analysis in barriers

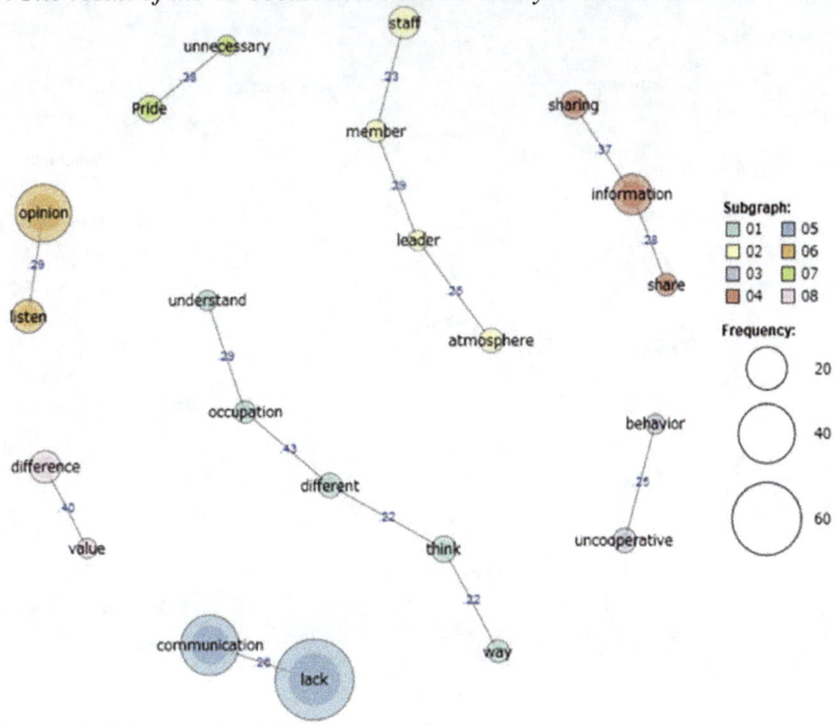

Note. This figure shows the results of the co-occurrence network for the respondents with Barriers.

However, the results of the co-occurrence network depict similar concepts as different concepts (e.g., sharing, sharing, etc.) because words with similar meanings but different parts of speech and words with similar meanings are also extracted as different words. Therefore, in order to simplify the co-occurrence network, draw the co-occurrence networks by concept domain, and clarify the concept of factors that promote or hinder IPC, coding was performed in the second step of the analysis. The secondary analysis results based on the coding classification by concept domain are presented (Figures 6 and 7).

Figure 6. The result of co-occurrence network analysis with coding

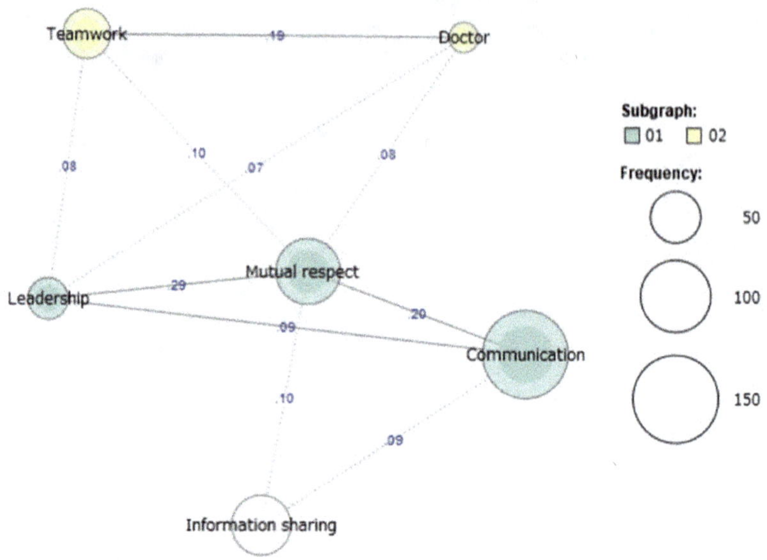

Note. This figure shows the results of the co-occurrence network for the respondents with Facilitators using Coding. In the concept domain co-occurrence network drawing, the facilitators were categorized into three major concepts group (described in the same color): "communication", "mutual respect", "leadership" and "teamwork", "Doctor", and" information sharing". The most co-occurring relationships were "mutual respect" and "leadership" (Jaccard coefficients =0.29), "communication, and 'mutual respect' (Jaccard coefficients =0.20).

Figure 7. The result of the co-occurrence network analysis with coding (barriers)

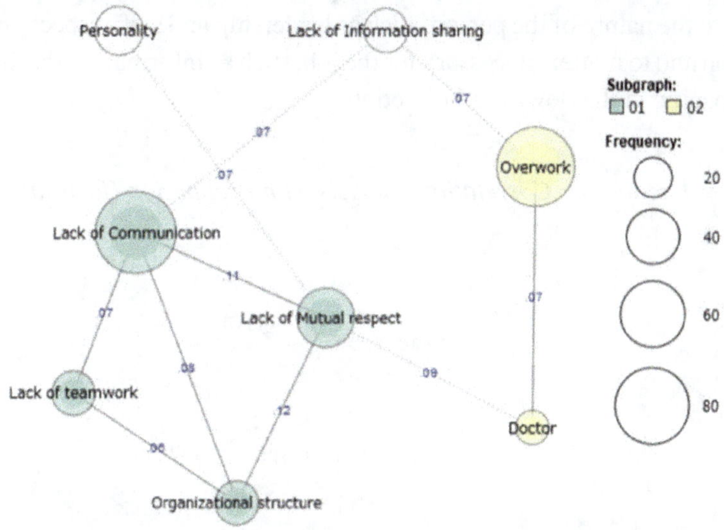

Note. This figure shows the results of the co-occurrence network for the respondents with Barriers using Coding. Barriers were categorized into four major concepts (described in the same color), but no highly co-occurring relationships were extracted.

According to the coding rules, 78.51% of the words for facilitators and 70.29% of the words for barriers could be classified into each concept domain. In the concept domain co-occurrence network drawing, the facilitators were categorized into three major concepts group (described in the same color): "communication", "mutual respect", "leadership" and "teamwork", "Doctor", and" information sharing." The most co-occurring relationships were "mutual respect" and "leadership" (Jaccard coefficients =0.29), "communication,", and "mutual respect" (Jaccard coefficients =0.20). Barriers were categorized into four major concepts (described in the same color), but no highly co-occurring relationships were extracted.

A correspondence analysis was also conducted to clarify how IPC was perceived according to job type and years of clinical experience. In the results of the correspondence analysis, using job title as an external variable, Facilitators indicated that nursing assistants viewed "information sharing" and capacity, physiotherapists viewed learning and capacity, and nurses viewed information sharing, capacity, and learning as concepts that facilitated collaboration. Physicians, medical radiology technicians, midwives,' medical technologist speech therapists, and clinical psychologists could be categorized into groups with similar co-occurrence. However, the former viewed leadership and mutual respect as Facilitators, while the latter viewed communication and patient-centeredness as Facilitators. In Figure 8, factor 1 was viewed in the upward direction as patient-centered and communication, and in the downward direction as representing medical technical aspects. Factor 2 was related to the nature of the person, such as leadership and self-respect, in the upward direction and to matters necessary for the job, such as information sharing, learning, and capacity, in the downward direction.

Figure 8. Facilitator: Correlation analysis with occupation (facilitators)

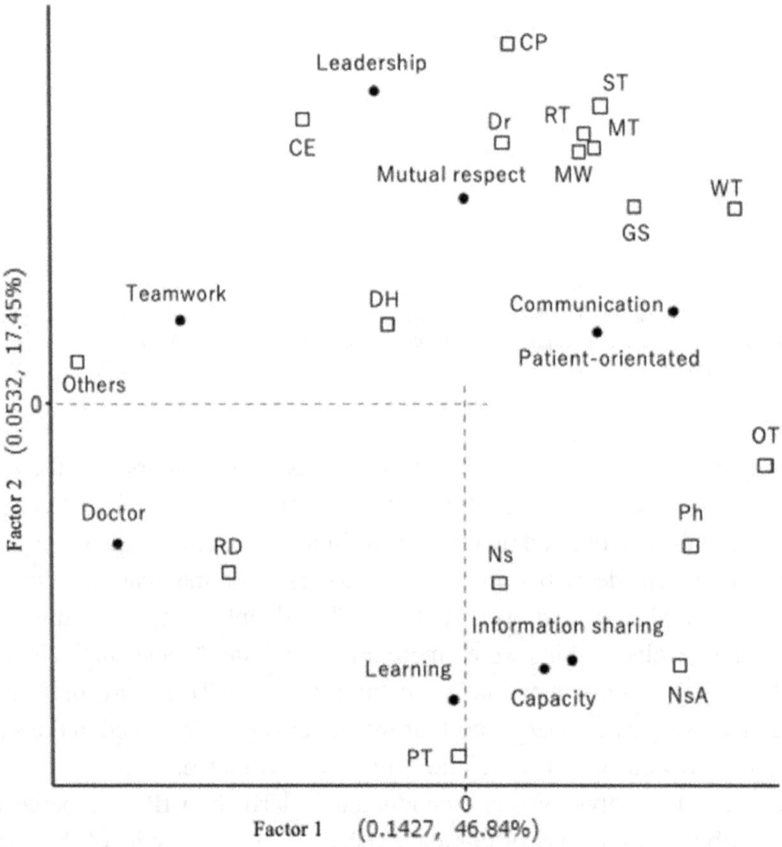

Note. This figure shows the results of the correlation analysis with occupation group with Facilitator. The closer the position of the occupations, the more similar concepts they had.

Regarding Barriers, nurses co-occurred with the concepts of lack of teamwork and lack of communication. At the same time, the groups of physiotherapists, nursing assistants, clinical research coordinator, and registered dieticians were associated with work overload and lack of information. Residents, and clinical psychologists were considered Barriers as Doctors. Speech therapists, pharmacists, medical radiology technicians, dental hygienists and clinical engineers were considered Barriers as Personality. Factor 1 in Figure 9 was considered to refer to psychological aspects such as psychological safety and mutual respect in the upward direction and patient-centeredness and communication in the downward direction.

Figure 9. Barriers: Correlation analysis with occupation

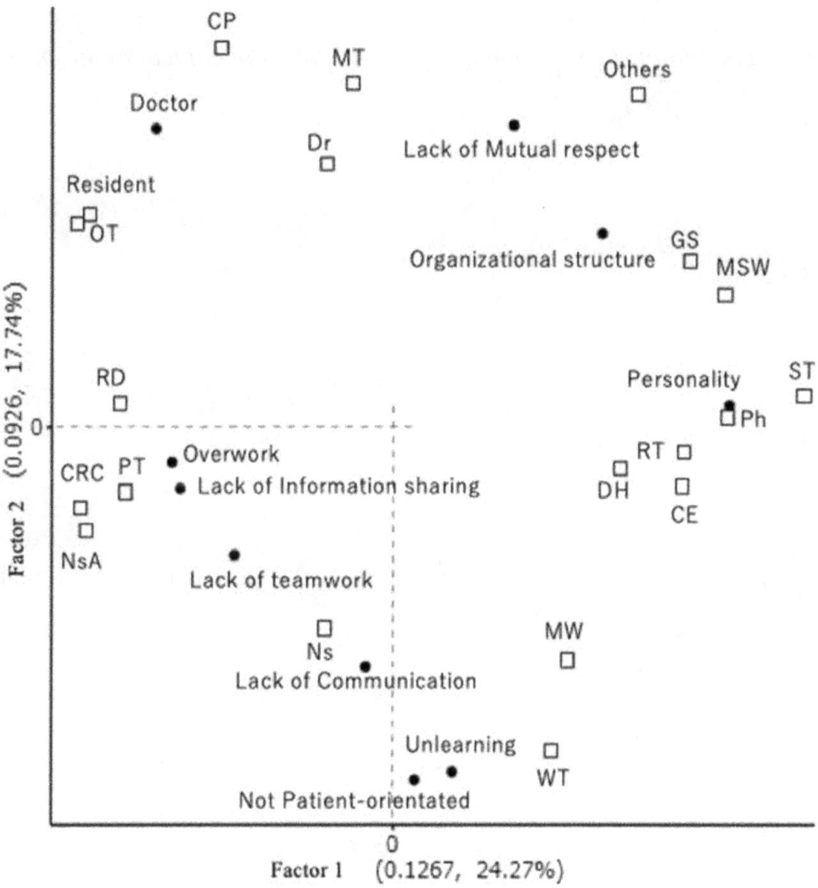

Note. This figure shows the results of correlation analysis with occupation with Barriers.

The further away from the origin, the more characteristic concepts co-occur for that occupation group. The closer the position of the occupations, the more similar concepts they had.

Using years of clinical experience as an external variable, the results revealed that among Facilitators, the 0-5 years of clinical experience group and the 5-10 years of clinical experience group placed more emphasis on information sharing, learning, and communication. Correspondence analysis revealed two groups, one with more than 20 years of clinical experience and one with less than 20 years, with the group having more than 20 years of experience viewing Facilitators as capacity and teamwork, and the group with less than 20 years viewing Facilitators as many factors (Figure 10).

Figure 10. Facilitator: Correlation analysis with years of clinical experience

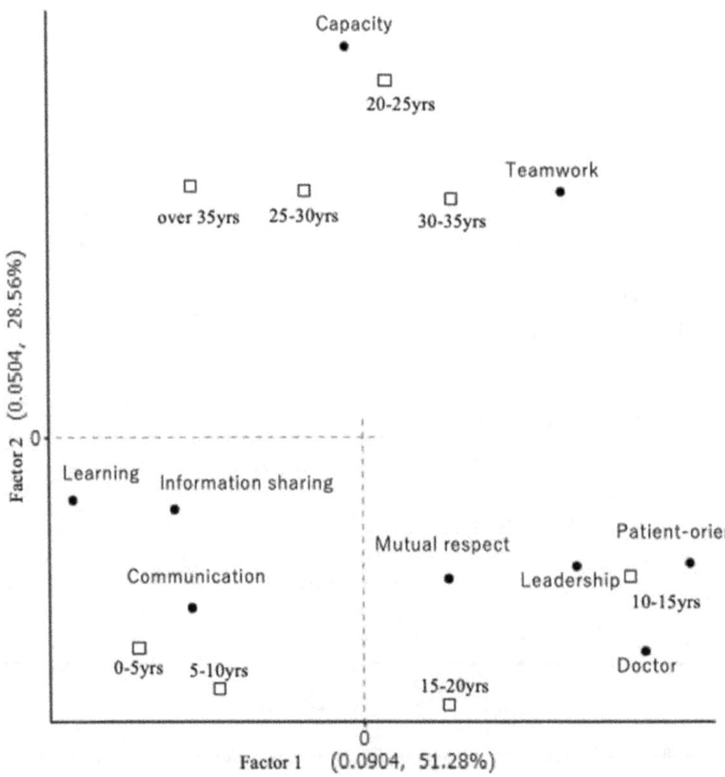

Note. This figure shows the results of correlation analysis with occupation with Facilitator. The further away from the origin, the more characteristic a concept co-occurs for a group of that number of years of experience. The closer the position of the groups, the more similar concepts they had.

Regarding Barriers, Factor 1 was viewed downward as status and organization in the workplace, such as Doctor and organizational structure, and upward as knowledge and information what the individual gains. Component 2 was viewed as organizational factors in the upward direction and individual factors in the downward direction. The 15-20 and 20-25 year groups saw the organizational structure as an impediment to collaboration; staff with five years or less associated lack of information sharing and lack of learning as impediments (Figure 11).

Figure 11. Barriers: Correlation analysis with years of clinical experience

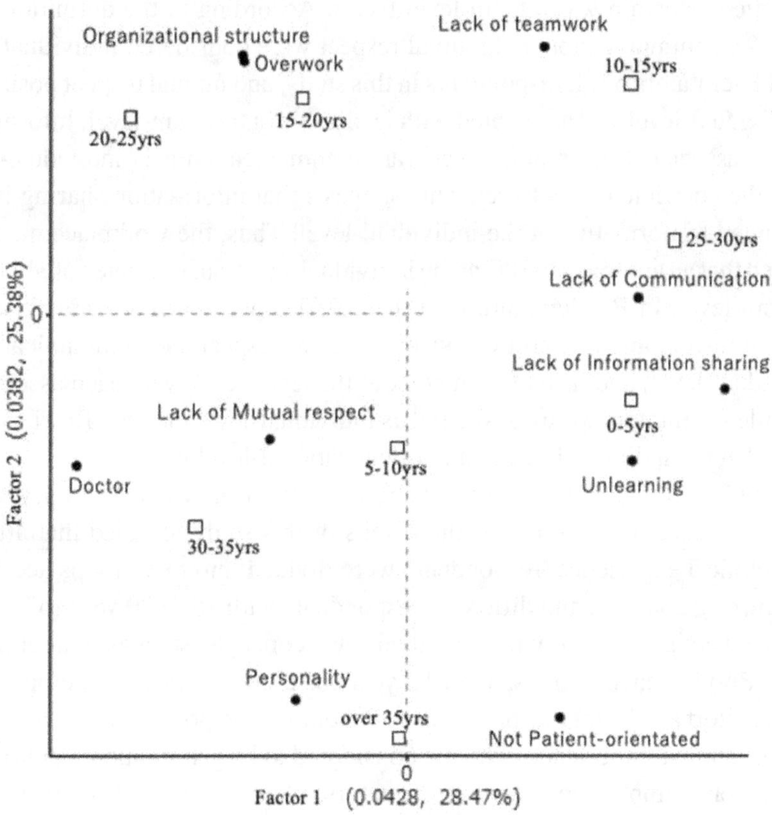

Note. This figure shows the results of correlation analysis with occupation with Facilitator. The further away from the origin, the more characteristic a concept co-occurs for a group of that number of years of experience. The closer the position of the groups, the more similar concepts they had.

DISCUSSION

The results of this post-coding co-occurrence network drawing revealed in Facilitators, that respondents in this study believed the presence of communication generated mutual respect. Furthermore, it was clear that leadership was perceived to emerge from mutual respect and promote IPC. Wei et al. (2022) found that individual-level Facilitators and barriers of IPC were related to interpersonal communication and relationships, while team-level factors were team member roles, resource allocation, clarification of roles, and hierarchical relationships among team members. In addition, organizational-level factors include work environment and conflicts of opinion. Communication and mutual respect were considered individual-level factors in this study, while leadership was a team-level factor. According to the definition (Wei et al., 2022), communication and mutual respect were considered individual-level factors of Facilitators by all respondents in this study, and mutual respect positioned at the individual-level was associated with leadership at the team-level. Information sharing was associated with mutual respect and communication at the individual-level, although the coefficient was lower. This suggests that information sharing is also an exchange of information at the individual-level. Thus, the workplace members recognized that an approach to IPC at the individual-level can promote collaboration at the team-level. In Barriers, although the coefficients were low, organizational structure at the organizational-level, lack of mutual respect and communication at the individual-level, and lack of teamwork at the team-level were each associated. Thus, while Facilitators were considered as individual-level matters, Barriers were considered at the individual, team, and organizational-level problems.

Next, we discuss the differences in the perception of IPC based on years of clinical experience. In Facilitators, the results of this study revealed that after 20 years of clinical experience, respondents were divided into two groups according to co-occurring concepts and differed. Respondents with 15 to 20 years of clinical experience were associated with individual-level concepts, such as mutual understanding. Respondents with less than 10 years of clinical experience emphasized individual effort as a factor that promotes collaboration; respondents with more than 10 years of clinical experience, who are considered to be getting more comfortable with their jobs, emphasized team-level factors; respondents with more than 15 years of clinical experience emphasized individual-level factors; respondents with more than 20 years of clinical experience emphasized both individual-level and team-level factors. This facility was a workplace where the number of people was divided exactly in half at the 20-year mark, with the percentage with less than 20 years of clinical experience and the percentage with more than 20 years of clinical experience being about 50%. However, it is fascinating to note that the perception of the factors promoting IPC was divided at precisely 20 years of clinical experience.

After 20 years of clinical experience, many members tend to be in management positions. While it is conceivable that they may have less contact with the primary workers in the field staff, they have more opportunities to discuss with many different professions at meetings and other occasions. Gradually, experience may narrow down what is needed for IPC while at the same time changing the idea that what is facilitated needs to be at both the individual and team-levels.

Regarding Barriers, respondents with 10 to 15 years cited team-level issues of lack of teamwork, while those with 15 to 25 years saw organizational-level issues (overwork and organizational structure) as Barriers. Respondents with five years or less and those with 25 to 30 years saw the disincentive to collaboration as an individual-level problem, while respondents with 5 to 10 years and those with more than 30 years saw both individual and team-level problems as Barriers. With years of clinical experience, the perception of disincentive changed from individual-level to individual and team-level to organizational level to individual-level to individual and team-level problems.

When considering both facilitating and inhibiting factors by years of clinical experience, respondents with 15 to 20 years of clinical experience, who are considered to play a central role in the organization, believed that the factors that promote collaboration are at the individual-level. On the other hand, respondents with 10-15 years of clinical experience viewed both Facilitators and Barriers as team-level issues. Respondents with less than five years of clinical experience tended to view Facilitators and Barriers as individual-level factors, and the causes of their inability to collaborate as individual problems. Thus, even when belonging to the same team, there were differences in the perception of factors that promote and inhibit collaboration depending on the years of clinical experience. It is important to bridge this gap within the organization.

In this study, the keywords "learning" and "unlearning" co-occurred, especially among staff with fewer years of clinical experience. It is generally believed that informal learning is necessary to promote IPC. For example, Wagter et al. (2012) found that 80% of critical skills in healthcare settings are acquired through daily informal interactions without formal education. Wagter et al. (2012) also stated that understanding the patterns of informal learning relationships can help create environments and conditions that strategically promote and support informal learning in the workplace. Schot et al. (2020) also indicate that much of the learning in healthcare settings occurs through personal experiences and daily interactions. What can be inferred from these studies is that learning in the medical field is primarily formal and informal and that what leads to informal learning is interaction and communication through individual-level dialogue. Montgomery et al. (2024) also discuss how informal communication, including gossip, is essential for sharing information about potential and actual adverse events. The present results also suggest that communication, information sharing, and learning are associated with communication, especially among staff with a few years of clinical experience, and informal communication is an essential channel for learning and information gathering. Burm et al. (2019) studied organizational and communication issues in an internal medicine unit and found that informal communication is important to support patient care. However, they stated that there is a systems gap behind this need and that change at the systems level is needed, rather than leaving it to informal communication arising from chance alone. While it is not wrong to view learning through informal interactions as facilitating IPC for less experienced staff, it is important not to rely on this alone, but to provide systemwide learning opportunities.

By occupation, most occupations viewed Facilitators as individual-level issues. However, within the same individual-level, they were divided into two categories: work-related issues such as information sharing, capacity, and learning, and individual-level issues related to human relations such as communication and mutual understanding. This might be due to differences in perception of whether IPC is facilitated by solving work-related problems at the individual level or from interactions among the various professions. In terms of specific occupations, nurses, nursing assistants, and physical therapists believed that Facilitators were at the individual level in terms of competence, information sharing, and learning. Bulduk et al. (2016) reported that nurses were more likely to consider gossip generated by informal conversations to be harmful to the organization. In the present study, communication did not emerge as Facilitators in nurses, suggesting that nurses considered the negative aspects of communication and did not view it as main Facilitators. In addition, Campbell et al. (2020) conducted a study to improve collaboration between registered nurses and nursing assistants in the delivery of nursing care in acute care settings and examined the effects of interventions on teamwork, communication, and appropriate delegation of authority from nurses to nursing assistants and described the need for appropriate delegation of authority from nurses to nursing assistants. The need for appropriate delegation of authority from nurses to nursing assistants was discussed. In the current study, the concepts of information sharing and learning co-occurred between nurses and nursing assistants. The co-occurrence of lack of information sharing was also evident in the nursing assistants, which predicts the possibility that the nursing assistants are seeking information and direction from the nurses.

A group consisting of physical therapists, nursing assistants, and others believed that busyness due to overwork and lack of information sharing led to Barriers. Some occupations believed that Barriers were due to individual-level problem such as personalities, while others believed that Barriers were both individual and organizational-level problems, such as organizational structure and mutual understanding. This also showed that levels of perceptions of Barriers varied by occupation.

Hall (2005) states that as professionalization increases in healthcare facilities, the knowledge and culture of each professional group can become a problem for effective interprofessional teamwork, and that identifying interprofessional issues can also help in the development of IPC educational methodologies. Thus, using text mining to analyze qualitative descriptions and identify attitudes toward interprofessional collaboration within organizations will help determine measures to promote collaboration. In this study, we found several experience year groups and occupations which considered Facilitators as individual-level of communication.

As a limitation of this study, the low response rate (29.1%) suggests that participants with a high awareness of interprofessional collaboration may have been more likely to respond actively. This low response raises the possibility of bias in the results and limits the generalizability of the findings. However, despite this, through text mining of participants' free-form responses, it became clear that there are differences in the elements necessary for IPC depending on job type and years of clinical experience. This study is considered to indicate the specific items necessary for AITCS, an existing evaluation scale.

Various qualitative research methods exist, such as interviews and interpretation of open-ended questionnaire responses. In the present study, words described by parts of speech were classified, and a network was constructed based on their frequency of occurrence in sentences. As a result, the attitudes toward team medicine in each group classified by age, affiliation, and years of clinical experience emerged. Analyzing free-text descriptions by differentiating them into parts of speech through text mining helped to objectify qualitative information. However, there are many challenges with this method. The free-text descriptions may be influenced by the mood of the surveyed person at the time of the survey. Also, there is no consistent way to define coding, and it is largely left to the researcher's judgment. It is necessary to devise a way to analyze the data as objectively as possible.

CONCLUSION

We conducted text mining based on participants' free descriptions of factors that promote and inhibit IPC, visualized qualitative information of how team members perceive IPC, and clarified the factors necessary for IPC. The co-occurrence network depiction in the primary analysis showed the co-occurrence of many words, making interpretation difficult. By using coding rules, it was possible to diagram the text analysis results in a simple form and clarify the concept of IPC in the workplace. Furthermore, by conducting a correspondence analysis, differences in the concept of IPC by job type and years of clinical experience emerged, and the concept of promoting and hindering diverse collaborative cooperation within the workplace was clarified. Ideally, these differences in perception should be applied to the education of multidisciplinary cooperation and collaboration in the workplace, leading to mutual understanding. Although there are some analytical issues with text mining, the results suggest that it can be a supplement to quantitative surveys, and further research development can be expected in the future.

REFERENCES

Bulduk, S., Özel, İ., & Dinçer, Y. (2016). Informal communication in healthcare (gossip and rumour): Nurses' attitudes. *Athens Journal of Health*, *3*(4), 23–29. DOI: 10.30958/ajh.3-4-3

Burm, S., Boese, K., Faden, L., DeLuca, S., Huda, N., Hibbert, K., & Goldszmidt, M. (2019). Recognizing the importance of informal communication events in improving collaborative care. *BMJ Quality & Safety*, *28*(4), 289–295. DOI: 10.1136/bmjqs-2017-007441 PMID: 30121585

Campbell, A. R., Layne, D., Scott, E., & Wei, H. (2020). Interventions to promote teamwork, delegation and communication among registered nurses and nursing assistants: An integrative review. *Journal of Nursing Management*, *28*(7), 1465–1472. DOI: 10.1111/jonm.13083 PMID: 32621342

Esperat, M. C., Hust, C., Song, H., Garcia, M., & McMurry, L. J. (2023). Interprofessional collaborative practice: Management of chronic disease and mental health issues in primary care. *Public Health Reports*, *138*(1, suppl), 29S–35S. DOI: 10.1177/00333549231155469 PMID: 37226954

Fukui, M., & Abe, H. (2013). The Graphic interpretation of the Co-occurrence Network Diagram in a different writing style. *Journal of Graphic Science of Japan, 47* (4), 3-9.

Hall, P. (2005). Interprofessional teamwork: Professional cultures as barriers. *Journal of Interprofessional Care, 19*(sup1), 188-196. https://doi.org/DOI: 10.1080/13561820500081745

Higuchi, K. (2017). A two-step approach to quantitative content analysis: KH coder tutorial using Anne of Green Gables (part II). *Ritsumeikan Social Sciences Review, 53*(1), 137. https://www.ritsumei.ac.jp/file.jsp?id=346128

Körner, M. (2010). Interprofessional teamwork in medical rehabilitation: A comparison of multidisciplinary and interdisciplinary team approach. *Clinical Rehabilitation*, *24*(8), 745–755. DOI: 10.1177/0269215510367538 PMID: 20530646

Lindqvist, S., Duncan, A., Shepstone, L., Watts, F., & Pearce, S. (2005). Development of the 'Attitudes to Health Professionals Questionnaire' (AHPQ): A measure to assess interprofessional attitudes. *Journal of Interprofessional Care*, *19*(3), 269–279. DOI: 10.1080/13561820400026071 PMID: 16029980

Miyoshi, Y., Yoshioka, S. I., & Yamamoto, M. (2024). Transferability of Effective Consultation Skills for Decision-Making Support in the Voluntary Surrender of Older Adult Drivers' Licences in Super-Aged Japan. *International Journal of Older People Nursing*, *19*(4), e12630. DOI: 10.1111/opn.12630 PMID: 38990513

Montgomery, A., Lainidi, O., & Georganta, K. (2024). Why talking is not cheap: Adverse events and informal communication. *Healthcare (Basel)*, *12*(6), 635. Advance online publication. DOI: 10.3390/healthcare12060635 PMID: 38540601

Morita, T., Irisawa,S., Nagashio, A., Nomura, K.,Tsukada, T.,Otsuka, H., & Sugita, H.(2012). An analysis on the image of the city by text mining using free answer data. *Japanese Journal of Japan Society of Civil Engineers*, 68(5), I_315-I_323. DOI: 10.2208/jscejipm.68.I_315

Orchard, C. A., King, G. A., Khalili, H., & Bezzina, M. B. (2012). Assessment of Interprofessional Team Collaboration Scale (AITCS): Development and testing of the instrument. *The Journal of Continuing Education in the Health Professions*, *32*(1), 58–67. DOI: 10.1002/chp.21123 PMID: 22447712

Reeves, S., Zwarenstein, M., Goldman, J., Barr, H., Freeth, D., Hammick, M., & Koppel, I. (2008). Interprofessional education: Effects on professional practice and health care outcomes. *Cochrane Database of Systematic Reviews*, (1). Advance online publication. DOI: 10.1002/14651858.CD002213.pub2 PMID: 18254002

Rosenman, E. D., Ilgen, J. S., Shandro, J. R., Harper, A. L., & Fernandez, R. (2015). A systematic review of tools used to assess team leadership in health care action teams. *Academic Medicine*, *90*(10), 1408–1422. DOI: 10.1097/ACM.0000000000000848 PMID: 26200585

Schot, E., Tummers, L., & Noordegraaf, M. (2020). Working on working together. A systematic review on how healthcare professionals contribute to interprofessional collaboration. *Journal of Interprofessional Care*, *34*(3), 332–342. DOI: 10.1080/13561820.2019.1636007 PMID: 31329469

Tsakitzidis, G., Timmermans, O., Callewaert, N., Verhoeven, V., Lopez-Hartmann, M., Truijen, S., Meulemans, H., & Van Royen, P. (2016). Outcome indicators on interprofessional collaboration interventions for elderly. *International Journal of Integrated Care*, *16*(2), 5. Advance online publication. DOI: 10.5334/ijic.2017 PMID: 27616961

Wagter, J. M., van de Bunt, G., Honing, M., Eckenhausen, M., & Scherpbier, A. (2012). Informal interprofessional learning: Visualizing the clinical workplace. *Journal of Interprofessional Care*, *26*(3), 173–182. DOI: 10.3109/13561820.2012.656773 PMID: 22332642

Wei, H., Horns, P., Sears, S. F., Huang, K., Smith, C. M., & Wei, T. L. (2022). A systematic meta-review of systematic reviews about interprofessional collaboration: Facilitators, barriers, and outcomes. *Journal of Interprofessional Care*, *36*(5), 735–749. DOI: 10.1080/13561820.2021.1973975 PMID: 35129041

Yasuda, H., Kawamukai, H., & Nishimura, H. (2021). Relationship analysis of failure risk factors in small and medium-sized company projects focusing on co-occurrence. *Journal of Japan Society of Information and Knowledge*, *31*(2), 181–185. DOI: 10.2964/jsik_2021_024

Zwarenstein, M., Goldman, J., & Reeves, S. (2009). Interprofessional collaboration: Effects of practice-based interventions on professional practice and healthcare outcomes. *Cochrane Database of Systematic Reviews*, (3). Advance online publication. DOI: 10.1002/14651858.CD000072.pub2 PMID: 19588316

Chapter 8
Collaboration and Ethics

Joyce Kathleen Engel
Brock University, Canada

ABSTRACT

Interprofessional collaboration includes relationships and decision making among health professionals, patients, families, and communities. Because its aim of high-quality care is consistent with acting in the best interest of patients, interprofessional collaboration is inherently ethical. Ethical knowledge is an important guidepost for interprofessional education, behaviors, and decision making. Interprofessional collaboration, however, also requires awareness of the impact of culture, context, emotion, disciplinary values and beliefs, and legal-centric views on the provision of ethical interprofessional, patient-centred care and on interprofessional relationships. This chapter discusses integration of ethics within interprofessional collaboration and decision making. Consideration is given to ethical theoretical frameworks and concepts and their application within interprofessional relationships and collaboration, as well as to the global predominance of traditional Western bioethics and informed consent and their limitations in selected cultural contexts.

INTERPROFESSIONAL COLLABORATION: ETHICAL KNOWING AND WORKING TOGETHER

Movement towards interprofessional care has been encouraged and promoted globally, nationally, and locally by health care experts and advocates as well as by organizations and regulatory bodies for health care disciplines. At a global level, the World Health Organization's (2018) *Framework for Action on Interprofessional Education* urges policy makers, organizations, community health leaders, and health care professionals (HCPs) to adopt the practice of interprofessional and collaborative health care. The practice of professionals working together collaboratively is en-

DOI: 10.4018/979-8-3693-2230-7.ch008

couraged as a strategy to address global shortages in health care workers by creating flexible teams with efficient and effective use of collective and diverse expertise.

Interprofessional practice is also encouraged as capable of producing high quality health outcomes and health care systems, despite funding issues and health care crises such as pandemics, natural disasters, and demographic shifts towards an aging population (World Health Organization [WHO], 2018). The effectiveness of interprofessional practice is related to professionals working together in teams and to its focus on collaboration and on optimal employment of unique and common skill sets and knowledge backgrounds of different health professionals in provision of quality health care, rather than on respective roles (Engel & Prentice, 2013). Rising complexities in health care delivery and aging populations suggest the collaborative combining and working together of various professional minds and skill sets is both relevant and timely.

Interprofessional collaboration and teamwork is inherently ethical because of its focus on results that ultimately promote the best interests of patients (Engel & Prentice, 2013), a perspective highlighted in a 2015 report by the Institute of Medicine [IOM]. The report also indicated that interprofessional education was instrumental to interprofessional collaboration and teamwork and by implication, to decreases in medical errors, increased patient safety, and lower costs in health care. This optimism was reflected in the work of an expert panel, initially composed of representatives from national organizations in the United States involved in the education of health care professionals including nurses, dentists, pharmacists, osteopaths, and public health practitioners. The panel identified core competencies for interprofessional education (Interprofessional Education Collaborative [IPEC], 2023) and incorporated competencies identified by IOM and ideas from WHO's framework on collaborative practice and interprofessional education (IPEC, 2023). Underlying this work was an assumption that a collaboration ready workforce begins with students in the various health professions who are exposed early to values and skills essential to interprofessional collaboration and teamwork (IPEC, 2023). Importantly, the IPEC panel specifically delineated the importance of ethics by including ethics and values as a core competency (IPEC, 2023). This competency emphasized values commonly associated with ethical behavior such as respect and compassion for others and maintenance of dignity, both within patient and caregiver relationships and within team relationships. Further, the need for ethical conduct and shared values among team members was outlined, which includes valuing the expertise of other health care professionals (IPEC, 2023), a perspective that reflects Kantian and ethical thought on the worth of persons (Oberle & Raffin Bouchal, 2009).

The IPEC documents are accepted widely in the United States and globally as a basis for regulatory and practice guidelines and program accreditation (IPEC, 2023). Recent revisions have incorporated ethical concepts such as social justice and health equity, based on feedback from various professionals and organizations, suggesting a rising pre-eminence of ethics. Farrell (2016), however, noted that the emergence of shared ethics and values as important in interprofessional collaboration continues to face challenges, including a medical hierarchy, that disregards expertise of other health professionals in decisions about what is best or right for patients and where safe spaces are too few in which to express differing values or ethical perspectives. Similarly, in a review of 501 articles, during which the term patient was examined within the context of interprofessional practice, Engel et al. (2019) suggested that while interprofessional practice involves patients, the primary thrust of articles about interprofessional collaboration is not the patient, but rather relationships among care providers. This finding underscores the probability that challenges, and wide gaps, still exist in interprofessional relationships, where values and beliefs define professional disciplines (Engel & Prentice, 2013) and resultant decisions both unify and divide professionals, as well as patients, families, and populations regarding what is best for the patient, or ethical (Engel & Prentice, 2013; Pakkanen et al., 2022; Wright & Brajtman, 2011).

Although studies investigating ethical and interprofessional decision making have typically involved nurses and physicians, health professionals from different disciplines, generally and perhaps even globally, share the ethical principle of beneficence (Oberle & Raffin Bouchal, 2009; Wright & Brajtman, 2011), which is foundational to the relationship with a patient and the raison d'etre for the relationship. Values, beliefs, and other concepts important to ethical behavior and decision making such as truth telling, importance of choice, respect for others, and duty of care have also been identified (Aveyard et al., 2005; Butcher & Mackie, 2021). Despite this shared basis, tensions arise in interprofessional care (Pakkanen et al., 2022) that involve clashes in values (Greenfield, 2007), determinations about what is best for a patient, and differing disciplinary interpretations and priorities related to ethical concepts (Wright & Brajtman, 2011), which can be further exacerbated by sociopolitical, organizational, and cultural factors (McAuliffe, 2022; Moore et al. 2014).

Concerns about what is right or wrong or the *ought* in clinical situations can be signalled at personal and emotive levels (Cook & Brunton, 2018) and, at the level of the profession itself, as evidenced through educational content and various documents such as clinical guidelines (Cyna & Simmons, 2017). The distress that occurs from differences about what *ought* to be done frequently evolves from breakdowns in communication among and between teams, which is also a factor in promoting misunderstandings and non-negotiation of beliefs, values, and attitudes stemming from the unique professional identities of team members (Engel & Prentice, 2013; Moore et al., 2014; Musto et al., 2023).

Ethics and Ethical Decision Making

Ethics is concerned with choosing options, judging the rightness of options, and justifying choices whereas law lays out societal expectations along with the consequences of acting in a way that is counter to what is expected (Johnstone et al., 2015; Oberle & Raffin Bouchal, 2009). As a field of study, ethics belongs to an area of philosophy known as moral philosophy, which systematically seeks to develop understanding about the good and to find answers to complex problems about what is considered morally right or morally wrong (Burkhardt & Nathaniel, 2013; Oberle & Raffin Bouchal, 2009). Debates about whether to use the term morals (or morality) or the term ethics suggest that the use of morals, which has a strong traditional association with religion, is sometimes more relevant when referring to a personal system of right and wrong (Burkhardt & Nathaniel, 2013; Oberle & Raffin Bouchal, 2009). Although morals and ethics are used interchangeably when questions of *ought* arise (Oberle & Raffin Bouchal, 2009), ethics often is used to refer more broadly to a study of what is right or wrong and to application of moral philosophy where social norms and practices are applied (Burkhardt & Nathaniel, 2013). Regardless of how ethics and morals are defined, they are considered central to the practice of health care professionals, as evidenced by the inclusion of ethics in recommendations about interprofessional education (IPEC, 2023) and in codes of ethics for various professional groups in health care. These codes, while criticized as being too general to be helpful in situated responses (Sturm et al., 2022), are public and normative statements (Oberle & Bouchal, 2009), which articulate values that professional groups consider as having priority. They are intended to provide guidance about how to engage with others, including colleagues, patients, the profession, and society (Burkhardt & Nathaniel, 2013) and identify expectations about ethical behaviors by members of professional groups (Oberle & Bouchal, 2009; Burkhardt & Nathaniel, 2013).

Dilemmas are thought to be particularly relevant to medical practice, where choices need to be made between mutually exclusive courses of action (Oberle & Raffin Bouchal, 2009). Oberle and Raffin Bouchal (2009), however, suggest that ethical decision making does not always involve dilemmas; instead, ethical decision making occurs in everyday practice and interactions and either define or are a consequence of interactions. For example, ethical choice making occurs when nurses need to determine which patient needs have priority among all urgent needs, or resources are limited to meet the needs of patients, or a patient refuses a medication that would be extremely helpful. Everyday ethics also arise in interprofessional interactions that fail to fully respect the opinions or expertise of other professionals or to listen attentively to the concerns of family members. Ethical decision making, whether in dilemmas or in everyday interactions include, but go beyond technical knowledge, and are different from legal obligations that unlike the should or *ought* of ethical obligation, indicate what a practitioner *must* do (Oberle & Raffin Bouchal, 2009).

Ethics and morals are rooted in beliefs and values (Greenfield, 2007; Oberle & Raffin Bouchal, 2009) and govern how we interact and behave in the world (Greenfield, 2007). Beliefs are defined as what is seen as truth, whereas values are beliefs that are considered significant or treasured (Oberle & Raffin Bouchal, 2009). Beliefs and values become deeply rooted from the time of birth and arise out of cultural, religious, socio-political, socio-economic, educational, professional, and legal experiences (Sturm et al., 2022). They are influenced by and often shared within networks of relationships, including families, communities, and societies. The influence of values and beliefs, both personal and professional, on behaviors and decisions is evidenced in a study of nurses in Dubai. Nurses from non-Western backgrounds were found to emphasize science and task over presence and caring, raising concern that care decisions did not adequately discern goals of patients, thus failing to fully support patient self-determination and autonomy and presenting barriers to teamwork and collaboration (Kuzemski et al., 2022). In a study of decisional relationships among physicians and a variety of other health disciplines, MacDonald et al. (2023) found that beliefs about hierarchy and the power of physicians determined behaviors as to how much and with whom knowledge was exchanged within the interprofessional team. The findings of these studies support other research that indicates the influence of existing personal and professional beliefs and values on care and teamwork, potentially involving ethical issues and decisions with colleagues and patients (Johnstone et al., 2015; Sturm et al., 2022).

Although highly influential, values and beliefs can be mediated through ethical knowledge, which offers choices and alternatives for ethical action (Lechausser et al., 2018) and increases the confidence needed to seek help or to have meaningful discussions with interprofessional team members in uncomfortable or tense situations (Brown Whitehead et al., 2020; Lechausser et al., 2018). To enable personal, professional, and interprofessional growth and facilitate collaborative problem solving, ethical knowledge in pre-licensure programs needs to go beyond introductory concepts (Brown Whitehead et al., 2020) and codes of ethics and standards, which prescribe behavior and thought but do not necessarily create understanding of their ethical foundations.

Ethical knowledge involves philosophical, theoretical, and practical knowledge (Lechausser et al. 2018). Key ethical categories of ethical theory such as deontology, consequentialism, and virtue ethics are considered normative because they attempt to identify and justify principles and rules or criteria for what is good or bad. These principles or rules guide how persons ought to behave (Burkhardt & Nathaniel, 2013; Oberle & Raffin Bouchal, 2009). The ideas of Immanuel Kant emphasize reason, autonomy of the individual and the freedom to make choices, and the obligation arise out of duty and have been especially influential in contemporary ethics and codes of conduct for health professionals (Burkhardt & Nathaniel, 2013). Kantian theory is concerned with how individuals conduct themselves and suggests that actions only have moral worth when they occur with the intention of goodwill or out of duty and in accordance with universal principles or rules. Universal principles and rules are established through rational thought and logic, rather than because of external influences, experience, fear of consequences, or emotions. According to Kant, the dignity and moral worth of the individual is maintained through the Practical Imperative, which involves the commitment to treat others always as the end and never as means to an end (Burkhardt & Nathaniel, 2013; Oberle & Raffin Bouchal, 2009). This rule assumes that persons should not be exploited or dominated by others and is based on the premise that humanity has absolute worth (Oberle & Raffin Bouchal, 2009). The premise of worth is foundational to respect for others and has significant implications for interactions between health professionals and patients, including provision of care that is free of exploitation for financial or legal gain (Sturm et al., 2022). Seeing others as having worth is also relevant to interactions among health professionals. This is evidenced, for example, when team members are treated as equitable contributors and collaborators in health care situations with valuable, although sometimes different, knowledge bases and intentions, rather than as persons with the capacity to exhibit unquestioning obedience to institutions and professionals with perceived power (Webster & Shirley, 2016).

The premises of deontology rest on pure reason and the nature of the act itself rather on concern for consequences or outcomes. This contrasts with utilitarianism or consequentialism, in which outcomes are emphasized and happiness is considered a moral good. Theorists such as John Stuart Mill and David Hume rejected the concept of universalism and instead, advanced the idea that good was based on what resulted in the greatest good for the greatest number (the Principle of Utility) or the usefulness of an action. Ethical motivation in utilitarianism arises out of the pursuit of pleasure and minimization of pain (Oberle & Raffin Bouchal, 2009), a view that is consistent with the desire of individuals and societies to achieve harmony and to consider the common good (Burkhardt & Nathaniel, 2013). Within organizations and societies, this view of ethics often becomes an important guideline when considering allocation of resources or implementation of public health practices to protect the majority, such as masking or immunizations. At the level of interprofessional collaboration, utilitarianism becomes a useful theory when considering what outcome would represent the greatest good for the client rather than what disciplinary perspective or individual interest should assume dominance in care decisions (Webster & Shirley, 2016).

Unlike deontology or consequentialism, which focus on action, virtue ethics is firmly centered in the nature of the agent and not on the act or on obligation

(Oberle & Raffin Bouchal, 2009). Virtue ethics draws on the writings of Aristotle and assumes that behavior is guided by good habits and excellence of character. For Aristotle, the basic question was not what one should *do*, but rather, what one should *be* (Burkhardt & Nathaniel, 2013; Webster & Shirley, 2016). Modern professional groups extol virtues such as trustworthiness, temperance, compassion, caring, and humility (Burkhardt & Nathaniel, 2013; Oberle & Raffin Bouchal, 2009; Webster & Shirley, 2016), all of which are conducive to ethical interactions with others. In situations, for example, such as discharge and disposition planning, the virtues of prudence, trustworthiness, vigilance, and courage may be particularly important within interprofessional teams and facilitate moving beyond established hierarchal relationships and institutional constraints (Webster & Shirley, 2016). Appropriate care for patients involves prudence or the capacity to discern what is important and what might be missing in care. This is best achieved through open discussion and trust in the expertise of various professionals who have professional knowledge and knowledge of the patient, as well as of the institution or community because of employment or partnering relationships. Both courage and vigilance are involved in speaking up when choices or recommendations for patient disposition potentially jeopardize the well-being and safety of patients and communities. Speaking up and speaking out for the greatest good is best accomplished when environments emphasize interprofessional inclusivity in decision making and respect for the knowledge and assessment skills of various disciplines (Webster & Shirley, 2016).

Biomedical ethics, proposed by Thomas Beauchamp and James Childress, involves principled reasoning. It was initially applied specifically to medicine but, as its influence broadened, became known as bioethics (Oberle & Raffin Bouchal, 2009). Bioethics reflects other normative ethical theories, including obligation or duty of care that was stressed by Kant and concern with good outcomes (Oberle & Raffin Bouchal, 2009) that was found in utilitarianism. The principles of autonomy, beneficence, nonmaleficence, and justice proposed by Beauchamp and Childress (1994) have been highly influential throughout the health professions (Moore et al.,2014), especially in the Western world, leading some writers to claim that bioethics *is* the ethical basis of health practice (Varkey, 2016).

Autonomy is often considered the central principle of bioethics (Oberle & Raffin Bouchal, 2009; Varkey, 2016). As in Kantian ethics, a key concept of autonomy is that persons have intrinsic worth and are capable of reason and of choice. Further, autonomy assumes that guilt and shame may be experienced when persons believe that they could have acted differently or made other choices (Beauchamp & Childress, 1994). The presence of guilt or shame is acknowledgement that persons are moral agents who are can and should be allowed to decide their own destiny. Hence, persons can be held responsible for their decisions and need to be able to exercise self-determination, providing they have the necessary information and the freedom to make other choices (Beauchamp & Childress, 1994; Oberle & Raffin Bouchal, 2009), concepts and contingencies essential to informed consent.

Beneficence, which may be the central principle in nursing (Oberle & Raffin Bouchal, 2009), reflects ideas of Hippocrates and the injunction to help and do what is right for the patient. It involves positive action such keeping promises, relieving or preventing pain or distress, and demonstrating respect, rather than avoiding negative actions or doing harm, which is conceptualized in nonmaleficence, a third principle (Burkhardt & Nathaniel, 2013; Oberle & Bouchal, 2009; Varkey, 2016).

When the intention of health professions to carry out positive actions takes precedence over the desires or goals of patients and their freedom to choose, then beneficence overrides autonomy and paternalism occurs (Varkey, 2021). In some situations, such as emergencies, where patients may be unresponsive and require immediate care, paternalism is an ethical behavior. Paternalism, however, can be insidious or even obvious and well accepted because of established practices or culture, as evidenced in debates over the use of lying with patients experiencing dementia to achieve care goals (Long et al., 2023), such as relieving distress or gaining compliance. In several European and Eastern settings, concealment of serious diagnoses by families and care providers is a culturally approved practice, despite studies suggesting that many patients in those settings may wish to know their diagnosis. Concealment arises out of beliefs, as in specific regions in India, that it represents family love and medical professionalism or in cultures influenced by Confucianism, that it is congruent with filial piety (Nilushi Holmes & Illing, 2021). Although a shared cultural background among health professionals, families, and patients can be determinant in making ethical decisions about concealment of a diagnoses, workload, lack of privacy, limited background in cultural aspects of care, and lack of clear formal or legal guidelines for health providers can promulgate non-disclosure in any setting (Nilushi Holmes & Illing, 2021). Concealment of diagnoses by health providers can arise out a duty of care, but this expression of paternalism can lead to internal conflict for the individual care provider and psychological exhaustion (Nilushi Holmes and Illing, 2021). Additionally, it can facilitate conflict and frustration within the interprofessional team (Moore et al., 2014) related to truth telling and honesty, which are widely shared values among health professionals. Partial or full concealment of factors and decisions in ethical dilemmas and situations, including those honoring cultural practices and contexts, can inhibit ongoing collaboration and discussion with interprofessional team members, leading to polarization and moral inaction (Moore et al., 2014) and jeopardize beneficence.

The principle of nonmaleficence, at a practical level, involves weighing burdens and benefits with the goal of relieving patients of unduly burdensome care (Varkey, 2016). Lying to those experiencing dementia and concealing serious diagnosis can be conceptualized as nonmaleficence if the harms of truth telling in these situations are considered. Correcting a patient who is markedly confused, for example, may cause distress that is seen as unwarranted and sharing a serious diagnosis with a patient may lead to loss of hope and abandonment of treatment, which are advanced as nonmaleficence and arguments against truth telling.

Justice is the fourth principle in bioethics and is primarily concerned with fairness. Distributive justice encompasses proper distribution of burdens and benefits in society, based on equal share, merit, need, effort, societal contribution, or fair market value (Oberle & Raffin Bouchal, 2009; Varkey, 2016). At the point of care, this can involve allocation of care to individual patients based on need. At system and global levels, this can include dissemination of health care technology and care providers based on merit, which is problematic when resources are limited or there are geopolitical circumstances such as war (Oberle & Raffin Bouchal, 2009). At a global level, Nortje et al., (2021) point out that the bias towards bioethics and its narrow view of context and autonomy has impacted the quality and type of health care that Indigenous peoples receive, which is, ironically, a matter of proper distribution of societal benefits and justice.

Two additional principles are often included in bioethics: fidelity or keeping promises and veracity or truth telling. Both are important components of a trusting relationship (Oberle & Raffin Bouchal, 2009) and are critical in the commitment to honor autonomy through processes such as informed consent, as well as in interprofessional collaboration, where trust among different disciplines is important in reaching decisions, whether at individual patient, system, or global levels.

Traditional Western ethical thought has emphasized the concept of the individual as a rational being who is able to make choices, which has influenced the predominance of logic and reason in Western health care. The importance of reason is reflected in the development of linear models for decision making in ethical situations; these models, however, do not necessarily guide *awareness* or *recognition* of ethical situations (Greenfield, 2007), which is a foundation of ethical sensitivity (Lechasseur et al., 2018). Recognition of ethical issues and concerns, however, may begin with emotive responses and not with rational thought. Findings of a large qualitative, international study with physiotherapists, found that the occurrence of emotions such as anger, frustration, and feeling threatened are important signals of clashes between personal and professional values and serve as important early warnings (Sturm et al., 2022) of potential ethical issues and dilemmas and the need to correct the wrong (Greenfield, 2007). Heightened ethical concern is influenced by interpretation and meaning making (Lechausser et al., 2018), which in turn, are influenced by particular differences in values and priorities among disciplines (Wright & Brajtman, 2011) and potentially by the differing emphases on autonomy in medicine and on beneficence in nursing.

Collaboration and Informed Consent

The deep roots of reason and autonomy in Western health care ethics are reflected in informed consent, seen both as a legal and a deeply moral obligation. Consent is a critical springboard to initiate interventions, but also guides and defines interactions and the care relationship between health care professionals and patients (Aveyard et al., 2022). Although generally accepted that informed consent enables persons to express their will, questions arise as to its purpose and the process of providing information to gain consent. Specifically, there are questions about whether information ensures sufficient understanding to actually consent or whether it is to authorize what is proposed and to comfortably predict the course of care (Aveyard et al., 2022), which is more pertinent to beneficence than to autonomy. Questions also arise such as who should be involved in the consent process, which highlights cultural differences in how autonomy is conceptualized, and how much information is necessary to observe both legal and ethical obligations.

Informed consent highlights how differing interpretations, understandings, and priorities in clinical application can challenge collaborative ethical reasoning within and among interprofessional teams. Anaesthetists, for example, have raised concerns about the rightness of disclosing all material risks to patients during the process of obtaining fully informed consent for regional anaesthesia (Cyna & Simmons, 2017), as required by their clinical guidelines. They suggest that the sharing of all possible risks can offer too much information without discernable benefit to the patient (Cyna & Simmons, 2017). Informing patients without understanding how patients may interpret information or what the patients really want to know may mitigate against the autonomy of patients, which is the very ethical foundation of informed consent. This perspective is echoed in a powerful narrative shared by Musto et al. (2023) in which a woman with longstanding mental health issues and a terminal cancer diagnosis agrees to MAiD (Medical Assistance in Dying). On the day scheduled for MAiD, the community nurse who had worked extensively with the woman, discovered this was not what the woman understood would happen or even desired, despite giving informed consent. This narrative has important implications: Information alone cannot assume consent or assure autonomy and needs to be titrated in language and concepts to what is meaningful to the patient. Further, breakdowns in interprofessional collaboration can compromise ethical care. It is a reminder that interprofessional collaboration is essentially relational and broadly includes "learners, practitioners, patients/clients/families" in "effective interpersonal relationships" (Canadian Interprofessional Health Collaborative [CIHC], 2010, p. 8) in the ethical development and delivery of care.

The influence of autonomy is not restricted to informed consent and to patient-provider relationships, but also affects interprofessional collaboration and relationships. In Canada, provincial laws, and to a lesser extent federal laws, outline what decisional and self-regulatory autonomy is accorded to various health professionals (Oberle & Raffin Bouchal, 2009). This autonomy represents societal agreement on expectations and accountabilities of health professionals but also belief in the worth and contributions of their disciplinary education and experience. Laws, however, do not ensure that autonomy and perceived credibility are present in interprofessional and intraprofessional collaboration. Instead, collaboration is also dependent on organizational structures and on belief in the worth and moral weight of care choices of individual members at the local team level, based on their disciplinary knowledge, evidence, and standards. Autonomy is honored, for both health professionals and patients, when different backgrounds and ways of thinking are acknowledged and valued (Burkhardt & Nathaniel, 2013). Honoring autonomy goes further than professionals acting independently for the patient based on the knowledge and evidence in their own discipline or proceeding with the assurance that only their knowledge can be considered 'right' for the patient (McAuliffe, 2022). It entails belief in the intrinsic worth of other professionals and underpins the respect and trust necessary for open dialogue about beliefs, values, information, and disagreement in choices, with the aim of enabling active participation in decision making and optimal utilization of disciplinary skills and knowledge for the benefit of the patient (Burkhardt & Nathaniel, 2013; McAuliffe, 2022).

The open dialogue within interprofessional teams necessary for ethical decision making in interprofessional teams is influenced by professional hierarchies, lack of knowledge or discussion about professional roles, and cultural practices and norms. For example, in Japan, a high context culture, behavior is guided by knowledge expected about non-explicit rules and avoidance of discussion of professional roles and responsibilities with other health team members, with reliance instead on situational knowledge (Haruta et al., 2018). Interprofessional relationships reflect adherence to a medical hierarchy, with "relationships not based on respect but on belonging" (Haruta et al., 2018, p. 325). These behaviors were highlighted in the Japanese translation, adaptation, and validation of the interprofessional facilitation scale (IPFS) (Haruta et al., 2018), which involved participants in various settings and represented 19 different types of health professionals. During the adaptation, it was noted that health professionals in Japan will need to practice explicit respect for members of the interprofessional team and overcome fears that active facilitation of relationships within the team will break existing relationships.

At a broader level, failure of systems to collaborate and sufficiently acknowledge, respect, and value health professionals and their expertise in discussions, decisions, and structures related to delivery of health care can negatively influence interprofessional relationships, including those with patients. In China, for example, physicians have been excluded from discussions to transform the health system to one more efficient, universal, and equitable in health care and inclusive of therapeutic relationships between all health providers and patients and those significant to them (Sun et al., 2021). Underfunding, workload, and changing expectations have facilitated a difficult transition for physicians in system reforms and contributed to diminished esteem and respect for physicians and deterioration in the relationships between patients and physicians, with accompanying potential for poorer care outcomes, which is an ethical concern (Sun et al., 2021).

Closely related to autonomy is the concept of personhood. Personhood is seen as a fundamental human right in many disciplines such as law, medicine, nursing, and anthropology and is fundamental to ethical reasoning and action (Young, 2019). Traditional Western ethics has been heavily influenced by a perspective of person as normatively unique and with capacity for self-centered decision making (McAuliffe,2022; Young, 2019). This view has been heavily influenced by Judeo-Christian thinking in which the individual was created prior to the creation of society, which exists primarily to satisfy human needs. When the good of society takes primacy over the needs of the individual, autonomy is seen as threatened (Hwang, 2015). This, however, contrasts with Eastern and Indigenous views of personhood in which connectedness and relationships are integral to ethical decision making (Nortje et al., 2021; Hwang, 2015). Within these systems, the individual self is highly interdependent and monistic or inseparable from the world or universe (Nortje et al., 2021; Hwang, 2015; McAuliffe); acting unethically or causing harm, harms not only others but those who harm (McAuliffe, 2022). Disclosure and decisions about illness or illness interventions are dependent on a web of interactions, including family and traditional healers or elders, rather than on legal-centric or medical direction (McAuliffe, 2023; Nortje et al., 2021) and promotion of individual self-determination is counterproductive (Nortje et al., 2021). Importantly, dignity or honoring the fullness and worth of persons in their context (Oberle & Raffin Bouchal, 2009) may be more significant than respecting autonomy (Nortje et al., 2021). Recognition of the inseparability of person and community is critical to health decisions in Indigenous and Eastern contexts and in interprofessional collaboration, where family members and traditional healers can be essential in ethical decision making (Nortje et al., 2021) and team members are also influenced Western, Eastern, or Indigenous beliefs and values.

CONCLUDING THOUGHTS

Ethics is typically considered important in decisions about patient care. It is equally relevant, however, in interprofessional collaboration and relationships. Recognition of the worth of the knowledge and expertise of other professionals and understanding of their roles, responsibilities, grounding beliefs and values, and priorities can facilitate the open dialogue necessary for ethical actions and decision making in interprofessional relationships.

REFERENCES

Aveyard, H., Edwards, S., & West, S. (2005). Core topics of health care ethics: The identification for interprofessional education. *Journal of Interprofessional Care, 19*(1), 63–69. DOI: 10.1080/13561820400021692 PMID: 15842081

Aveyard, H., Kolawole, A., Gurung, P., Cridlund, E., & Kozlowska, O. (2022). Informed consent prior to nursing care: Nurses' use of information. *Nursing Ethics, 29*(5), 1244–1252. DOI: 10.1177/09697330221095148 PMID: 35724324

Beauchamp, T., & Childress, J. (1994). *Principles of biomedical ethics*. Oxford University Press.

Brown Whitehead, P., Swope, M. G., & Ferren Carter, K. (2020, Spring-Fall). Impact of a team-based, interprofessional, clinical ethics immersion on moral resilience. *Teaching Ethics, 20*(1-2), 65–74. Advance online publication. DOI: 10.5840/tej202132585

Burkhardt, M., & Nathaniel, A. (2013). *Ethics and issues in contemporary nursing*. Delmar Cengage Learning.

Butcher, L., & Mackie, E. (2021). *Ethics frameworks: an annotated bibliography*. Retrieved from https://healthethics.ca

Canadian Interprofessional Health Collaborative. (2010). *A national interprofessional competency framework*. Retrieved from https://health.ubc.ca/sites/health. ubc.ca/files/documents/CIHC_IPCompetencies_Feb1210.pdf

Cook, C., & Brunton, M. (2018). The importance of moral emotions for effective collaboration in culturally diverse healthcare teams. *Nursing Inquiry, 25*(2), e12214. Advance online publication. DOI: 10.1111/nin.12214 PMID: 28730736

Cyna, A. M., & Simmons, S. W. (2017). Guidelines on informed consent in anaesthesia: Unrealistic, unethical, untenable…. *British Journal of Anaesthesia, 119*(6), 1086–1089. DOI: 10.1093/bja/aex347 PMID: 29028983

Engel, J., & Prentice, D. (2013). The ethics of interprofessional collaboration. *Nursing Ethics, 20*(4), 426–435. DOI: 10.1177/0969733012468466 PMID: 23329780

Engel, J., Prentice, D., & Hicks, R. (2019). Where does the patient fit? An analysis of word use within the context of interprofessional collaborative care. *Global Qualitative Nursing Research, 6*, 2333393619889353. Advance online publication. DOI: 10.1177/2333393619889353 PMID: 31840037

Farrell, C. (2016). The ethics and value of true interprofessionalism. *AMA Journal of Ethics, 18*(9), 887–890. DOI: 10.1001/journalofethics.2016.18.9.fred1-1609

Greenfield, B. (2007). The role of emotions in ethical decision making: Implications for physical therapist education. *Journal, Physical Therapy Education, 21*(1), 14–21. DOI: 10.1097/00001416-200701000-00003

Haruta, J., Breugelmans, R., & Nishigori, H. (2018). Translation and cultural adaptation of the Japanese version of the interprofessional facilitation scale. *Journal of Interprofessional Care, 32*(3), 321–328. DOI: 10.1080/13561820.2017.1398720 PMID: 29161176

Hwang, K. (2015). Morality 'East' and 'West': cultural concerns. In Wright, J. (Ed.), *International Encyclopedia of the Social and Behavioral Sciences* (pp. 806–810). Elsevier. DOI: 10.1016/B978-0-08-097086-8.64005-9

Institute of Medicine. (2015). *Measuring the impact of interprofessional practice on collaborative practice and patient outcomes.* National Academies Press.

Johnstone, M., Hutchinson, A., & Peter, E. (2015). Moral distress' – time to abandon a flawed nursing construct? *Nursing Ethics, 22*(1), 5–14. DOI: 10.1177/0969733013505312 PMID: 24311238

Kuzemski, D., Thirlwall, A., Brunton, M., & Brownie, S. (2022). I speak a little Arabic: Nursing communication in a cross-cultural context. *Journal of Clinical Nursing, 31*(1-2), 145–157. DOI: 10.1111/jocn.15891 PMID: 34263493

Lechasseur, K., Caux, C., Dolle, S., & Legault, A. (2018). Nursing ethics: An integrative review. *Nursing Ethics, 26*(6), 694–706. DOI: 10.1177/0969733016667773 PMID: 27694548

Long, S., Irving, K., & Murphy, C. (2023). Is therapeutic lying contradictory to person-centred care? Toward understanding the connection. *Aging & Mental Health, 28*(3), 520–530. DOI: 10.1080/13607863.2023.2202632 PMID: 37139937

McAuliffe, D. (2022). *Interprofessional ethics: collaboration in the social, health and human sciences.* Cambridge University Press.

Moore, J., Engel, J., & Prentice, D. (2014). Relational ethics in everyday practice. *Canadian Oncology Nursing Journal = Revue Canadienne de Nursing Oncologique, 24*(1), 31–34. DOI: 10.5737/1181912x2413134 PMID: 24707705

Musto, L., Starzomski, R., Rodney, P., & Dodek, P. (2023). Nurses and health care providers as moral agents: from moral distress to moral action. In (R. Starzomski, J. Storch, & P. Rodney, Eds.) *Towards a moral horizon: nursing ethics for leadership and practice* (pp. 225-266), University of Victoria Libraries ePublishing Services.

Nilushi Holmes, S., & Illing, J. (2021). Breaking bad news: Tackling cultural dilemmas. *BMJ Supportive & Palliative Care, 11*(2), 128–132. DOI: 10.1136/bmjspcare-2020-002700 PMID: 33762267

Nortje, N., Jones-Bonofiglio, K., & Sotomayor, C. (2021). Exploring values among three cultures from a global bioethics perspective. *Global Bioethics = Problemi di Bioetica, 32*(1), 1–14. DOI: 10.1080/11287462.2021.1879462 PMID: 33658749

Oberle, K., & Raffin-Bouchal, S. (2009). *Ethics in Canadian nursing practice: navigating the journey*. Pearson Prentice Hall.

Pakkanen, P., Haggman-Laitila, A., & Kangasniemi, M. (2022). Ethical issues identified in nurses' interprofessional collaboration in clinical practice: a meta-synthesis. *Journal of Interprofessional Care, 36*(5), 725-734. Doi: . 1892612epub. DOI: 10.1080/13561820.2021

Sturm, A., Ager, A., & Roth, R. (2022). Western ideals and global realities – physiotherapists' views on factors that play a role in ethical decision-making: an international qualitative analysis. *European Journal of Physiotherapy, 26* (1), 12-24. Doi: . 2022.2155.240.DOI: 10.1080/21679169

Sun, T., Wang, J., Zhang, S., Shi, Y., Liu, B., & Wang, X. (2021). Status, causes and consequences of physicians' self-perceived reputation damage in China: A cross-sectional survey. *BMC Health Services Research, 21*(1), 344. DOI: 10.1186/s12913-021-06306-6 PMID: 33853589

Varkey, B. (2021). Principles of clinical ethics and their application to practice. *Medical Principles and Practice : International Journal of the Kuwait University, Health Science Centre, 30*(1), 17–28. DOI: 10.1159/000509119 PMID: 32498071

Webster, L., & Shirley, J. (2016). No need to object: Ethical obligations for interprofessional collaboration in emergency department discharge planning. *Annual Review of Nursing Research, 34*(1), 183–XI. DOI: 10.1891/0739-6686.34.183 PMID: 26673382

World Health Organization. (2018). Health professions networks: nursing and midwifery human resources: Framework for action on interprofessional education and collaborative practice. *https://interprofessional.global/wp-content/uploads/2018/11/WHO-2010-WHO-framework-for-action-on-interprofessional-education-collaborative-practice.pdf*

Wright, D., & Brajtman, S. (2011). Relational and embodied knowing: Nursing ethics within the interprofessional team. *Nursing Ethics*, *18*(1), 20–30. DOI: 10.1177/0969733010386165 PMID: 21285194

Young, G. (2019). Personhood across disciplines: Application to ethical theory and mental health ethics. *Ethics, Medicine, and Public Health*, *10*, 93–101. DOI: 10.1016/j.jemep.2019.100407

Chapter 9

Transformational Leadership Effect on Human Resource Management Through Organizational Culture in the Healthcare Sector of Ethiopia

Wako Jio
https://orcid.org/0009-0003-6192-459X
Bule Hora University, Ethiopia

Shashi Kant
https://orcid.org/0000-0003-4722-5736
Bule Hora University, Ethiopia

Hirut Assegid
https://orcid.org/0009-0003-6192-459X
Bule Hora University, Ethiopia

Kenenisa Lami
Jimma University, Ethiopia

DOI: 10.4018/979-8-3693-2230-7.ch009

ABSTRACT

The chapter studies how transformational leadership influences Human Resource Management practices within the organizational culture of Ethiopian healthcare. With data from 385 healthcare practitioners the research uses quantitative methods to analyze the connections between transformational leadership methods while studying human resource management and organizational culture. The Kaiser-Meyer-Olkin (KMO) test shows ideal data suitability for factor analysis. The research validates transformational leadership and organizational culture constructs through Confirmatory Factor Analysis to verify they produce reliable and valid results. Our SEM analysis with AMOS measures how transformational leadership affects HRM success paths mediated by organizational culture. Our analysis shows that when leaders embrace transformational behaviors they help HR practices with support cultures which create better employee work results and higher satisfaction. HRM systems in healthcare organizations and provides needed guidance for Ethiopian health care administrators.

INTRODUCTION

Global businesses now use transformational leadership methods because these methods strongly affect how well organizations perform especially in healthcare settings (Rojak et al., 2024). Global healthcare systems need strong leadership now more than ever because they must enhance their services while boosting workplace productivity and inspiring their employees. In the 1970s James MacGregor Burns founded transformational leadership by showing how leaders stimulate followers past their personal needs for the organization's benefit (Eaton et al., 2024). In healthcare this approach works best because people matter most and cultural values directly shape how teams work.

Research proves transformational leadership produces better organization results such as higher employee happiness rates and keeps staff engaged while improving total performance (Rojak et al., 2024). Research indicates that groups led by transformational leaders create an environment where people trust each other more while working together to develop fresh solutions that help healthcare organizations respond to their fast-changing environment. The healthcare system in Ethiopia faces everyday operational problems including shortages of resources, people leaving their jobs plus few chances to train new people properly. Many research gaps exist between transformational leadership and HRM because scholars have not yet thoroughly studied how these fields work together in Ethiopian medical organizations.

This chapter studies the influence of transformational leadership in collaboration with organizational culture and HRM practices (Riani, 2024).

The research question guiding this study is: "***What effects does transformational leadership create on HRM systems through organizational culture in Ethiopian healthcare facilities?***" Our research aims to show future researchers and government officials what transformational leadership needs to succeed in healthcare organizations. Our research aims to help Ethiopia create better health policies by showing how transformational leadership makes better organizational performance and culture.

BACKGROUND OF THE STUDY

Current changes in international healthcare demand top quality leadership to achieve better patient care outcomes while keeping employees satisfied. When healthcare professionals practice transformational leadership they motivate their teams to produce better results and work together. Implementing transformational leadership in developing areas of Ethiopia faces difficult hurdles for study (Rojak et al., 2024). The Ethiopian Ministry of Health trains leaders to enhance healthcare delivery services. Despite its target to develop transformational leadership in healthcare managers the program encountered major difficulties (Eaton et al., 2024). Healthcare system leaders stuck to old-fashioned top-down management methods despite challenges to change. At rural healthcare facilities insufficient equipment made it difficult for leaders to put their new strategies into action effectively. The majority of employees resisted new approaches because normal organizational values put hierarchy ahead of partnership working.

The Ethiopian government implemented its Health Extension Program to show how transforming healthcare delivery needs local health worker support and community services. Despite positive early results the Health Extension Program failed to sustain its impact because health administrators at higher levels did not demonstrate transformational leadership (Rojak et al., 2024). Health extension workers abandoned their roles and became burnt out because leadership teams without transformational traits failed to spur worker motivation. Shifts in program effectiveness revealed that the program needed transformational leaders who build positive workplace culture (Eaton et al., 2024).

Our case examples show how organizations in Ethiopia encounter real-world difficulties when trying to use transformational leadership in healthcare (Rojak et al., 2024). Leadership development problems linked to poor training programs faces cultural barriers and lack of available resources. Understanding these issues helps us build better strategies that improve leadership techniques at hospitals to get better HRM results and enhance patient health. Our research analyzes the challenges in healthcare leadership implementation to show how these difficulties can be addressed by policy leaders and medical care executives (Riani, 2024).

STATEMENT OF THE PROBLEM

Ethiopia's healthcare sector faces a critical moment because strong leadership must help HRM teams build better workplaces to deliver better care (Riani, 2024). Transformational leadership should create an organization that empowers employees to work better together for better healthcare results. Healthcare organizations across Ethiopia currently demonstrate a large gap between leadership standards and real operational procedures (Febrian & Solihin, 2024). Research findings about transformational leadership producing good results differ across industries but remain uncertain for Ethiopian hospitals (Eaton et al., 2024). Research shows both that transformational leadership raises employee happiness but also proved hard to implement due to cultural and organizational barriers. Studies have yet to clearly demonstrate how transformational leadership changes HR practices and shapes workplace culture since research has not fully explained these relationships (Rojak et al., 2024).

Research shows transformational leadership works best in Western organizations but studies rarely test its effectiveness in Ethiopian socio-cultural settings (Rojak et al., 2024). The existing research about Ethiopian healthcare leaders remains incomplete because it does not analyze their unique resource limitations, high employee turnover and cultural barriers when undergoing changes. Simple problems like poor leader training and no established methods to bring about transformation make these problems worse.

This research explores the relationship between transformational leadership in care settings with Ethiopian healthcare organizational culture and human resource management. Using both number-based research methods and real-world examples this study will show us how these ideas work together. The study provides actionable direction for healthcare leaders and policy makers to develop transformational leadership methods that match local practices and traditions. This research aims to help leaders and policy-makers develop better ways to lead their workforce and produce improved healthcare results in Ethiopia.

THEORITICAL FOUNDATION

Transformational Leadership Theory: According to James MacGregor Burns' transformational leadership theory from the 1970s effective leaders motivate their staff by helping them achieve organizational goals that benefit everyone (Eaton et al., 2024). Leadership approaches depend heavily on vision development and effective communication as well as emotional insight. Healthcare settings require leaders who create mutual respect so everyone feels free to take initiative together as a team. The theory highlights four dimensions: The four basic traits of transformational leadership include idealized influence, inspirational motivation, intellectual stimulation, and individualized consideration. These qualities establish a positive work culture while improving staff commitment and help organizations understand healthcare leadership better (Rojak et al., 2024).

Organizational Culture Theory: This theory studies the common values and working methods that direct how staff members behave in their organization (Ezra & Charles, 2023). According to research pioneers like Edgar Schein organizational culture theory shows that shared values create systems which control how organizations work while shaping employee work behavior. A positive health care environment benefits employee motivation while delivering better treatment results and speeding up the use of new techniques. Leading organizations to success relies on combining good leadership with healthy organizational cultures to help teams adopt transformational practices properly (Febrian & Solihin, 2024).

Human Resource Management (HRM) Theory: HRM theory covers a range of procedures and guidelines pertaining to personnel management in a business (Papsiene, 2024). It highlights the significance of promoting employee development, performance management, and employee relations as well as the strategic alignment of HRM with business goals (Bauwens et al., 2024). Effective HRM is essential for drawing in and keeping qualified workers in the healthcare industry. By emphasizing how leadership styles may influence HRM procedures and eventually result in increased employee performance and satisfaction, this theory enhances the transformational leadership paradigm (Riani, 2024).

Social Exchange Theory: According to social exchange theory, social conduct results from an exchange process that aims to reduce costs and maximize benefits (Ong et al., 2024). It implies that more organizational loyalty and staff engagement might result from effective leadership practices in the workplace. A sense of reciprocity and trust is fostered in the healthcare industry when transformative leaders connect with employees in a way that is empowering and encouraging. By focusing on the relationship dynamics between leaders and employees, this theory deepens our knowledge of how transformational leadership affects HRM and organizational culture (Febrian & Solihin, 2024).

DEFINITIONS AND ORIGINS OF TERMS

Transformational Leadership: The leadership style known as the Transformation Leadership encourages and inspires followers to achieve great results, supporting development at both individual and professional levels (Rojak et al., 2024). The idea that goes back to the fact that James McGregor is at work at the end of the 20th century underlines how leaders can influence the goals and ideals of their followers. Characteristics of this style include charm, intellectual stimulation, inspiring motivation, and personalized attention, all of which contribute to increased levels of performance and participation in companies (Eaton et al., 2024).

Human Resource Management (HRM): The strategic approach to managing an organization's personnel in order to maximize performance and accomplish organizational objectives is known as human resource management (Riani, 2024). Recruitment, training, performance management and employee relations are only some of the many tasks it includes (Bauwens et al., 2024). At the beginning of the 20th century, the expression "human resources" was invented, and to the conventional objective of managing people with a more strategic function which prioritizes the culture of the company and the development of employees. HRM is essential for the development of trained managers and managed personnel, especially in sectors such as healthcare, where service delivery is primarily dependent on human capital (Riani, 2024).

Organizational Culture: The common values, attitudes, customs, and behaviors that define an organization and shape the interactions of its members are referred to as its organizational culture (Febrian & Solihin, 2024). Edgar Schein and other organizational theorists used the phrase, which had its roots in anthropology. Organizational culture influences how workers view their workplace and directs their actions. A strong, positive culture is essential to the success of health care organizations because it may result in better patient care, more teamwork, and higher employee morale.

Social Exchange Theory: According to social psychology, social conduct may be explained as a sequence of trades in which people try to maximize advantages and reduce disadvantages (Ong et al., 2024). George Homans initially proposed the idea in the 1950s, and Peter Blau and others later developed it. According to this idea, constructive interactions between managers and staff members in organizational settings cultivate commitment and trust, which can improve output and motivation. The use of Social Exchange Theory in the healthcare industry clarifies the relationship dynamics between transformational leaders and their teams, emphasizing the need of encouraging interactions in creating a productive workplace (Ong et al., 2024).

EMPIRICAL LITERATURE REVIEW

Transformational Leadership and Human Resource Management

Numerous studies on transformational leadership and human resource management (HRM) have shown how much of an influence it has on different HRM procedures and organizational results (Rojak et al., 2024). The ability of leaders to inspire and encourage followers to achieve extraordinary performance via a shared vision and dedication to corporate goals is the fundamental characteristic of transformational leadership (Eaton et al., 2024). According to empirical research, transformational leaders create an atmosphere that supports creativity, flexibility, and employee involvement all of which are essential elements of successful human resource management (Riani, 2024). Job satisfaction and staff motivation are two important areas where transformational leadership affects HRM (Eaton et al., 2024). According to studies, transformative leaders use specialized consideration, offering mentorship and assistance that is specific to each employee's requirements. This strategy not only boosts staff morale but also increases dedication to the company and work satisfaction. For example, a research in the healthcare industry discovered a significant correlation between transformational leadership and increased work satisfaction among nurses, which in turn led to better retention rates and lower turnover. The significance of leadership styles in influencing HRM results in hospital settings is shown by this research. Furthermore, the development of a healthy corporate culture—a critical component of successful HRM—has been associated with transformational leadership (Rojak et al., 2024). According to research, leaders that embrace a transformational approach are more likely to foster an environment of open communication, cooperation, and trust. Because workers feel appreciated and empowered to participate in decision-making, such a culture fosters the success of HRM practices (Riani, 2024). For instance, research conducted in a healthcare business found that transformational leadership enhanced a collaborative culture, which promoted cooperation and raised the standard of patient care overall (Eaton et al., 2024). This emphasizes how corporate culture and transformative leadership are mutually dependent, highlighting the importance of leadership in efficient HRM (Febrian & Solihin, 2024).

Transformational leadership is essential for promoting organizational development and change in addition to encouraging motivation and a healthy culture (Eaton et al., 2024). According to empirical data, transformational leaders are better at putting HRM approaches into practice that support corporate objectives, especially while things are changing (Riani, 2024). For example, it was discovered that transformational leaders were able to successfully convey the goal and justification for the changes during the adoption of new healthcare policies, which led to a more seamless implementation and increased employee support. According to studies, transformational leaders' companies are better able to adjust to changes in the external environment, which is crucial for maintaining a competitive edge in the fast-paced healthcare industry (Febrian & Solihin, 2024). Additionally, studies have shown that transformational leadership plays a mediating role in the connection between organizational performance and HRM strategies (Riani, 2024). Through alignment with the organization's vision and values, transformational leaders improve the efficacy of HRM procedures including hiring, training, and performance management (Bauwens et al., 2024). One research, for example, found that transformational leaders who actively participate in the hiring process not only draw in talent that aligns with the company culture, but also support workers' long-term growth through focused training programs (Eaton et al., 2024). Since workers are more likely to be engaged, productive, and dedicated to accomplishing the organization's goals when leadership and HRM practices are in sync, organizational performance eventually improves (Riani, 2024).

H1: Transformational leadership and Human Resource Management have empirical association

Transformational Leadership and Organizational Culture

Organizational culture currently depends on transformational leadership, in particular in dynamic and difficult conditions, such as the health care industry (Rojak et al., 2024). The ability to inspire and encourage followers to pass the organizational needs in advance is the basis of transformational leadership (Eaton et al., 2024). The four main factors of this style of leadership are intellectual stimulation, individual care, stimulating motivation, and idealized influence. As empirical research has shown several times, these aspects of transformative leadership are necessary to create a superior corporate culture that promotes creativity, teamwork and employee engagement (Rojak et al., 2024). The development of the general vision and a set of values among employees is one of the most important consequences of transformative leadership over corporate culture (Ferian and Solihin, 2024). Research shows that change leaders are successfully communicating a compelling vision that addresses the values and objectives of team members. For example, studies in health conditions show that managers who express a convincing vision inspire employees and contribute to a feeling of loyalty and belonging to the company. Employees are more inclined to cooperate with common objectives in a cohesive culture created by this common vision, which improves the results of companies as a whole (Eaton et al., 2024). Additionally, transformational leaders cultivate an atmosphere of transparency and trust, two qualities that are essential to a positive corporate culture (Febrian

& Solihin, 2024). According to empirical research, transformational leadership is linked to higher levels of trust amongst followers and team members (Rojak et al., 2024). For instance, research conducted in a hospital environment discovered that transformational leaders who uphold ethical decision-making and openness foster a culture of trust in which staff members feel free to voice their opinions. Employees are more willing to take chances and be creative when there is trust, which is crucial for adjusting to the quick changes that are frequently observed in healthcare settings (Febrian & Solihin, 2024).

One of the main components of transformational leadership, intellectual stimulation, improves company culture by fostering workers' creativity and critical thinking (Eaton et al., 2024). According to research, managers that encourage creative thinking and question the status quo foster an environment where staff members feel free to provide fresh concepts and solutions. This is especially important in healthcare companies as executives work to continuously enhance patient care while navigating difficult obstacles. One research study, for example, showed how transformational leaders who push employees to challenge established procedures foster an innovative culture that enhances patient outcomes and service delivery (Febrian & Solihin, 2024). Additionally, the focus placed by transformational leadership on individual attention helps firms foster a culture of growth and support (Rojak et al., 2024). An atmosphere where people feel appreciated and acknowledged is created by leaders who take the time to learn about the specific needs and strengths of their staff. Because employees are more inclined to remain with a company that supports their professional and personal development, empirical data indicates that this individualized strategy improves employee satisfaction and retention. This dedication is essential in healthcare environments as better patient care and organizational efficacy are strongly correlated with high staff engagement levels (Febrian & Solihin, 2024). Even while transformational leadership has a good effect on corporate culture, there are always issues, especially in industries like healthcare (Rojak et al., 2024). According to certain empirical research, hierarchical systems and prevailing cultural norms may make transformative leadership less successful. For instance, transformational leaders may find it difficult to enact cultural changes in companies with strict hierarchies, which might result in opposition from staff members used to conventional leadership philosophies. This emphasizes how important it is for leaders to not only exhibit transformative traits but also understand and successfully negotiate the current culture (Febrian & Solihin, 2024).

H2: Transformational leadership and Organizational Culture have empirical association.

Organizational Culture and Human Resource Management

Human resource management (HRM) techniques and results are significantly shaped by organizational culture, which also affects how businesses recruit, nurture, and retain talent (Riani, 2024). HRM techniques function within an organization's culture, which is defined as the common values, attitudes, and behaviors that define it. A strong organizational culture has been shown to improve employees, satisfaction and performance. This has a beneficial effect on overall company efficiency (Fefian & Solihin, 2024). Meanwhile, low moral spirit, high renewal and poor performance among employees may be the result of a culture that does not correspond to the principles of HRM. Sets and choices are two important areas where corporate culture influences HRM (Riani, 2024). Research shows that companies with a well-defined culture are more likely to attract candidates whose beliefs and actions correspond to their beliefs in the company. For example, research shows that firms with a strong cultural identity have a higher probability that combines well with current structures, increase employee satisfaction and reduce turnover. This alignment makes it fluid as people associated with growing your business are likely to stay, but also increases the chances of employee retention. Organizational culture also has a big influence on HRM training and development procedures (Febrian & Solihin, 2024). Research indicates that a culture that places a high value on learning and development creates an atmosphere where workers are more likely to pursue ongoing professional development. For example, companies that contribute to innovative culture and knowledge exchange encourage employees to work with colleagues in search of training opportunities. Research conducted in the healthcare industry shows that institutions with a culture that prioritizes professional growth were highly involved with high personnel and efficient involvement, directly related to the best patient care outcomes. This highlights how important it is to align education initiatives with the company's cultural values.

Another important HRM field that is influenced by corporate culture is the management of efficiency (Riani, 2024). Research shows that the culture of determining employee prioritization participation, feedback, and confirmation leads to more successful effectiveness management procedures. Employees are likely to actively participate in the process of checking effectiveness, contribute to an environment of responsibility and constant development when they feel valued and encouraged. According to this study, companies with open communication and retro action cultures have the happiest employees satisfied with their performance magazines, improving personal and business goal alignment (Bauwens et al., 2024). Organizational culture also affects HRM conflicts and employee relationship resolution procedures (Ferian and Solihin, 2024). Conflicts are processed constructively, and not in defense in cultures that value cooperation and respect for each other. According to empirical studies, companies with these cultures better contribute to a conflict, which increases moral spirit and cooperation. However, companies with a hierarchical or competitive culture can struggle to resolve conflicts, increasing tensions and reducing employee engagement. This highlights how important it is to have an organizational culture that values good employee interaction as a basis for effective talent management (Riani, 2024). Nonetheless, there are certain difficulties in the link between HRM and corporate culture (Febrian & Solihin, 2024). Potential discrepancies between an organization's professed culture and workers' real experiences are also highlighted by empirical research. For example, research found that companies may promote values like cooperation and teamwork but neglect to put these principles into effect through HRM procedures. Employee disenchantment and a decline in organizational commitment may result from this separation. Therefore, in order to create a supportive and cohesive work environment, it is imperative that firms make sure that their HRM practices are continuously in line with their cultural values (Riani, 2024).

H3: Organizational Culture and Human Resource Management have empirical association.

Transformational Leadership, Human Resource Management and Organizational Culture Mediation

In empirical literature, the relationship among transformational leadership, HRM, and organizational culture has received a lot of attention, especially in relation to how these dimensions impact one another and enhance overall organizational success (Rojak et al., 2024). A supportive corporate culture is frequently seen as being fostered by transformational leadership, which is defined as inspiring and encouraging staff to put the needs of the firm ahead of their own (Febrian & Solihin, 2024). In turn, this culture plays a crucial mediating role that improves the efficacy of HRM procedures. Through the examination of these connections, scholars have shed light on how transformative leadership, viewed through the prism of organizational culture, may result in better HRM results (Riani, 2024). Organizational culture development has been demonstrated to be significantly impacted by transformational leadership (Rojak et al., 2024). An atmosphere that fosters common ideals and objectives is produced by leaders that exhibit transformational traits like idealized influence and inspiring motivation. According to empirical research, transformational leaders are more likely to foster an environment in their firms that values cooperation, trust, and creativity. For instance, studies in a number of industries, such as healthcare and education, have shown that transformational leaders who successfully convey a compelling vision encourage staff members to adopt company values, creating a unified culture that supports strategic goals. Since employee engagement and dedication are key elements of effective HRM and are increased by a strong company culture, this alignment is crucial (Riani, 2024). It is also notable that organizational culture plays a mediating role in the interaction between HRM practices and transformational leadership (Febrian & Solihin, 2024). According to empirical data, a good corporate culture improves the execution and efficacy of HRM efforts in addition to reinforcing the benefits of transformational leadership (Rojak et al., 2024). Organizations with a culture that encourages learning and growth, for example, are better able to take advantage of transformational leadership's motivating qualities (Eaton et al., 2024). Research indicates that when leaders support professional development and ongoing improvement, staff members are more likely to participate in HRM activities like skill development and training, which improves organizational performance (Rojak et al., 2024). This emphasizes how crucial it is to cultivate a culture that supports transformational leadership techniques in order to optimize HRM efficacy (Riani, 2024).

Furthermore, organizational culture frequently acts as a mediator in the link between transformational leadership and HRM outcomes like job satisfaction and employee retention (Febrian & Solihin, 2024). According to research, employees are more committed to the company and have better job satisfaction when transformational leaders foster a culture of appreciation and support. For instance, a research study conducted in the healthcare industry found that decreased turnover rates among nursing personnel were the consequence of transformational leadership approaches combined with a supportive corporate culture (Rojak et al., 2024). This research highlights the crucial role that organizational culture plays as a mediating element, indicating that transformational leadership's positive effects on HRM outcomes are enhanced when leadership techniques and the organization's underlying culture are strongly aligned (Riani, 2024). However, when transformative leadership and the current corporate culture are not aligned, problems may occur (Febrian & Solihin, 2024). According to empirical research, there are situations in which leaders may advocate for transformational principles but the dominant culture may be reluctant to change, which might result in disputes and employee disengagement (Eaton et al., 2024). For instance, transformational CEOs may find it difficult to enact cultural shifts that encourage cooperation and creativity in companies with strict hierarchical systems. The efficacy of HRM procedures may be hampered by this mismatch as workers may feel cut off from the objectives of the company (Riani, 2024). Therefore, for leaders looking to successfully apply transformational approaches, it is crucial to comprehend the mediating function of corporate culture (Febrian & Solihin, 2024).

H4: Transformational leadership, Human Resource Management and Organizational Culture mediation have empirical association.

CONCEPTUAL FRAMEWORK

Figure 1. Conceptual Framework

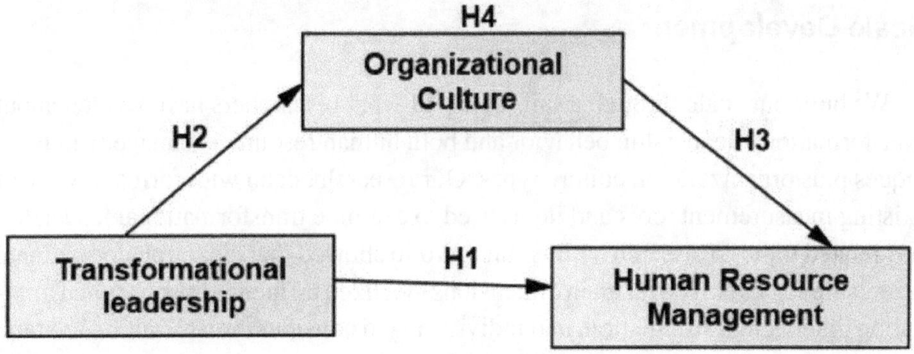

RESEARCH METHODOLOGY

In this study, this research adopts a numerical approach to understand how transformational leadership and human resources affect healthcare organizational culture in Ethiopia (Liang et al., 2024). We chose 390 participants by random selection based on organized groups to make our findings represent all healthcare settings. Our methodology allowed us to study multiple organizational contexts and gather complete data on their operational elements. Our study gathered necessary information using a structured survey tool to examine transformational leadership, HRM practices, and organizational culture as its research components. Each response option for the questionnaire offered a five-point scale between disagree and agree while letting participants describe their level of agreement (Kariuki et al., 2024). The research tested sampling suitability and examined measurement instrument reliability through Kaiser-Meyer-Olkin (KMO) and Bartlett's Test of Sphericity (Civelek, 2018). These tests showed the data needed factor analysis and confirmed that our sample size was adequate plus our data quality for further analysis. Through Exploratory Factor Analysis we identified the main components of our constructs and improved our measurement scales. The EFA results helped us build a better measurement model by showing how items relate to each other and suggesting which factors need merging or removing (Civelek, 2018). After performing the EFA test we employed AMOS to study transformational leadership connections to HRM and organizational culture. Through SEM analysis all associated relationships could be studied at once to show clear pathways between different elements. Standard statistical tests measured the quality of our model design by analyzing Chi-square statistics along with CFI and RMSEA outputs to verify that our research aligns with theory and produces meaningful results (Civelek, 2018).

Scale Development

We built our scale through a full review of what researchers have written about transformational leadership behavior and both human resources management techniques plus organizational culture types. Our research began with formal review of existing measurement tools and items used to examine transformational leadership and related topics. Research by Bass and Avolio showed that clear transformational leadership scales exist with main dimensions idealized influence, inspirational motivation, intellectual stimulation, and individualized consideration (Gachira & Ntara, 2024). Research by Becker and Huselid formed our selection criteria to measure HRM practices including hiring, training, evaluating and dealing with employees. The organizational culture scale emerged from Schein's and Denison's research models which examined adaptability of employees, their level of involvement and their understanding of the company's mission. The research team modified measurement tools to apply directly to Ethiopian healthcare settings but stayed true to their basic purpose. A small group of healthcare professionals tested the items before research started to make them easier to understand and better match the subject. Our modified scale includes clear dimensions for each measure so we can accurately monitor the research connections. Through extensive scale development steps researchers built proper tools to measure all relevant aspects of transformational leadership HRM practices and organizational culture in their specific environment (Gachira & Ntara, 2024).

DATA ANALYSIS

Table 1. KMO and Bartlett's Test

Kaiser-Meyer-Olkin Measure of Sampling Adequacy.		**.906**
Bartlett's Test of Sphericity	Approx. Chi-Square	2095.96
	Df	126
	Sig.	.000

Source: Authors

Table 1 shows the data's suitability for factor analysis through Kaiser-Meyer-Olkin (KMO) and Bartlett's Test of Sphericity results. The sample hearing quality stands strong for factor analysis because the 0.906 KMO value shows good relations among variables with a minimum requirement of 0.6. Our dataset's high KMO value shows that the variables hold enough joint variance to make effective factor analysis possible. Bartlett's Test of Sphericity shows our data is ready for factor analysis because the Chi-Square approximation result is 2095.96 with 126 free dimensions that produce a p-value of 0.000. Our results show a significant pattern of correlations between variables because the p-value is below 0.05 which means we must reject the identity matrix assumption. Our results demonstrate a clear link between variables which makes them suitable for additional analysis. Our research shows that this dataset can detect hidden factor patterns reliably which makes it suitable for research on studied constructs.

Table 2. Total Variance Explained

C	Initial Eigenvalues			Extraction Sums of Squared Loadings			Rotation Sums of Squared Loadings		
	Total	% of Variance	Cumulative %	Total	% of Variance	Cumulative %	Total	% of Variance	Cumulative %
1	4.1	32.5	32.5	4.1	32.5	32.5	3.0	21.1	21.1
2	1.7	9.7	42.2	1.7	9.7	42.2	2.6	15.1	36.2
3	1.7	9.7	51.0	1.7	9.7	51.0	1.8	14.8	51.0
4	.99	6.2	57.2						
5	.81	6.3	64.5						
6	.73	5.9	69.4						

Extraction Method: Principal Component Analysis.
Source: Authors

The table 2 shows the results from our Principal Component Analysis which includes the eigenvalues before extraction and after rotation. Our results show six significant factors that explain 51% of the dataset variance. Our study reveals that the first factor explains 32.5% of the variance through its 4.1 eigenvalue whiles the 1.7 eigenvalues from factors two and three combine to account for 9.7% more. These three identified constructs explain 51% of all variances seen in the dataset. After extraction the first three components held their strengths consistently with the first factor explaining 32.5% of the variance and second and third factors keeping their respective contributions. After rotation the three main factors explain 21.1%, 15.1% and 14.8% of the total variance. The results show that the initial factor dominates the analysis yet reveals important connections between the data's different elements. Factors four, five, and six display eigenvalues under 1.0 which reduces their importance in explaining measurement constructs. Our analysis identifies six key factors that collectively explain 69.4% of the data variance in a structured way.

Confirmatory Principle Component Examination

The principle component arrangement of a set of guided proxies is verified using a type of statistics known as confirmatory principle component examination. Based on the underlying frame job and correlatives among observed proxies, investigations can evaluate hypotheses utilizing CFA. To evaluate the hypothesis that there is a association among the proxies that are being steered and the latent conceptions that underpin them, the inquiry employed CFA under table 3.

Table 3. Covariances

Covariance			Estimate	S.E.	C.R.	P	Hy.
Organizational Culture	**<-->**	**Transformational leadership**	**.274**	**.032**	**8.073**	**.00**	**H2**
Organizational Culture	<-->	Human Resource Management	.303	.029	7.989	.00	**H3**
Transformational leadership	<-->	Human Resource Management	.254	0.34	7.741	.00	**H1**

Source: Authors

Our results show the strength and direction between Organizational Culture Transformational Leadership and Human Resource Management through Table 3's statistics. The covariance results from our analysis show how strongly and what direction these organizational elements attach to each other. Our analysis shows a 0.274 relationship between Organizational Culture and Transformational Leadership with a measurement uncertainty of 0.032. The findings show a powerful relationship between Organizational Culture and Transformational Leadership since the result of 8.073 matches our H2 hypothesis. An organizational culture's positivity directly links to transformational leadership behaviors when leaders make their culture support engagement. The relationship between these elements shows a 0.303 match with a 0.029 standard error. The relationship between organizational culture and transformational leadership practice shows strong results through 7.989 in critical ratio and 0.00 p-value which backs Hypothesis 3 (H3). When organizations build cultures that focus on employee growth they will naturally improve their HRM practices. Our results show that the connection between Transformational Leadership and Human Resource Management activities generates a 0.254 covariance value with a 0.034 standard error. The results show a statistical connection between the investigated areas which backs our first hypothesis (H1). When leaders influence positively their teams they make a difference in HRM strategies outcomes.

Table 4. Validity Concern

	CR	AVE	MSV	MaxR(H)	*TL*	OC	HRM
TL	0.732	0.643	0.219	0.852	**0.654**		
OC	0.758	0.657	0.132	0.763	0.171	**0.665**	
HRM	0.793	0.603	0.274	0.797	0.383	0.193	**0.684**

Note: TL= Transformational leadership; OC= Organizational Culture; HRM= Human Resource Management
Source: Authors

Table 4 shows validity information about how TC, OC, and HRM models measure Transformational Leadership (TL), Organizational Culture (OC), and Human Resource Management (HRM). It displays Composite Reliability (CR), Average Variance Extracted (AVE), Maximum Shared Variance (MSV), and Maximum Reliability (MaxR(H)) results. The test results help assess if our measurement scales accurately represent both their internal coherence and their correlation to true constructs. The tests show all three measurement areas have acceptable internal consistency standards in place. For total labor the Composite Reliability score is 0.732 while OC shows 0.758 and HRM reaches 0.793 reliability. The measurement scales achieve better reliability compared to industry standards because their values exceed 0.7. Both the Average Variance Extracted results indicate proper measurement of our study's main elements. The measurement scale show that TL reports an AVE of 0.643, OC reports an AVE of 0.657, and HRM reports an AVE of 0.603. When constructs explain more than 50% of indicator variation they demonstrate valid measurement properties according to AVE values. Shared variance ratings show that TL differs most from other constructs while HRM stands apart least. These low MSV values show that the investigated constructs stand apart because they do not share excessive variance in their elements which is vital for proving discriminant validity. The measurement reliability of our constructs shows strong results. TL scores 0.852, OC scores 0.763, and HRM scores 0.797 on the MaxR(H) assessment.

Mediating Examination

Figure 2. Structural Equation Model

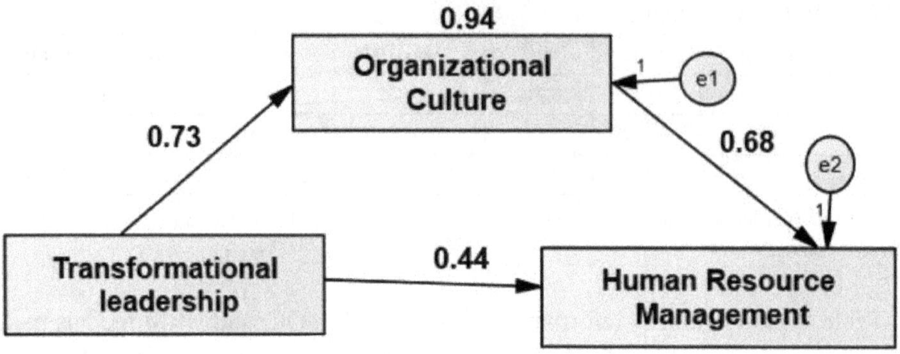

Model Fit Indices

Table 5. indices for Model Fit

Sig.	Chi-Sq	RMR	Fitness Goodness	Fitness Confirmatory	TLI	RMSEA
0.006	1.073	.036	0.930	0.912	0.911	.028

Source: Authors

In Table 5 we present SEM model fit indices to show how well the proposed design matches with actual data results. The measurements confirm our model has statistically important fit since Significance equals 0.006. Standard social science modeling of human behaviors delivers imperfect results reflected in low p-values. The Chi-Square result comes out at 1.073 with a low value showing the model's good match with real-world evidence. A fitting model shows up with a low Chi-Square value but its impact depends on the Degrees of Freedom figure which the results do not provide. Data shows a good match between the model and the observations since our Root Mean Square Residual value is 0.036 below the standard threshold of 0.08. Standard model fitness measurements (Fitness Goodness Index and Fitness Confirmatory Index) show values of 0.930 and 0.912 respectively which exceed the recommended threshold benchmark of 0.90. The results from these indices confirm that the model matches the data structure very well. The model's fit is proven once again by a Tucker-Lewis index score of 0.911 which goes beyond the required 0.90 benchmark. Our model achieves high quality matching through the RMSEA result of 0.028 since it remains considerably more manageable than the standard allowable threshold of 0.06. The RMSEA shows excellent model match with readings from 0.05 to 0.08.

Table 6. Regression Examination

Relative			**Approx.**	**S.E.**	**C.R.**	**P**	**Ass.**
Organizational Culture	**<---**	**Transformational leadership**	**.864**	**.143**	**7.583**	**.00**	**H2**
Human Resource Management	<---	Organizational Culture	.328	.131	2.853	.00	H3
Human Resource Management	<---	Transformational leadership	.957	.192	7.958	.00	H1

Source: Authors

Table 6 shows the findings of our statistical analysis on the interconnections between Transformational Leadership, Organizational Culture, and Human Resource Management. The table displays estimated parameters alongside their respective standard errors C.R. values P-values and corresponding Hypothesis tests. Our research shows that Transformational Leadership impacts Organizational Culture with a determined path from 0.864 to 0.00 (CR = 7.583, S.E. = 0.143). The 0.00 p-value proves a strong connection that backs up H2. Organizations with more effective transformational leaders experience stronger positive cultural outcomes according to our study. Our findings show Organizational Culture enhances Human Resource Management practices with a 0.328 impact and 2.853 critical ratio. The p-value measurement of 0.00 shows a strong link between Leadership Transformation and H3 results. Well-constructed organizational cultures enhance the results HRM delivers because organizations with solid support systems tend to perform stronger HR strategies. Our analysis shows Transformational Leadership directly affects Human Resource Management performance with a statistical effect of 0.957 and 7.958 times the standard error. The evidence confirms Hypothesis 1 because the p-value remains zero throughout our analysis. Our analysis shows that leaders who use transformational leadership styles help both create supportive company cultures and improve HRM practices.

Table 7. Mediating role Effect

	Influence	Worth	Path Influence
Transformational leadership → Human Resource Management	Direct Influence	.44	Direct influence stated
Transformational leadership → Organizational Culture → Human Resource Management	Indirect Influence	.73*.68=.49	Indirect Influence Ensued
	Whole influence	.94	Partial mediation

Source: Authors

Table 7 shows how Organizational Culture acts as an intermediary in the bond between Transformational Leadership and Human Resource Management. The table shows you both main effects and secondary impacts to teach you about their working methods. Transformational Leadership's direct impact on Human Resource Management measures up to 0.44 showing strong independent effects. Leaders who use transformational methods create real HR improvements without needing other supporting elements. Our calculations show Organizational Culture partly connects Transformational Leadership to Human Resource Management. The indirect impact stands at 0.49 due to 0.73 influence of Transformational Leadership on Organizational Culture and 0.68 effect of Organizational Culture on Human Resource Management. Much of how transformational leadership affects HRM happens because of its impact on organizational culture. Our analysis shows that Transformational Leadership produces a strong impact on Human Resource Management through both direct and indirect relationships with a combined effect of 0.94. The analysis shows that both Organizational Culture and Transformational Leadership affect HRM but Organizational Culture works as a partial mediator between them.

DISCUSSION

The findings of this study shed important light on how organizational culture, human resources management, and transformative leadership are interrelated. The prominent links found between these variables highlight how critical and powerful leadership influences organizational dynamics and improved HRM procedures. The leaders who demonstrate transformational characteristics, such as inspiration, motivation and support are crucial to create a favorable cultural atmosphere, in accordance with a significant favorable effect of transformational leadership on organizational culture. This corresponds to previous studies, which emphasizes the importance of leadership in the development of the environment at work, which contributes to the cooperation and involvement of employees. Furthermore, the results show that organizational culture plays a critical role in mediating relationships between human resource management and transformational leadership. The idea that a leader-created cultural environment has a major impact on HRM practice is also confirmed by the large indirect impact of transformative leadership on HRM through organizational culture. HRM outcomes like employee happiness, retention, and performance are likely to increase for companies that place a high priority on an inclusive and encouraging culture. This research supports the claim that organizational culture has a significant role in influencing the formulation and application of HRM strategies rather than just serving as a background. In addition, the direct effect of transformational leadership on HRM shows that successful HRM initiatives can be caused by good leadership, even if there is a strong cultural intermediary. This implies that although culture has a great influence, the characteristics of leadership are what really matters with regard to HRM. Even in various cultural contexts, managers can use solutions and actions to make appropriate changes and apply working HRM methods. Emphasizing the complex links between these concepts, the findings of the research add to the broader conversations about management and leadership. To obtain the best results of HRM, organizations must focus on creating a reliable organizational culture that supports their strategic objectives in addition to training in transformation leaders. Organizations can have a synergistic effect which promotes the overall performance and well-being of employees, developing both strong leadership and a culture of support. Future studies will explore this dynamic in more detail in the context of other organizations and examine the potential impact of external variables on these connections.

CONCLUSION

The conclusions of the study emphasize the important interactions that exist between organizational culture, human resources management and transformational leadership. According to the facts, the leaders of the transformation have a great influence on the growth of a healthy corporate culture which improves HRM procedures. The results show that although HRM is directly influenced by transformative leadership, this effect is amplified by corporate culture and that a supportive cultural background is essential to optimize the effectiveness of HRM. These observations have practical applications for businesses that are aiming to enhance HR planning. Organizations may establish a favorable atmosphere for employee engagement and performance by making investments in transformational leadership development and cultivating a robust organizational culture. In the end, this study advances knowledge of how culture and leadership interact together to influence HRM results, offering a foundation for further organizational development research and practice. Companies need to integrate effective leadership and strong culture as companies continue to negotiate and change to achieve long-term success and competitive advantage.

MANAGERIAL IMPLICATIONS

In the conclusion of this study, there are a number of important consequences for managing companies that strive to improve their HRM procedures thanks to strong organizational culture and leadership. First of all, companies need to pay attention to their leaders' priorities and develop transformative leadership skills. Workshops and training courses that highlight abilities such as staff support, motivation, and clarification of vision will help leaders develop a healthy workplace culture. By promoting these characteristics, managers can motivate staff, increase engagement and improve production. The report also emphasizes how important it is to match company culture with strategic objectives. A collaborative, innovative, and inclusive culture should be actively evaluated and fostered by managers. Initiatives such as employee feedback systems, cultural notes, and compensation programs can help. Organizations can ensure that HRM procedures are not only successful, but also appeal to employees by creating a solid cultural foundation. Additionally, managers should use an integrated approach to organizational development, taking into account the dual impact of organizational culture and transformational leadership on HRM. Instead of viewing culture and leadership as individuals, they must acknowledge the extent to which they are interdependent and try to include management in their plans. This leveling can facilitate the use of HRM practice, which are accepted by employees at all levels and are not only descending mandates.

PRACTICAL IMPLICATIONS

The research conclusions include applications that are important for businesses that aim to improve operational efficiency using the best HRM (HR Management). Organizations must first and foremost create meticulous programs for the development of leadership. This should highlight the qualities of transformative leadership. Offering managers the tools they need to encourage and inspire their teams, these programs can contribute to the climate of trust and cooperation. In addition to improving management skills, these investments in leadership contribute to a productive and happy workplace, which increases the involvement of employees. Organizations also need to pay great attention to the evaluation and development of their organizational culture. This means that culture responds to the organization's mission and values, and conducting frequent cultural audits. Pragmatic behaviours may include creating mentoring programs, providing platforms for staff deposits, and rewards and stimuli for cultural deposits. The company demonstrates its commitment to a comfortable work environment and is actively involved in cultural projects. Furthermore, it is extremely important to include organizational culture and transformative leadership in the usual HRM procedures. Managers are responsible for ensuring that HR programs and politicians respond to leadership and cultural values. For example, efficiency management systems can be created to encourage actions that demonstrate transformational leadership, and hiring procedures can be created to attract candidates who share the organization's cultural values.

THEORETICAL IMPLICATIONS

The conclusions of this study make a significant theoretical contribution to knowledge about the link between organizational culture, human resource management (HRM), and transformational leadership. This study adds to current theory of leadership and management, showing that transformative leadership directly and indirectly affects HRM through organizational culture. This supports the idea that good leadership is a complex concept that involves organizational culture and the ability to influence HRM procedures. Furthermore, discussions on the importance of cultural factors in organizational success reach a depth of awareness of organizational culture as intermediaries in this respect. This emphasizes how important it is for future studies to investigate the ways in which certain cultural traits—like diversity, flexibility, and creativity—interact with leadership philosophies to influence HRM results. According to the findings, these characteristics are not separate phenomena but rather interrelated components that work together to influence performance, therefore researchers should take this into account when creating models of organizational behavior. This study also highlights the need for a theoretical framework for a more integrated approach to leadership and culture. We encourage scientists to examine how transformational leadership and organizational culture can work together to increase organizational efficiency and demonstrate synergistic relationships. This perspective promotes a complete understanding of management theory and leads to additional research into the cultural and leadership dynamics in various contexts and organizational industries.

RECOMMENDATIONS

The research conclusions allow us to develop many proposals for businesses seeking to improve HRM procedures using corporate culture and effective leadership.

First of all, businesses should give top priority to the transformational leadership development of their management teams. Targeted programs that highlight key leadership skills such as emotional intelligence, efficient communication, and motivational approaches will support this. Organizations can develop more ambitious and involved jobs and have these capabilities in their managers. It is also recommended that companies regularly evaluate their organizational culture to identify their advantages and disadvantages. Employing equipment such as focus groups, employee surveys, and cultural audits gives you important information about the current state of the culture and how well it fits with the company's goals. Organizations should create programs that contribute to the culture of cooperation, diversity and creativity in the light of these assessments. This can lead to the creation of forums for the contribution of staff, to the honor and to the celebration of cultural contributions and to the development of the atmosphere, which contributes to an open dialogue. In addition, companies wish to include organizational culture and transformational leadership concepts in their HRM procedures. This implies a comparison of presumed leadership and cultural characteristics with the processes of hiring, teaching and evaluation of efficiency. For instance, hiring procedures might concentrate on drawing applicants who share the organization's cultural values in addition to having the requisite abilities. Likewise, it is possible to create performance management systems that incentivize actions that demonstrate transformational leadership and foster a great workplace culture. Finally, it is important to always evaluate these efforts. Organizations need to establish measures to assess how cultural efforts and leadership development affect HRM outcomes. Organizations can modify data from their strategy and maintain their effectiveness in creating a positive work environment, regularly assessing these measures.

FUTURE DIRECTIONS

To expand the knowledge gathered in this study, future research in the fields of organizational culture, transformational leadership and human resource management (HRM) should study a certain number of important subjects. First, longitudinal studies can be performed to see how these measurements change over time. Such research will help researchers better understand how culture and leadership are dynamic factors that influence HRM practices. This allows businesses to change their plans as conditions change. Future research can also examine how external factors such as market dynamics, economic situations, and technological events influence how transformative leadership, organizational culture, and how HRM interact. Organizations may create more robust and flexible HRM strategies by comprehending the interactions between these external factors and internal dynamics. Examining how various corporate cultures affect the efficacy of transformational leadership is another exciting avenue for future study. Researchers can study how different types of cultures, such as clans, adchocracy, markets, and hierarchies, influence employee participation, retention, and performance outcomes. This complex approach can provide infiltration information for modifying HRM and steps for developing leadership according to a particular cultural context. Furthermore, comparative research in the context of many organizations, including public sector organizations, multinational corporations, and nonprofit organizations, improves an understanding of how organizational culture and change leadership differs between contexts. Such research identifies best practices and tactics that work well in a particular situation, providing useful information for managers and managers. Finally, including qualitative approaches into next studies may provide deeper, more contextualized understandings of workers' and leaders' real-world experiences. The nuances of the daily interactions between organizational culture and transformational leadership may be revealed through case studies, ethnographic research, and interviews, which would further improve HRM procedures.

REFERENCES

Bauwens, R., Audenaert, M., & Decramer, A. (2024). Performance management systems, innovative work behavior and the role of transformational leadership: An experimental approach. *Journal of Organizational Effectiveness: People and Performance*, *11*(1), 178–195. DOI: 10.1108/JOEPP-03-2022-0066

Civelek, M. E. (2018). Essentials of Structural Equation Modeling. In *Zea Books*. DOI: 10.13014/K2SJ1HR5

Eaton, L., Bridgman, T., & Cummings, S. (2024). Advancing the democratization of work: A new intellectual history of transformational leadership theory. *Leadership*, *20*(3), 125–143. DOI: 10.1177/17427150241232705

Ezra, W., & Charles, M. (2023). Organizational Culture Among Religious Founded Schools in Enhancing Teachers' Performance: A Case Study of Bishop Willigers Secondary School in Bugweri District, Eastern Uganda. *Research and Advances in Education*, *2*(9), 61–73. DOI: 10.56397/RAE.2023.09.06

Febrian, W. D., & Solihin, A. (2024). Analysis of Improving Organizational Culture Through Employee Engagement, Talent Management, Training and Development Human Resources. *Siber Journal of Advanced Multidisciplinary*, *1*(4), 185–195. DOI: 10.38035/sjam.v1i4.86

Gachira, J. N., & Ntara, C. (2024). Effect of Transformational Leadership on Organisational Performance of Top 100 SMEs in Nairobi, Kenya. *Journal of Human Resource & Leadership*, *8*(2), 82–99.

Kariuki, B. W., Gichuhi, D., & Mwaura, P. (2024). Influence of Corporate Culture on the Implementation of Change Initiatives in Kirinyaga County Government, Kenya. *African Journal of Empirical Research*, *5*(4), 957–965. DOI: 10.51867/ajernet.5.4.78

Liang, Z., Zhao, Y., Yu, H., Habibi, M., & Mahmoudi, T. (2024). Artificial neural networks coupled with numerical approach for the stability prediction of non-uniform functionally graded microscale cylindrical structures. *Structures (Oxford)*, *60*, 105826. DOI: 10.1016/j.istruc.2023.105826

Ong, A. K. S., German, J. D., Dangaran, P. C., Paz, J. J. B., & Macatangay, R. R. G. (2024). Service quality and customer satisfaction analysis among motorcycle taxi transportation in the Philippines through SERVQUAL dimensions and social exchange theory. *Case Studies on Transport Policy*, *15*, 101139. DOI: 10.1016/j.cstp.2023.101139

Papsiene, P. (2024). Theoretical modeling of organizational reflex in human resource management from the perspective of organizational biological approach. *Humanities & Social Sciences Communications*, *11*(1), 1–13. DOI: 10.1057/s41599-024-02644-y

Riani, D. (2024). Reimagining Human Resource: Redefine Human Resource Management Practices for the Future. *Jurnal Riset Bisnis Dan Manajemen*, *17*(1), 149–157. DOI: 10.23969/jrbm.v17i1.12997

Rojak, J. A., Sanaji, S., Witjaksono, A. D., & Kistyanto, A. (2024). The influence of transformational leadership and organizational culture on employee performance. *EDUKASIA: Jurnal Pendidikan Dan Pembelajaran*, *5*(1), 977–990. DOI: 10.62775/edukasia.v5i1.926

KEY TERMS AND DEFINITIONS

Cultural Assessment: Our cultural assessment tool helps us examine and study how work happens in our company today. Our team studies employee responses through several methods to understand their work benefits and critical areas while matching them to business targets.

Employee Engagement: When employees give both their psychological heart and soul to their organization's strategic vision. When employees become engaged they work better and feel more motivated while helping the organization reach its goals.

Human Resource Management (HRM): HRM uses workforce administration methods from staff hiring through training and performance tracking to connect well with employees. Human Resource Management ensures employees perform their best work while matching their skills precisely to company objectives.

Leadership Development: Organizations use this method to teach leadership principles and build individual performance skills across their teams. Our leadership development efforts feature different types of learning opportunities including professional development programs, mentorship partnerships, and instructor-led coaching for better results.

Organizational Culture: The collective set of values and customs that define how employees behave and think inside their organization. The state of an organization shows in how tasks get carried out and determines how people in the company interact while creating the work setting.

Performance Management: We track employee metrics and skills development against business targets through an ongoing system. Employers lead performance development by clearly stating what they expect, sharing feedback, and watching the results to help employees mature while making the business thrive.

Transformational Leadership: A transformational leader with the power to motivate teams to outstanding work results and develop their skills (Eaton et al., 2024). Leaders who transform values motivate their team through planned goals and friendly interactions.

Chapter 10
Evidence-Based Management in Healthcare Companies:
Strategic Model for Effective Multidisciplinary Collaboration

Alba Maria Gallo
https://orcid.org/0009-0007-1987-5252
Giustino Fortunato University, Italy

Ubaldo Comite
https://orcid.org/0000-0002-9801-9601
Giustino Fortunato University, Italy

ABSTRACT

The paper examines the adoption of Evidence-Based Management (EBM) as a fundamental model in healthcare management, emphasising evidence-based principles to address organisational strengths and weaknesses. EBM enables managers to navigate complex healthcare systems by systematically observing phenomena, formulating hypotheses and collecting data. It promotes effective multidisciplinary collaboration through mutual trust, psychological safety, clear objectives and meaningful work. By promoting social capital, organisational learning and collaborative leadership, EBM addresses systemic challenges, improves the quality of decision-making and aligns with sustainability principles, ensuring a dynamic and ethical response to the demands of the healthcare sector.

DOI: 10.4018/979-8-3693-2230-7.ch010

THE HEALTH COMPANY IN ITALY

The public health institution is structured through a set of organizational processes that facilitate the adoption of strategic and operational decisions aimed at optimizing productivity. The interconnection between corporate vision and operational effectiveness is essential, being closely linked to the development of certain mechanisms such as quality management systems, information systems, performance evaluation systems, planning systems, management control and accounting systems.

These instruments play a fundamental role in the functioning of health care companies and take the form of:

- Tools that enhance corporate leadership roles, stimulate motivation and promote active management in governance functions. For example, district commissioning budgets not only define the role of the professionals involved but also guide the strategic orientation and definition of specific directives (Funari et al., 2019).
- Vectors that catalyze cultural change within the organization, introducing innovative practices that replace traditional ones (Lai & Gomes, 2018), promoting a substantial renewal of operational methodologies (Di Cagno et al., 2019). For example, the integration of elements such as the ability to promote collegial decision-making in the evaluation process facilitated the creation of new values, consequently stimulating the emergence of an organizational culture inclined towards participation.

These essential factors of the corporatization process function as instruments through which operational processes not only replace old practices but also shift the focus of organizations from a predominantly political influence to one based on sound management principles (Vicarelli, 2004). Therefore, the main functions, operational mechanisms and techniques used to give body and substance to the corporate dimension in the public health sector are of fundamental importance.

The term 'healthcare enterprise' refers to the complex array of resources, technologies, services and professionals that is oriented towards the achievement of objectives aimed at public health. These objectives facilitate the delivery of health care, playing an important role in defining the mission and vision of such entities (League, 2013). Healthcare organizations are committed to the protection of collective health and pursue objectives of health promotion, disease prevention and, more generally, improvement of the quality of life.

The prevailing organizational culture in health care companies places the importance of human health at the center (Borgonovi, 2004). The operators of these institutions, both managers and staff, are dedicated to satisfying the needs of patients and rewarding their achievements. Within these organizations, the concept of excellence translates into a continuous effort to exceed expectations through high standards of work, demonstrating that the work performed in a healthcare context is extremely varied and complex.

Healthcare facilities are characterized by a highly variable and complex working environment (Burns et al., 2012). This variety and complexity results from the interaction between different organizational functions reflected in both a hierarchical and sectoral structure. Operations within healthcare facilities require management that effectively harmonizes all areas of activity, from clinical practice to logistics, in order to efficiently respond to different operational and clinical needs (Del Gesso, 2014).

A historical excursus is necessary to fully understand the task of public enterprises today. According to early theories in the field of economic and business doctrine, public enterprises had the task of satisfying certain basic needs of citizens, a responsibility that could not be transferred to private entities (D'Amico, 2009). Initially, enterprises were considered private productive entities exempt from entrepreneurial risk. However, the legal conception of public enterprises has evolved to require specific requirements, both subjective and objective, which not only imply managerial autonomy and durability of the institution, but also responsibility towards the entire community (Onesti & Angiola, 2009).

Social and economic changes have raised doubts about the validity of traditional management principles, affecting the prerogatives and role of citizens and institutions. In this context, citizens are no longer seen as mere passive recipients of administrative decisions, but as active participants in shaping them and analyzing their results.

In more recent years, the progressive decline in the availability of public goods and services and the persistent reduction in economic resources, aggravated by the various economic crises, have directed public management towards an increasingly stringent use of corporate-derived principles, methods and tools for impact assessment and collective improvement.

In this perspective, reforms do not only pursue efficiency and management effectiveness but also aim to increase the country's competitiveness. The focus has therefore shifted not only to strengthening performance, in terms of efficiency and cost-effectiveness, but also to broadening the impetus given to national competitiveness (Lega, 2023).

Recently, numerous studies have focused their attention on the public sector, in particular examining auditing as an essential tool for governance, planning and control, cost accounting, financial capacity and investment management, and information systems. These analyses lay the foundation for the design of strategic interventions to strengthen the structure and efficiency of the public sector.

In the context of progressive outsourcing and deregulation of the public sector, outlined by the concept of New Public Management (NPM) (Hood, 1991), later followed by Public Governance, significant transformations have occurred. The NPM paradigm induced significant changes in the dynamics of corporate management, planning, programming, control and decision-making processes, overcoming the inefficiencies generated by a bureaucratic model centered on compliance with rigid procedures. Thus, there has been a shift from procedure-oriented administration to administration focused on results. At the same time, privatization reforms, as suggested by Hood (1991), have emphasized the importance of professional management, the use of performance evaluation tools and an increased focus on results. This led to the integration of operational units within the administrations themselves and the adoption of a managerial approach typical of business, which cannot be reduced to mere bureaucracy.

These changes, consistent with some mega-trends identified in the specialist literature, are also believed to be related to the quality and quasi-privatization of public services, with a renewed interest in the concept of 'subsidiarity' in their provision. In addition, a significant development of automation, particularly of information and communication technologies (ICTs), has been observed to influence both the production and distribution of public services.

There is also evidence of an increase in internalization programs focusing on general public management issues. Following subsequent empirical analyses, Jones and Mussari (2000) redefined NPM using a model based on the five 'Rs', outlining a more structured approach to public management and its regulatory and operational evolution:

- Reorganization: involves the elimination of non-essential components within the organization that do not contribute to the value creation of the services offered.
- Reconfiguration: suggests the modification of activities, favoring the adoption of innovative rather than marginal solutions, designing processes from scratch to increase the satisfaction and quality of services provided.
- Renewal: involves the development of new or renewed methodologies for service delivery.
- Harmonization: involves aligning the organizational structure with the strategy to achieve stability objectives.
- Reconsideration: accelerates analysis and feedback processes to achieve quick adjustments and solutions.

New Public Management (NPM) thus integrates the principles of business management in the public sector, with the aim of developing organizational processes that are more aligned with current changes, market needs and stakeholder expectations. A crucial role is played by management systems, which, being linked to the NPM reforms, include:

- Quality management systems, e.g. Total Quality Management and quality certifications (ISO 9000);
- Personnel management systems, such as the implementation of performance-based pay systems and mechanisms for recruitment and career progression;
- Planning and control systems, such as the introduction of budgeting or public policy impact assessment practices (Borgonovi et al., 2013)
- The adoption of these management processes and logics has emerged as a necessity to ensure the long-term sustainability of the public sector, facilitated by the decentralization of power and greater management autonomy.

The following chapter will be devoted exclusively to an in-depth discussion of Evidence-Based Management (EBM) within public health organizations, an approach that emphasizes the importance of basing management decisions on hard data and scientific evidence. This discussion is essential in the context of New Public Management (NPM), which has introduced a set of business principles into the public sector aimed at optimizing performance, increasing efficiency and improving the quality of services provided.

Understanding the NPM is crucial to understanding the importance and urgency of adopting an evidence-based approach. Indeed, the NPM emphasized the need for more strategic and results-oriented management in public institutions, thus paving the way for the implementation of EBM. The adoption of evidence-based strategies and decisions not only corresponds to the ideals of transparency and accountability promoted by the NPM, but is also a direct extension of them, aiming at a more informed and methodologically rigorous management.

The chapter aims to delve into the key components of the public health institution, accessing advanced concepts that guide strategies and reveal the importance of Evidence-Based Management and strategic management.

HIGH-QUALITY SERVICES IN THE HEALTH SECTOR

Tackling the analysis of the theme of excellence in the health care business entails embarking on a path not without obstacles. Many are the critical elements that emerge under different profiles: considerations relating to the protection of the right to health and issues concerning the identification of corporate and managerial elements bearers of excellence (Borgonovi, 2021). An in-depth reflection on excellence in healthcare organizations can therefore represent a significant contribution to the construction of structured pathways that guarantee high quality performance.

The decisive contribution to the definition of excellence can be found in the scientific literature and was made by Donabedian in his study 'Donabedian model' (Donabedian, 1985).

The author divides the concept into three main aspects:

- The general structure, which refers to the organizational configuration of the entity.
- The activities performed for patient care, essentially related to the quality of the service provided.
- The results obtained regarding the consequences of the treatment on the patient's health (Castriota et al., 2023).

From the results one can deduce the degree of patient satisfaction, it is crucial to assess whether the care provided was effective in mitigating or eliminating risk factors or, on the contrary, contributed to undesirable effects. It is therefore essential to identify the elements within the organization that relate directly to excellence, such as good management practices, effective clinical processes and procedures that aim to optimize patient service. This implies not only the valorization of experience, but also the ability to adapt models and best practices in order to continuously excel, representing the real challenge for a healthcare organization of excellence.

Initially, attention to the peculiarities of the concept of 'good health' and its relevance within the socio-economic landscape of each nation emphasizes the importance of continuous quality improvement within the corporate environment (Barnato et al., 2017). The goal of continuous quality improvement within the corporate environment should be the primary objective of every healthcare company.

According to the Donabedian model, there are two basic pillars: the first refers to the organizational structure, understood as continuous investment in staff training to raise the level of performance. The second concerns the technical nature, which includes the procedures and execution of clinical disciplines, seen as a set of practices necessary to achieve operational excellence. This macro-area approach facilitates the identification of several determining factors in evaluating the performance of a healthcare organization, such as the competence and managerial preparedness of staff, effectiveness, i.e. the ability to rapidly achieve high quality results, and timeliness in activating resources in critical situations, maximizing the benefits of preventive interventions. A personalized service that ensures respect and effectively responds to individual needs is fundamental to creating business dynamics that consistently raise the standard of healthcare (Ferretti et al., 2014).

In this context, 'Clinical Governance' acquires particular importance, as illustrated in the study 'A First Class Service: Quality in the new NHS'.[1] which emphasizes the need to combine the quality of healthcare services with continuous performance improvement, thus highlighting the critical importance of these practices in the context of corporate quality assessment. Primary importance is attached to the continuous improvement of performance, whereby scientific information on the effectiveness of interventions becomes the core of the evaluation of decisions made by the business administration. However, this construction clashes with the need to create a healthcare environment in which the traditional clinical approach gives way to management and organizational requirements, thus promoting an in-depth reading of the performance achieved in the light of multidisciplinarity. In this scenario, the Evidence-Based Management approach, discussed in the next section, emerges as a potential solution.

EVIDENCE-BASED MANAGEMENT

Evidence-based management is a business management model that adopts scientific evidence-based criteria applied to management, which is particularly relevant in healthcare organizations. In the current medical context, this approach is increasingly used to guide and support professionals in implementing best practices. The concept of evidence-based, in the broadest sense, is based on the systematic observation of a phenomenon, the formulation of several operational hypotheses and the collection of data and information useful to confirm or not the initial hypothesis (Kovner et. al, 2000). It is undisputed that, just as it is essential for physicians to take scientific evidence into account when treating patients, it is likewise indispensable for strategic business decisions to be based on clear evidence of the effectiveness of the choices made in the organizational context (Pfeffer & Sutton, 2006).

Managers do not always assess the strengths and weaknesses of their companies in a structured and analytical manner; they rarely use scientifically based organizational analysis tools (Rundall, 2007). It is at this point that the application of Evidence-Based Management comes into action, i.e. the model that seeks to integrate the principles of evidence-based medicine into the management of healthcare companies. This model constitutes a guide to adopt a management style based on objective and measurable evidence, i.e. on incontrovertible data and information.

In essence, the decision-making process of managers (Lai et al., 2015) of a healthcare company can be based on:

- Results derived from scientific research (Francesconi, 2007).

- Demonstration of the benefits obtained through the application of evidence-based interventions (Ferrari, 2014).
- Comparison with the results of similar healthcare companies in different contexts (Ballini, 2014).

The adoption of scientifically based organizational interventions has the advantage, on the one hand, of increasing the likelihood of success and, on the other hand, of reducing the risk of failure by preventing inadequately thought-out interventions from having negative effects on the entire company (Lega & Vendramini, 2008).

Clinical Governance is a useful tool in this area. It represents a managerial approach that enhances the joint work between healthcare and management professionals (Brennan & Flynn, 2013), promoting the improvement of the business organization.

The approach adopted goes beyond the mere improvement of operational efficiency, extending attention to the overall effectiveness of corporate performance. It is therefore a strategy that imposes an obligation on public health institutions to pursue continuous improvement in the quality of the services offered and to ensure, through regular monitoring, that high standards of care are maintained. This process encourages the development of an environment that supports the dissemination of professional excellence. It is important to emphasize that the effectiveness of Clinical Governance is closely influenced by its ability to penetrate all levels of the healthcare organization, with particular emphasis on the evaluation of structures, organizational processes, funding mechanisms, performance and the ongoing training of staff, both clinical and administrative.

Clinical Governance, therefore, is proposed as a strategic guide for healthcare organizations, orienting them towards continuous improvement. In particular, it takes on the task of promoting a proactive role in the definition of quality standards, which can serve as clear and achievable objectives for professionals.

There are two main objectives:

(1) A holistic management of healthcare companies, integrating quality of care with greater efficiency in terms of economic sustainability;
(2) Reduce the operational difference between clinical professionals and management.

In the context of clinical risk management, the process begins with the analysis of errors or events that have occurred in specific departments, in order to identify systemic solutions that improve business processes. This is pursued by ensuring greater safety and promoting effective communication to external stakeholders.

This approach aims to develop more efficient healthcare policies and to increase the resilience and operational capacity of healthcare organizations. Organizations implementing such systems have reported, in the medium to long term, significant improvements in internal processes and business operations, as well as showing significant managerial results (Freedman, 2002).

The innovation implemented in managerial processes is crucial for the future prospects of healthcare companies that, through such strategies, can address and mitigate manifestations of organizational immobility and rigidity.

EVIDENCE-BASED STRATEGIC MANAGEMENT IN HEALTHCARE COMPANIES

The adoption of a strategic management approach in healthcare companies manifests itself in the implementation of performance leadership, which results directly from positive interactions between actors inside and outside the organization. To understand the scientific debate on this topic, the authors conducted a systematic literature review. The work adopts an interdisciplinary approach based on the literature review. The database used was Scopus, with an initial search based on the keywords Evidence-Based Management and Collaborative Models. However, this search did not return any direct results. To explore the topic further, a broader search limited to the areas of Business, Management and Accounting and Economics, Econometrics and Finance was then conducted, using only the keyword Evidence-Based Management. The selection is summarized within the PRISMA.

All 33 articles were analyzed manually, and from each of them a clear link between Evidence-Based Management and effective and strategic collaboration between employees and other organizational actors emerges. Although the literature does not explicitly treat the topic as a stand-alone, it is frequently considered as a key element within broader discussions on evidence-based management. This therefore highlights a significant gap: the topic of collaboration within evidence-based management is not addressed as a stand-alone phenomenon, but rather integrated into other study contexts. Although it is recognized as a key element within evidence-based management, it is not the subject of an independent systematic analysis, but is treated as a cross-cutting aspect within other organizational and strategic dynamics. However, studies such as Rangachari's (2020) show that collaboration and knowledge sharing between professionals are central aspects in the successful implementation of evidence-based practices. In particular, the model of knowledge-sharing networks in complex professional systems highlights how EBM is not only a data-driven decision-making approach, but a collective process that requires continuous interactions between stakeholders, managers and healthcare professionals. These findings underline the importance of greater theoretical and applicative attention to the collaborative dimension of EBM, so that it is recognized as an area of study in its own right and not just a secondary aspect of general organizational dynamics.

Managers in the healthcare sector, operating in a complex environment, must possess and utilize all the necessary resources to achieve strategic corporate objectives. Consequently, effective collaboration with all stakeholders is very important for the achievement of these goals (Marks, 2020). Indeed, the collaborative approach is crucial in strategic decision-making, as it allows for the collection of different forms of evidence, including data from scientific literature, practical experience and stakeholder involvement (Del Grosso & Van Roey, 2024).

The modern managerial paradigm within healthcare companies, which emerged in the second half of the last century, began to receive managerial notions from business schools, integrating this knowledge with other disciplines (Salvioni, 2007). This approach led to the emergence of the concept of 'strategic management'. During the evolution of strategic management, various business theories have been adopted that have profoundly influenced organization and business progress, as can be seen from the extensive literature on the subject. Only organizations that are able to adapt to change are destined to survive and grow in every respect (Bianchi Martini, 2013).

This underlines the importance of adopting a dynamic and future-oriented strategic management to drive the company towards success through well-structured strategic planning. To this end, the use of HR Analytics proves crucial in gathering data on organizational health and employee well-being, contributing to an evidence-based approach to human resource management and business performance improvement (Lathabhavan, 2024).

It is therefore useful to briefly recall the strategic planning process. This process essentially consists of five main stages (Prenestini, 2012):

1. Identification of organizational purposes.
2. Preliminary assessment and drafting of SMART (Specific, Measurable, Achievable, Relevant, Temporary) objectives.
3. Formulation of the organization's internal strategies.
4. Definition of general tactics.
5. Completion of the strategic plan.

Leadership and strategic management within healthcare structures play an essential role in outlining the future of the organization, defining the objectives to be achieved, formulating implementation strategies, establishing operational methodologies and, finally, determining how resources and rewards are allocated. In this context, the adoption of EBMgt+, which introduces a more rigorous analysis of available data and evidence, enables managers to make more informed and data-driven decisions (Weber et al., 2024).

Harrison and Thompson (2014), exploring the topic of strategic management in healthcare facilities, argue that in order to make informed decisions, it is essential to have access to accurate information and to use strategic intelligence. Strategic intelligence enables evidence-based decision-making by collecting and analyzing data about the organization, leadership, available resources and key stakeholders, as well as the external context in which the healthcare company operates. This methodology aligns with the concept of Evidence-Based Management, which emphasizes the use of reliable information to reduce uncertainty in decisions and improve operational efficiency (Criado-Perez et al., 2024).

A holistic approach to strategic planning includes:

- The analysis of the organization, its stakeholders and the external context.
- The collection and effective communication of the strategic information needed to define the key elements for business performance.
- The evaluation of strategic alternatives to arrive at the definition and implementation of coordinated actions.
- The formulation of implementation plans.

It is essential that the planning process is long-term oriented and aimed at ensuring that all necessary elements are identified and properly evaluated. The adoption of a collaborative model, in which relevant information is shared among all parties involved, promotes more effective decision-making and greater organizational transparency (Kelstrup, 2024).

Strategic thinking in healthcare organizations requires that relevant information is shared through a system that ensures its complete availability. In this way, the public health organization can make the most of all available opportunities and formulate innovative strategies that contribute to the realization of its primary objectives. The integration of EBM and collaborative models ensures a structured approach to resource management, allowing quantitative and qualitative data to be combined to make more informed and targeted decisions (Bosquillon et al., 2024).

These aspects, combined with a broader and more diverse testimonial evidence, make it possible to build a more robust health management, based on reliable data and effective interaction between the parties involved in the decision-making process (Del Grosso & Van Roey, 2024).

STRATEGIC MANAGEMENT

The strategic direction of healthcare companies can be defined as the mission and vision of the organization towards which it is directed in order to achieve predefined goals (Harrison, 2013). Healthcare structures possess their own organizational identity, formed by both internal and external elements, this orientation is defined and implemented through defined instruments, in fact the strategic management of a public healthcare organization uses fundamental tools such as mission statements, value statements and codes of ethics to clearly define its objectives. However, it is crucial to distinguish between the formal documentation of these policies and their actual implementation in practice. A strategic guide that is effectively integrated into planning processes provides employees and managers with precise indications for informed decisions and proactive actions, thus helping to consolidate the trustworthiness and reputation of the institution in its operational context.

The involvement of internal and external stakeholders is crucial to ensure that the adopted strategy is effectively accepted and sustained over time, thereby increasing the likelihood of long-term success of the strategic direction set (Coronella et al., 2016).

The three fundamental areas that contribute to the definition of corporate strategy include resources, stakeholders, and external forces, all of which are crucial in influencing the strategic direction of a healthcare organization. These components, when coordinated effectively, can clearly define and utilize the organization's mission and vision, which are essential for appropriately assessing opportunities and making informed decisions. In addition to guiding internally, these concepts also facilitate communication with the users of healthcare services.

STRATEGIC BUSINESS ANALYSIS

Within the framework of strategic business analysis, taking into account the previously mentioned elements, assessments can be conducted that enable healthcare companies to make accurate and targeted decisions, enhancing innovation and business transformation (Coda et al., 2017). Through an organizational analysis that examines direction, purpose, resources and key stakeholders, companies can make the best use of available resources to generate added value for the organization (Cassano, 2013). In particular, the strategic use of resources, such as the implementation of computerized electronic health record systems, can significantly improve business operations. The effective management and exploitation of resources contributes not only to the generation of value, but also to the maximum utilization of systemic capabilities, making it essential to identify resources that can offer lasting competitive advantages (Ciambotti, 2015).

Consequently, it is very important to identify the resources that can form the basis for a sustainable competitive advantage in order to maximize opportunities and counter threats from the external environment. Many organizations have structured resources or highly specialized health departments (Comite, 2022); in these cases we speak of competitive parity, where no entity loses a clear advantage. Conversely, if an organization possesses a unique and particularly relevant resource, this becomes an essential source of competitive advantage.

In the specific context of a healthcare company, corporate strategy should be based not only on what the organization is able to achieve better than its competitors, but also on the ability to harness and exploit specific resources to build a future competitive advantage.

Ultimately, it can be argued that strategic analysis is crucial to support leadership and management in clearly identifying how corporate actions can be effectively directed to improve competitiveness. This process can positively influence the value creation system or limit its potential, secondly when resources are managed to maximize competitive advantage (Salvatore, 2022).

CONCLUSIONS AND FUTURE PROSPECTS

It is evident, in light of the literature analyzed and the operational dynamics within healthcare organizations, that they are constantly challenged to operate in an environment characterized by increasing complexity and dynamism. In this context, the need for continuous performance improvement emerges as an inescapable imperative. The adoption of EBM is therefore a fundamental strategy that integrates the most effective practices and accumulated scientific evidence into daily management, resulting in more informed decisions. However, as highlighted in the literature, the effectiveness of EBM cannot be separated from an organizational model that favors collaboration between the various actors involved, allowing transparent access to information and reducing the risks of data distortion for strategic purposes (Ganz, 2020).

Looking ahead, it is essential that healthcare institutions deepen the integration of EBM into their management systems. This implies not only a more extensive use of data and research to guide clinical and administrative decisions, but also an ongoing investment in staff training on these principles. It is also crucial to foster an organizational culture that promotes critical thinking and continuous learning, which are decisive factors for preserving organizational agility and adapting effectively to the new challenges of the healthcare sector (Rangachari, 2020). In this context, HR Analytics emerge as a crucial element to foster the adoption of EBM and improve the performance of healthcare organizations. According to McCartney and Fu (2021), access to advanced HR analytics technologies enables the collection of strategic data that, when used correctly, facilitate evidence-based decision-making and directly improve organizational performance. This is particularly relevant in the healthcare sector, where HR analytics can be used to monitor staff satisfaction, prevent burnout and optimize the allocation of human resources. The literature points out that the success of EBM depends not only on the availability of data, but also on the ability to share them effectively and without internal barriers between the different decision-making levels. The collaborative approach is therefore essential to prevent actors involved, such as managers or healthcare professionals, from altering or selecting data in order to protect their own interests, as demonstrated by Ganz's (2020) research on the use of organizational experiments.

Concrete examples confirm the benefits of such collaboration. Kovner et al. (2000) report that multidisciplinary teams composed of clinicians, administrators and data analysts worked together to analyze hospital readmission data and redesign discharge planning protocols, resulting in a measurable reduction in avoidable readmissions. Similarly, McCartney and Fu (2021) describe how the joint implementation of HR analytics involving both nursing staff and medical leadership led to better workforce planning, reduced staff turnover, and enhanced patient care. Moreover, the integration of advanced technologies such as artificial intelligence and big data analysis, in particular telemedicine, represents a significant opportunity to further refine EBM. These technological advances improve the ability of healthcare organizations to anticipate outcomes and optimize the allocation of resources by facilitating more precise and evidence-based management. However, this technological progress must be balanced with rigorous ethical evaluation and the implementation of policies that ensure the protection of patient privacy and equitable access to care.

The implementation of EBM goes beyond the use of information and research to guide clinical and management decisions: it requires a continuous investment in staff training and the dissemination of an organizational culture based on collaboration, critical thinking and continuous learning. These elements are essential to preserve the flexibility of healthcare organizations and their ability to adapt to the challenges of the field. Healthcare companies that adopt a strategic approach based on EBM, supported by a collaborative model and the use of HR Analytics, are better prepared to manage uncertainty and ensure high quality services, while responsibly responding to the needs of the population. This model not only provides effective operational guidance, but also outlines a sustainable path for the evolution of the healthcare sector. However, the literature review revealed a significant gap; that is the link between EBM and collaborative models is not treated as a central discussion, but rather as an integrated element in other contexts. This approach is limiting, as collaboration is not only a marginal aspect of EBM, but an indispensable factor for its real effectiveness. Therefore, future studies should focus directly on analyzing the link between EBM and collaborative models, moving beyond the approach that considers it a secondary element. This topic must become an independent object of study, with the aim of developing evidence-based healthcare management models that are truly applicable and sustainable.

REFERENCES

Ballini, L. (2014). *Governance in health systems innovation*. Il Pensiero Scientifico Editore.

Barnato, A. E., Moore, R., Moore, C. G., Kohatsu, N. D., & Sudore, R. L. (2017). Financial incentives to increase advance care planning among medicaid beneficiaries: Lessons learned from two pragmatic randomized trials. *Journal of Pain and Symptom Management, 54*(1), 85–95. DOI: 10.1016/j.jpainsymman.2017.02.016 PMID: 28450218

Bianchi Martini, B. (2013). Corporate development strategies, corporate governance processes and value creation. In *Theories, empirical analyses and experiences in comparison*. Franco Angeli Editore.

Borgonovi, E. (2004). Corporateisation and clinical governance. In *MECOSAN, 49*, 2-6.

Borgonovi, E. (2021). *Gestione per la salute. Scienza, diritti, responsabilità sociale, efficienza*. Franco Angeli.

Borgonovi, E., Fattore, G., & Longo, F. (2013). *Management of public institutions*. Egea.

Bosquillon, C., Cujko, L., Gautel, G., Di Pippo, S., & Vittori, E. (2024). Is the lunar economy solely for the space industry? Opportunities for nonspace companies in lunar infrastructure leveraging technological synergies. *New Space, 12*(3), 174–187. DOI: 10.1089/space.2023.0057

Brennan, N. M., & Flynn, M. A. (2013). Differentiating clinical governance, clinical management and clinical practice. *Clinical Governance, 18*(2), 114–131. DOI: 10.1108/14777271311317909

Burns, L. R., Bradley, E. H., Weiner, B. J., & Shortell, S. (2012). *Shortell and Kaluzny health management: organisation, design and behaviour*. Delmar Cengage Learning.

Cassano, R. (2013). *Accountability and stakeholder relations in public enterprises*. Franco Angeli Editore.

Castriota, S., Delmastro, M., & Tonin, M. (2023). National or local infodemic? The demand for news during the COVID-19 pandemic. *International Journal of Health Economics and Management, 23*(4), 507–536. DOI: 10.1007/s10754-023-09350-3 PMID: 37069418

Ciambotti, M. (2015). *Topics and research in business economics: firms, entrepreneurship, human capital.* Franco Angeli publisher.

Coda, V., Invernizzi, G., & Russo, P. (2017). *Business strategy*. McGraw Hill Education.

Comite, U. (2022). The hospital company in the perspective of process reengineering: between health services and care profiles. In Teliti, E., & Laghi, P. (Eds.), *Process, processes and the technological revolution*. Cedam.

Coronella, S., Risaliti, G., & Verona, R. (2016). Fiscal policy in the doctrine of business economics: critical reflections. In Il governo tra tradizione e innovazione, edited by M. Luciano, R. Lombardi, L. Anselmi. Milan: Franco Angeli editore.

Criado-Perez, C., Jackson, C., Minbashian, A., & Collins, C. G. (2024). Cognitive reflection and decision-making accuracy: Examining their relation and boundary conditions in the context of evidence-based management. *Journal of Business and Psychology*, *39*(1), 249–273. DOI: 10.1007/s10869-023-09883-x

D'Amico, E. (2009). *Evolution of planning and managerial controls in central state administrations*. Wolters Kluwer.

Del Gesso, C. (2014). The systemic view of the public health enterprise. Evolutionary trends of organisation, management and detection in the health protection system. Milan: Franco Angeli editore.

Del Grosso, P., & Van Roey, K. (2024). Diversifying evidence in evidence-based management. *Philosophy of Management*, *23*(4), 439–460. DOI: 10.1007/s40926-024-00318-y

Di Cagno, N., Adamo, S., & Giaccari, F. (2019). The company. Purpose-structure-administration. In *Collana di Studi Aziendali, Serie Studi Istituzionali*. Cacucci publisher.

Donabedian, A. (1985). *The Methods and Findings of Quality Assessment and Monitoring: An Illustrated Analysis*. Health Administration Press.

Ferrari, F. (2014). Evidence-based management. In *Rivista di Management per le professioni sanitarie*. Maggioli Editore.

Francesconi, A. (2007). *Organisational and technological innovation in health care. The role of health technology assessment*. FrancoAngeli Editore.

Freedman, D. B. (2002). Clinical governance: Bringing together management and clinical approaches to quality in the UK. *Clinica Chimica Acta*, *319*(2), 133–141. DOI: 10.1016/S0009-8981(02)00034-7 PMID: 11955490

Funari, A., Lecci, F., & Ricci, A. (2019). Middle management in public health companies: national census and analysis of empowerment and empowerment mechanisms. In Report, O. A. S. I. (Ed.). EGEA.

Ganz, S. C. (2020). Hyperopic search: Organisations learning about managers learning about strategies. *Organization Science*, *31*(4), 821–838. DOI: 10.1287/orsc.2019.1330

Harrison, J. S., & Thompson, S. (2014). *Strategic management of healthcare organisations: A stakeholder management approach.* Business Expert Press.

Hood, C. (1991). A public management for all seasons? *Public Administration*, *69*(1), 3–19. DOI: 10.1111/j.1467-9299.1991.tb00779.x

Jones, L. R., & Mussari, R. (2000). Public management reform in the United States and Italy: Accounting, measurement and finance. *International. Public Management Review*, *1*(1), 56–83.

Kelstrup, J. D. (2024). Understanding the role of practical knowledge in evidence-based welfare reform-a three-stage model. *Humanities & Social Sciences Communications*, *11*(1), 1438. DOI: 10.1057/s41599-024-03937-y

Kovner, A. R., Elton, J. J., & Billings, J. (2000). Evidence-based management. *Frontiers of Health Services Management*, *16*(4), 3–24. DOI: 10.1097/01974520-200004000-00002 PMID: 11183283

Lai, A., & Gomes, D. (2018). Accounting in different cultures and from different perspectives. In *Accounting and business culture*. Franco Angeli publisher.

Lai, A., Lionzo, A., Stacchezzini, F., & Rossignoli, F. (2015). *From enterprise to network. Governance profiles and business models*. FrancoAngeli Editore.

Lathabhavan, R. (2024). Mental well-being through HR analytics: Investigating an employee supportive framework. *Personnel Review*, *53*(5), 1110–1128. DOI: 10.1108/PR-11-2022-0836

League, F. (2013). *Healthcare management: Essential frameworks and recent developments in healthcare and business*. EGEA.

Lega, F. (2023). *Economia e management sanitario. Settore, sistema, aziende, protagonisti* (3rd ed.). EGEA.

Lega, F., & Vendramini, E. (2008). Budgeting and performance management in the Italian National Health Service (NHS): Assessment and constructive criticism. *Journal of Health Organization and Management*, *22*(1), 11–22. DOI: 10.1108/14777260810862371 PMID: 18488516

Marks, L. (2020). From crisis to sustainable development: The role of measurement and control systems. *Management Control*, *3*, 5–16.

McCartney, S., & Fu, N. (2021). Bridging the gap: Why, how and when human resource analysis can impact organisational performance. *Management Decision*, *60*(13), 25–47. DOI: 10.1108/MD-12-2020-1581

Onesti, T., & Angiola, N. (2009). *Il controllo strategico nelle amministrazioni pubbliche*. Franco Angeli.

Pfeffer, J., & Sutton, R. (2006). *Hard facts, dangerous half-truths and total nonsense: Making money from evidence-based management*. Harvard Business Press.

Prenestini, A. (2012). The formation of strategies in public health companies. In *Strategia e performance management nelle Aziende pubbliche, 19.33*. EGEA.

Rangachari, P. (2020). Understanding the implementation of evidence-based practice (EBP) in HCOS through the lens of organisational theory. *Health Leadership Journal*, *12*, 35–48. PMID: 32607042

Rundall, T. G. (2007). Evidence-based management. *Hospitals & Health Networks*, *81*(11), 72. PMID: 18175596

Salvatore, F. P. (2022). *Management and performance in healthcare: economic and business aspects of healthcare companies*. Giuffrè Francesco Lefebvre.

Salvioni, D. (2007). Corporate governance, control and transparency. Milan: Franco Angeli editore.

Vicarelli, G. (2004). Corporateisation and management in the evolution of the Italian health system. In Health and society. Milan: Franco Angeli editore.

Weber, E., Wyverkens, A., & Leuridan, B. (2024). Rethinking evidence-based management. *Philosophy of Management*, *23*(1), 59–84. DOI: 10.1007/s40926-023-00236-5

ENDNOTE

1 Department of health, A first class service: quality in the new NHS, in The National Archives, 1998.

Chapter 11
Beyond Systems: Rethinking Integrated Healthcare With Team-Based Approaches, AI, and Dynamic Capabilities

Antonio Pesqueira
https://orcid.org/0000-0003-1530-6451
ISCTE-IUL, Portugal

Dora Almeida
https://orcid.org/0009-0009-1891-2861
Dynamic Capabilities Operational Progressive Institute, Switzerland

Noah Barr
https://orcid.org/0009-0008-1777-2599
DCOPI, Switzerland

ABSTRACT

The rapid advancement of Artificial Intelligence (AI) and the increasing complexity of healthcare systems necessitate a shift from system-centric models to dynamic, team-based approaches for integrated healthcare. This chapter introduces a conceptual and theoretical framework that merges AI capabilities, team-based healthcare models, and dynamic capabilities to create sustainable, patient-centered healthcare systems. It explores the role of AI in enhancing collaboration, decision-making, and operational efficiency while addressing the challenges of siloed healthcare practices.

DOI: 10.4018/979-8-3693-2230-7.ch011

INTRODUCTION

The complexities of modern healthcare systems demand a shift from traditional, siloed structures to more integrated, dynamic approaches capable of addressing multifaceted challenges. Rapid advancements in technology, particularly in Artificial Intelligence (AI), present transformative opportunities for healthcare delivery. However, the full potential of these technologies remains untapped due to entrenched systemic inefficiencies, lack of coordination among healthcare providers, and the absence of frameworks that promote adaptability and sustainability. This chapter proposes reimagining healthcare systems by integrating team-based approaches, AI, and dynamic capabilities to foster a patient-centered, sustainable future (Ball, 2021).

Team-based approaches promote shared accountability, diverse expertise, and improved communication—all critical for addressing the increasing complexity of patient needs. By fostering a culture of collaboration, these models help eliminate silos, reduce redundancies, and enhance the overall efficiency of healthcare delivery. These models inherently align with the integration of AI, which can catalyze enhancing coordination, operational efficiency, and decision-making. AI-driven decision support tools can provide clinicians with evidence-based recommendations, reducing diagnostic errors and improving treatment outcomes (Dillard-Wright, Shields-Haas, 2021). Additionally, AI can optimize resource allocation, ensuring that healthcare organizations make the most efficient use of their limited resources. However, integrating AI into healthcare systems is not without challenges, including ethical concerns, data privacy, and the need for interoperability. The ethical considerations surrounding algorithmic biases, transparency, and accountability must be addressed to ensure equitable access to AI-driven solutions. Despite these hurdles, AI has the potential to bridge gaps in healthcare delivery by facilitating seamless communication, reducing cognitive overload, and empowering healthcare teams with data-driven insights. Dynamic capabilities enable healthcare organizations to anticipate emerging trends, mobilize resources effectively, and reconfigure structures to remain adaptable in a rapidly evolving environment. Sensing involves identifying opportunities and threats in the healthcare landscape, such as advancements in AI technologies or shifts in patient demographics. Seizing entails capitalizing on these opportunities by adopting innovative tools and processes, such as AI-powered platforms for care coordination. Transforming refers to the ability to realign organizational structures and workflows to integrate new technologies and practices seamlessly. These capabilities are essential for leveraging AI to its fullest potential while ensuring that healthcare systems remain resilient and responsive to external and internal challenges. By embedding dynamic capabilities into their operational strategies, healthcare organizations can foster a culture of continuous improvement and innovation (Ebrahimi & Bridgelall, 2021).

This chapter introduces a conceptual framework that integrates team-based healthcare, AI, and dynamic capabilities to address systemic inefficiencies and promote sustainability. By aligning interdisciplinary collaboration with cutting-edge technology and adaptive organizational strategies, the proposed framework aims to create a roadmap for integrated healthcare systems that are both innovative and patient-centered. This framework emphasizes the importance of a holistic approach to healthcare delivery, where technology and human expertise are harmoniously blended to achieve optimal outcomes. In doing so, it seeks to address critical gaps in current healthcare delivery while paving the way for a more equitable and sustainable future.

BACKGROUND

Team-Based Healthcare Models: Foundations and Evolution

The complexities of healthcare delivery have led to an increasing recognition of the limitations inherent in traditional, siloed models of care. These isolated systems often struggle to meet the demands of modern healthcare, characterized by fragmented services, inefficiencies, and an inability to address the multifaceted needs of patients. In response, team-based healthcare has emerged as a transformative approach, emphasizing collaboration, shared accountability, and integration. By uniting diverse expertise within cohesive teams, this model aims to enhance healthcare systems' quality, efficiency, and sustainability (Jacob et al., 2022). The origins of team-based healthcare can be traced to the early twentieth century when multidisciplinary approaches were employed to address pressing public health crises. For instance, during tuberculosis outbreaks, the integration of medical, nursing, and public health expertise demonstrated the effectiveness of collaborative efforts in improving patient outcomes. The theoretical underpinnings of team-based healthcare are deeply rooted in interprofessional collaboration and systems theory. Interprofessional collaboration emphasizes the integration of diverse professional perspectives to achieve comprehensive and patient-centered care (ElBaih, 2023).

One of the most significant advantages of team-based healthcare is its ability to improve patient outcomes. By fostering collaboration among healthcare providers, teams can develop more comprehensive care plans that address the multifaceted needs of patients. Research has shown that team-based models are particularly effective in managing chronic conditions, reducing hospital readmissions, and enhancing patient satisfaction. Integrating diverse expertise allows for a more nuanced understanding of patient needs, ensuring that care is personalized and evidence-based. This approach not only improves clinical outcomes but also strengthens the patient-provider relationship, fostering trust and engagement (Javaid et al., 2023).

In addition to improving patient outcomes, team-based healthcare enhances operational efficiency. Traditional healthcare models often suffer from redundancies and fragmented workflows, leading to delays and resource wastage. Team-based approaches streamline these processes by promoting coordination and information sharing among providers. For example, care coordination teams can ensure that all providers have access to the same patient information, reducing the likelihood of duplicate tests or conflicting treatments. This optimization of resources is particularly crucial in resource-constrained settings, where efficiency can significantly impact the quality and accessibility of care. Healthcare providers working within team-based models also report higher levels of job satisfaction. The collaborative nature of these models fosters a sense of collective purpose and shared responsibility, which can alleviate the stress and burnout often associated with traditional healthcare environments. Improved communication and mutual support among team members contribute to a more positive work environment, enhancing provider well-being and, by extension, the quality of care delivered to patients (Kouba et al., 2023).

Despite its numerous advantages, implementing team-based healthcare is not without challenges. Cultural barriers, such as entrenched professional hierarchies and resistance to change, can impede the adoption of collaborative practices. Overcoming these barriers requires a cultural shift that values teamwork and interdisciplinary cooperation. This shift must be supported by training programs that equip healthcare providers with the skills needed to work effectively in team-based settings (Masih, 2022). Unfortunately, many healthcare professionals receive limited training in teamwork and communication, creating a gap that must be addressed through interprofessional education initiatives. Resource constraints also pose significant challenges to the implementation of team-based healthcare. Developing and sustaining interdisciplinary teams often requires additional time, personnel, and technology, which may be difficult to secure in underfunded or resource-limited settings. These constraints underscore the importance of strategic planning and investment to ensure the successful integration of team-based models into healthcare systems. Policymakers and administrators must prioritize the allocation of resources to support these initiatives, recognizing their potential to transform healthcare delivery (Vallentin et al., 2023).

The Patient-Centered Medical Home (PCMH) provides a compelling example of the principles of team-based healthcare in practice. Originating in the United States, the PCMH model emphasizes coordinated, patient-centered care delivered by interdisciplinary teams. These teams, which often include primary care physicians, nurses, social workers, and specialists, work collaboratively to develop comprehensive care plans tailored to the unique needs of each patient. Enhanced communication is facilitated by electronic health records and regular team meetings, ensuring that all providers are aligned in their approach to care. Studies have demonstrated that the PCMH model improves health outcomes, reduces healthcare costs, and increases patient satisfaction, highlighting its potential as a scalable and effective approach to team-based care (Wamba et al., 2023). Looking ahead, the future of team-based healthcare lies in its integration with emerging technologies and adaptive organizational frameworks. AI offers significant opportunities to enhance collaboration and decision-making within healthcare teams. AI-powered tools can provide real-time insights and recommendations, enabling teams to respond more effectively to patient needs. Similarly, the integration of dynamic capabilities into team-based models can enhance their adaptability and resilience, allowing healthcare organizations to navigate changing circumstances and emerging challenges (Vlasta, 2023).

Team-based healthcare also has a critical role to play in addressing global health challenges. As populations age and the prevalence of chronic diseases increases, the demand for coordinated and patient-centered care will continue to grow. Collaborative models can be scaled to meet these demands, ensuring that healthcare systems remain responsive and sustainable. Furthermore, team-based approaches can contribute to global health equity by promoting the efficient use of resources and improving access to quality care in underserved communities (Bhattamisraet al.,2023). Team-based healthcare represents a paradigm shift in the delivery of care, offering a holistic and collaborative approach to addressing the complexities of modern healthcare systems. By drawing on the principles of interprofessional collaboration and systems theory, these models enhance patient outcomes, improve efficiency, and foster a culture of shared accountability. However, their successful implementation requires overcoming cultural, educational, and resource-related challenges. As healthcare systems continue to evolve, the integration of team-based approaches with emerging technologies and adaptive frameworks will be essential for creating sustainable, patient-centered solutions that meet the needs of diverse populations (Yulianti & Sulistyawati, 2021).

The Role of Artificial Intelligence in Integrated Healthcare

AI has emerged as a transformative force in healthcare, redefining how systems operate, decisions are made, and care is delivered. As the complexity of modern healthcare grows beyond the capacities of traditional methods, AI offers unparalleled opportunities to enhance precision, efficiency, and patient outcomes. This section explores the evolution of AI in healthcare, emphasizing its theoretical underpinnings, practical applications, and the ethical challenges it faces. By highlighting AI's role in creating sustainable and adaptive healthcare systems, this analysis presents a comprehensive view of its transformative potential. In integrated healthcare systems,

AI has found applications across both clinical and operational domains. Predictive analytics exemplifies its ability to transform population health management. By analyzing historical and real-time data, AI systems can identify at-risk populations, predict disease outbreaks, and optimize care pathways. These predictive tools help healthcare providers anticipate patient needs, allocate resources more effectively, and reduce disparities in care by targeting underserved communities. This ability to leverage data for proactive decision-making has made predictive analytics an indispensable component of modern healthcare (Wani et al., 2022).

AI has also revolutionized diagnostic precision. Through its capacity to process medical images, genomic data, and other complex datasets, AI systems have achieved diagnostic accuracy that often surpasses that of human clinicians. For example, algorithms designed to detect conditions such as diabetic retinopathy and breast cancer have demonstrated reliability in accelerating diagnostic processes and minimizing errors. The integration of these tools into clinical workflows empowers healthcare providers with actionable insights, enabling more informed decisions and ultimately improving patient outcomes. Moreover, AI has been pivotal in advancing personalized medicine, where treatment plans are tailored to individual patients based on their genetic, environmental, and lifestyle factors (Patil et al., 2022). Machine learning models analyze multifaceted datasets to identify the most effective interventions for specific patient profiles. In oncology, for instance, AI-driven systems guide the selection of targeted therapies based on the genetic composition of tumors, significantly enhancing the efficacy of treatment. This shift toward personalized medicine underscores AI's role in enabling precision healthcare that caters to the unique needs of each patient. Beyond its clinical contributions, AI has had a profound impact on the operational efficiency of healthcare systems. By automating repetitive tasks and optimizing resource allocation, AI streamlines workflows and reduces administrative burdens. Natural language processing tools, for instance, simplify clinical documentation by transcribing and organizing notes, allowing providers to focus more on patient care. Predictive algorithms further enhance efficiency by managing hospital bed occupancy, staff scheduling, and supply chain logistics. These operational improvements not only lower costs but also ensure that resources are utilized effectively, enhancing the overall quality of healthcare delivery.

Despite its transformative potential, the integration of AI into healthcare presents significant ethical and practical challenges. Data privacy is a critical concern, as the sensitive nature of healthcare information requires compliance with stringent regulations such as the General Data Protection Regulation (GDPR) in Europe and the Health Insurance Portability and Accountability Act (HIPAA) in the United States. While these frameworks protect patient data, they also pose challenges to data sharing and interoperability, which are essential for maximizing the utility of AI systems (Secinaro et al., 2021).

Algorithmic transparency is another pressing issue. Many AI models, particularly those based on deep learning, function as "black boxes," providing little insight into their decision-making processes. This lack of interpretability can erode trust among clinicians and patients, raising concerns about accountability and the validity of AI-generated recommendations (Tariq et al.,2022). To address these concerns, researchers are increasingly focused on explainable AI (XAI), which aims to enhance the transparency of algorithms while maintaining their predictive power. Achieving interpretability is vital to integrating AI seamlessly into clinical workflows and ensuring it complements human expertise. Bias in AI systems further complicates its adoption in healthcare. If training datasets are not representative of diverse populations, the resulting algorithms may perpetuate existing inequalities. For instance, AI models trained predominantly on data from high-income countries may perform poorly in resource-limited settings, exacerbating disparities in healthcare access. Addressing such biases requires the development of more representative datasets and rigorous validation protocols to ensure equitable performance across diverse populations.

The future of AI in healthcare lies in its alignment with the principles of integrated care, which emphasize adaptability, sustainability, and patient-centeredness. Emerging technologies such as federated learning, edge computing, and quantum computing hold immense promise for advancing AI's role in healthcare. Federated learning facilitates collaborative model training while preserving data privacy, addressing one of the most significant barriers to AI implementation. Edge computing enhances real-time decision-making by processing data closer to its source, a capability that is particularly valuable in critical care settings (Kaplan & Hays, 2022). Quantum computing, though still in its infancy, offers the potential to solve complex problems in drug discovery and genomics, opening new frontiers in personalized medicine. Realizing this vision requires a multidisciplinary approach that brings together clinicians, data scientists, policymakers, and ethicists. Education and training programs are essential to equip healthcare professionals with the skills needed to integrate AI effectively into their practice. Robust governance frameworks must be established to oversee the ethical deployment of AI, ensuring that innovation aligns with the principles of equity and transparency. By fostering a culture of collaboration and addressing the challenges of privacy, transparency, and bias, healthcare systems can unlock the full potential of AI, creating a future that is both technologically advanced and deeply human-centered. AI represents a profound opportunity to reimagine healthcare by enhancing precision, efficiency, and personalization. However, its integration demands careful navigation of ethical and technical challenges. By aligning AI with the goals of integrated care, healthcare systems can achieve a transformative shift toward inclusivity, equity, and sustainability. This convergence of technology and humanity marks a pivotal moment in the evolution of healthcare, where innovation becomes a bridge to a more compassionate and effective system (Pereira et al., 2021).

In the rapidly evolving landscape of healthcare, adaptability, and sustainability are imperative for addressing complex challenges such as demographic shifts, technological disruptions, and global health crises. Healthcare organizations operate in environments characterized by high complexity, uncertainty, and interdependence. Integrated healthcare systems aim to provide seamless, coordinated, and patient-centered care by aligning services across various providers and settings. Future research and practice should focus on identifying strategies to overcome these barriers and enhance the operationalization of dynamic capabilities in healthcare. This includes developing tools and frameworks for assessing dynamic capabilities, fostering leadership that prioritizes adaptability and innovation, and creating incentives for organizations to invest in long-term transformation initiatives. Additionally, the integration of emerging technologies such as AI and machine learning can enhance the effectiveness of dynamic capabilities by providing real-time insights, predictive analytics, and decision support tools. These technologies not only complement dynamic capabilities but also enable healthcare organizations to address challenges with greater precision and agility (Kendzerska et al., 2021).

Moreover, fostering a culture of continuous learning and improvement is critical for embedding dynamic capabilities within healthcare organizations. This involves creating environments where experimentation is encouraged, failures are viewed as opportunities for growth, and cross-disciplinary collaboration is prioritized. By aligning organizational culture with the principles of dynamic capabilities, healthcare systems can build the resilience and adaptability needed to navigate future challenges effectively. As healthcare continues to navigate unprecedented challenges and opportunities, dynamic capabilities will remain central to shaping a future that is both innovative and sustainable. By aligning these capabilities with emerging technologies and fostering a culture of continuous improvement, healthcare organizations can build systems that are not only efficient and adaptive but also deeply attuned to the needs of the communities they serve (Shiwlani et al., 2023).

Linking Dynamic Capabilities with Organizational Theory in Healthcare

Dynamic capabilities, with their focus on sensing, seizing, and transforming, do not exist in isolation. These adaptive mechanisms are deeply intertwined with foundational principles of organizational theory, providing a lens through which healthcare organizations can understand and address their evolving challenges. By situating dynamic capabilities within the broader context of organizational frameworks, we uncover their critical role in fostering resilience and innovation in healthcare systems. This exploration not only establishes the theoretical underpinnings of dynamic capabilities but also highlights their practical applications in overcoming the multifaceted challenges inherent in healthcare delivery. Organizational theory has long served as a cornerstone for analyzing the structure, behavior, and evolution of healthcare systems. Within this domain, perspectives such as resource dependency theory, institutional theory, and systems thinking offer valuable frameworks for understanding how healthcare organizations function and adapt. Dynamic capabilities, when aligned with these theoretical constructs, emerge as a natural extension of organizational adaptability, offering a practical roadmap for navigating uncertainty while fostering growth and sustainability (Amini & Jahanbakhsh Javid, 2023).

The resource dependency perspective emphasizes the strategic importance of securing critical resources to maintain stability and ensure survival. In the context of healthcare, these resources include financial capital, skilled personnel, cutting-edge technologies, and reliable supply chains. Dynamic capabilities complement this perspective by focusing on the proactive identification and strategic mobilization of resources. Sensing capabilities enable organizations to detect shifts in external environments, such as emerging technological innovations or changes in policy. Seizing capabilities involves the strategic allocation of resources to capitalize on these shifts, ensuring that organizations remain competitive and relevant (Amini & Jahanbakhsh Javid, 2023). Transforming capabilities enable healthcare providers to optimize their operations, enhancing efficiency and resilience. For instance, during the COVID-19 pandemic, healthcare systems that effectively leveraged dynamic capabilities demonstrated an acute awareness of resource gaps, implemented innovative solutions to address these challenges, and restructured their processes to optimize resource utilization. This alignment underscores the synergy between dynamic capabilities and resource dependency theory, illustrating their combined potential to foster organizational stability under volatile conditions (Haleem et al., 2022).

Institutional theory offers another lens for understanding dynamic capabilities in healthcare. This perspective highlights the influence of regulatory environments, societal expectations, and cultural norms on organizational behavior. Healthcare organizations must navigate a dense web of institutional pressures, balancing compliance with regulatory standards, adherence to ethical practices, and responsiveness to patient needs. Dynamic capabilities provide a mechanism for reconciling these often-competing demands. Sensing capabilities allow organizations to identify shifts in institutional expectations, such as new privacy regulations or evolving patient preferences. Seizing capabilities enable them to adapt their practices, integrating innovations that meet both regulatory and societal requirements. Transforming capabilities ensure that these adaptations are embedded within organizational processes, creating a culture of continuous compliance and innovation. For example, the rapid adoption of telemedicine required healthcare providers to address not only technological and operational challenges but also ethical considerations such as patient confidentiality and equitable access. By leveraging dynamic capabilities, organizations successfully navigated these complexities, aligning their practices with institutional norms while driving forward innovative care models (Pesqueira & Sousa, 2022).

Additionally, systems thinking provides a holistic framework for analyzing the interconnected nature of healthcare organizations and their environments. This perspective emphasizes the dynamic interplay between various components of the healthcare ecosystem, from policy frameworks to patient behaviors. Dynamic capabilities resonate strongly with systems thinking, offering a structured approach to managing interdependencies and anticipating systemic disruptions. Healthcare organizations with robust dynamic capabilities are better positioned to align their internal processes with external demands, fostering collaboration across diverse stakeholders. For instance, integrated healthcare systems that utilize dynamic capabilities can address complex challenges such as care fragmentation by enhancing coordination, streamlining workflows, and improving communication among providers. These efforts create synergistic outcomes that benefit patients while improving the overall efficiency and resilience of the healthcare system (Bouguerra et al., 2022).

The interplay between dynamic capabilities and organizational theory underscores the necessity of contextualizing adaptability within a structured theoretical framework. Healthcare organizations must not only react to external pressures but also cultivate the capacity to anticipate, interpret, and respond to these pressures in ways that align with their strategic objectives and societal roles. This requires a deep understanding of their organizational environment and the ability to navigate its complexities with precision and foresight. Dynamic capabilities extend the relevance of organizational theory by bridging the gap between abstract constructs and actionable strategies. They provide healthcare organizations with a robust toolkit for enhancing adaptability and resilience, addressing both immediate challenges and long-term objectives. By integrating dynamic capabilities into their strategic frameworks, healthcare organizations can navigate the complexities of modern healthcare with greater agility, ensuring their relevance and sustainability in an ever-changing landscape. This integration fosters a proactive approach to healthcare management, enabling organizations to remain resilient in the face of evolving challenges while seizing opportunities for innovation and growth (Pesqueira, Sousa, 2022).

Moreover, the application of dynamic capabilities in healthcare extends beyond individual organizations to influence broader systemic outcomes. By aligning with the principles of resource dependency, institutional theory, and systems thinking, dynamic capabilities provide a holistic framework for navigating the complexities of healthcare delivery. This alignment enables healthcare systems to address systemic inefficiencies, foster innovation, and ensure sustainability at both organizational and systemic levels. For example, regional healthcare networks that leverage dynamic capabilities can coordinate resources more effectively, optimize patient outcomes, and enhance their capacity to respond to public health crises. These outcomes underscore the transformative potential of dynamic capabilities in creating adaptive and resilient healthcare ecosystems (Cifuentes-Faura, 2022).

The integration of dynamic capabilities into organizational theory enriches our understanding of these adaptive mechanisms while providing actionable insights for their application in healthcare. By contextualizing dynamic capabilities within established theoretical frameworks, healthcare organizations gain the tools needed to navigate an increasingly complex and uncertain environment. This alignment underscores the critical role of dynamic capabilities in driving innovation, fostering resilience, and ensuring the sustainability of healthcare systems in an era of unprecedented challenges and opportunities.

Table 1. Overview of dynamic capabilities and organizational theory in healthcare

Aspect	Dynamic Capabilities	Organizational Theory in Healthcare
Definition	Dynamic capabilities involve sensing opportunities, seizing them, and transforming organizational processes.	Organizational theory examines structures, behaviors, and systems shaping healthcare delivery.
Theoretical Foundation	Rooted in the resource-based view (RBV), focusing on adaptive processes for competitive advantage.	Draws from frameworks like resource dependency, institutional theory, and systems thinking.
Core Process 1	Sensing: Identifying opportunities and threats in the external environment.	Emphasizes the importance of aligning with environmental demands and resource availability.
Core Process 2	Seizing: Mobilizing resources and strategies to capture opportunities effectively.	Focuses on decision-making structures and strategies for resource optimization.
Core Process 3	Transforming: Reconfiguring internal structures to sustain innovation and adaptability.	Examines structural changes within healthcare organizations to meet evolving demands.
Focus	Proactive adaptation to environmental changes and innovation.	Understanding internal and external influences on organizational efficiency.
Application in Healthcare	Facilitates rapid adoption of technologies, resource management, and organizational restructuring.	Provides frameworks for understanding behaviors under regulatory and societal pressures.
Institutional Alignment	Adapts to norms, regulations, and cultural expectations while maintaining flexibility.	Explores the impact of institutional pressures on compliance and performance.
Systems Perspective	Integrates holistic views of interconnected processes for organizational success.	Emphasizes interconnectedness within healthcare ecosystems and multi-level interactions.

continued on following page

Table 1. Continued

Aspect	Dynamic Capabilities	Organizational Theory in Healthcare
Technology Integration	Drives adoption of AI, telemedicine, and digital platforms for operational efficiency.	Explores the role of technology in shaping healthcare delivery frameworks.
Resilience Building	Enhances agility and preparedness for crises like pandemics or resource shortages.	Provides insights into organizational adaptability under stress.
Key Challenge	Balancing innovation with compliance and long-term sustainability.	Managing resistance to change and aligning diverse stakeholder interests.
Ethical Considerations	Focuses on transparency, fairness, and equitable resource distribution.	Examines the role of ethics in decision-making and regulatory compliance.
Scalability	Supports scaling of innovations across systems while maintaining organizational coherence.	Analyzes how systems can adapt and expand within theoretical constraints.
Future Directions	Emphasizes continuous improvement, AI-driven insights, and cross-disciplinary collaboration.	Calls for integration of dynamic theories with practical implementation for better outcomes.

Source: the authors

The Intersection of Technology and Human Capital in Dynamic Capabilities

The relationship between technology and human capital forms a foundational element of dynamic capabilities in healthcare. Together, these forces enable organizations to sense, seize, and transform in response to rapid and often unpredictable changes in their environment. Technology provides the tools necessary for operational efficiency and decision-making based on vast datasets, while human capital offers the creativity, expertise, and judgment required to apply these tools effectively. This interplay fosters adaptability and innovation, positioning healthcare organizations to thrive in a competitive and complex landscape. By examining the synergistic relationship between technology and human capital, we gain insight into their combined roles in shaping and sustaining dynamic capabilities (Gebhardt et al.,2022).

Technology acts as a catalyst for dynamic capabilities, equipping healthcare organizations with the tools to anticipate and respond to challenges while capturing new opportunities. Advanced tools such as AI, machine learning, and predictive analytics empower organizations to process extensive datasets, recognize patterns, and generate actionable insights. For instance, AI diagnostic tools are capable of detecting diseases at earlier stages with remarkable accuracy, while predictive models forecast resource needs, guiding efficient planning and allocation. These technological advancements not only enhance decision-making processes but also support the integration of innovative practices into healthcare delivery systems, bridging gaps in efficiency and care quality. The adoption of digital platforms further illustrates technology's role in fostering dynamic capabilities. Systems such as electronic health records (EHRs) and telemedicine platforms streamline communication and coordination among providers, enabling more effective and integrated care delivery. Emerging technologies, including blockchain and the Internet of Things (IoT), offer additional opportunities to enhance transparency, security, and efficiency in operations. These tools empower healthcare organizations to respond proactively to environmental shifts, creating systems that are both resilient and sustainable. Such innovations underscore the potential of technology to not only address immediate needs but also anticipate future challenges, ensuring long-term adaptability (Kant & Anjali, 2021).

Human capital, however, remains the driving force behind the effective application of these technological tools. Healthcare professionals bring the expertise, empathy, and critical thinking skills necessary to translate technological innovations into meaningful patient outcomes. Dynamic capabilities are intrinsically tied to a workforce that is technically proficient, collaborative, and equipped with the leadership skills to navigate complex and evolving healthcare environments. Investment in workforce development, therefore, becomes a cornerstone of enhancing dynamic capabilities. Training initiatives that emphasize interdisciplinary collaboration, technical expertise, and adaptive leadership prepare healthcare professionals to maximize the potential of available technologies while driving organizational transformation. Organizational culture plays a critical role in harnessing the power of human capital (Mele et al., 2023). A culture that values continuous learning, innovation, and adaptability motivates employees to embrace change and contribute to the organization's evolution. By fostering an environment of trust and empowerment, healthcare organizations enable their workforce to lead transformative efforts. For instance, interprofessional education initiatives that bring together clinicians, administrators, and IT professionals bridge gaps in understanding and foster cohesive strategies with shared goals. This alignment of culture and capability ensures that human capital is fully leveraged to drive dynamic and sustainable organizational outcomes, reinforcing the broader objectives of adaptability and innovation. The intersection of technology and human capital creates a synergistic relationship that elevates dynamic capabilities. When healthcare professionals are equipped with advanced technological tools, they can make better-informed decisions, improve patient outcomes, and streamline operations. For example, clinicians using AI-driven decision support systems can diagnose conditions more accurately and develop targeted treatment plans, while administrators employing predictive analytics can optimize staffing, inventory, and resource allocation. These applications highlight how technology, when effectively integrated with human capital, revolutionizes healthcare delivery by enhancing its precision, efficiency, and responsiveness (Kotcher et al., 2021).

Team-based care models provide a practical illustration of this synergy. Interdisciplinary teams that integrate technology into their workflows improve coordination, reduce inefficiencies, and deliver patient-centered care. Digital platforms that facilitate real-time communication and data sharing further enhance these capabilities, ensuring that care plans are consistent, comprehensive, and aligned with patient needs. Such collaboration underscores the importance of aligning technological investments with workforce development initiatives, ensuring that employees are not only equipped to use new tools but also actively engaged in their design and implementation. This engagement fosters a sense of ownership and aligns technological innovation with practical, real-world applications. However, realizing the full potential of this intersection requires addressing several challenges. Resistance to change often poses significant barriers, particularly in healthcare environments where established routines and practices are deeply entrenched. Overcoming this resistance necessitates effective change management strategies, including transparent communication, stakeholder engagement, and demonstrable benefits. Additionally, ethical considerations surrounding data privacy, algorithmic fairness, and equitable access to technology must be addressed to maintain trust and integrity in healthcare delivery. Healthcare organizations must balance the pursuit of technological innovation with the imperative to uphold ethical standards and ensure inclusivity in their workforce strategies (Mostafiz et al., 2022).

Another critical challenge lies in fostering workforce inclusivity and equity in a technology-driven environment. Training and development initiatives must ensure that all employees, regardless of their role or background, have access to the resources and education needed to thrive. By prioritizing inclusivity, organizations not only support equity but also harness diverse perspectives and talents, driving innovation and adaptability. These efforts help build a workforce that is prepared to navigate the complexities of healthcare delivery, ensuring that technological advancements benefit all stakeholders. The future of dynamic capabilities in healthcare will increasingly depend on the seamless integration of technology and human capital (Junaid et al., 2023).

Emerging innovations, such as AI-powered digital twins and advanced robotics, promise to revolutionize care delivery and organizational adaptability. At the same time, human capital will remain central to this evolution, with a growing emphasis on interdisciplinary collaboration, emotional intelligence, and lifelong learning. To maximize these advancements, healthcare organizations must adopt a holistic approach that aligns technological investments with workforce strategies, fostering a culture of innovation and prioritizing ethical considerations. By doing so, organizations can build dynamic capabilities that drive adaptability, resilience, and sustainability in a complex and competitive environment (Kwok & Treiblmaier, 2023).

The relationship between technology and human capital lies at the heart of dynamic capabilities, forming a synergistic foundation for adaptability and innovation. While technology provides the tools for operational efficiency and transformative practices, human capital brings the judgment, creativity, and collaboration necessary to implement these tools effectively. Together, they enable healthcare organizations to respond proactively to challenges, seize opportunities, and sustain innovation in an ever-changing landscape. By investing in both technological advancements and workforce development, organizations can harness the full potential of dynamic capabilities, ensuring their relevance and success in a rapidly evolving healthcare sector. As the healthcare landscape continues to evolve, the integration of these elements will remain essential for building systems that are both forward-thinking and deeply attuned to the needs of patients and providers alike (Ullah et al., 2023).

A Comprehensive View of Enterprise Architecture Transition in Healthcare

Figure 1 highlights the multi-layered progression across the business, application, and technology domains. The evolution of healthcare enterprise architecture from its current state to a future, target-oriented model underscores the necessity for a structured approach to innovation and transformation. By mapping the current state, transitional phases, and future architecture, this model provides a roadmap for healthcare organizations to achieve adaptability, resilience, and sustainability (Kasneciet al., 2023).

Each layer—business, application, and technology—is tightly interconnected, showcasing dependencies and mutual reinforcement at every stage (Eager & Brunton, 2023). The "Current State" architecture reflects the as-is scenario of healthcare systems. Business capabilities at this stage are predominantly reactive, reflecting traditional care delivery models with limited integration of advanced technologies or team-based approaches. Silos between departments hinders collaboration, leading to inefficiencies in patient care. For example, resource shortages or unexpected patient influxes are often managed reactively rather than proactively.

The business culture in this state emphasizes maintaining the status quo rather than fostering adaptability or innovation. Application capabilities in the current state are primarily functional but lack depth and integration. Telemedicine and other digital platforms are either absent or implemented on a small scale, reducing their impact on accessibility and care delivery. The technology layer in the current state is characterized by outdated or legacy systems with limited interoperability and scalability. Manual processes dominate both administrative and clinical workflows, increasing inefficiencies and errors. There is little adoption of advanced tools such as AI or the IoT, and data management practices often fail to meet the demands of modern healthcare environments. This state underscores the need for foundational changes to prepare for future transformations (Jalil et al., 2023).

Figure 1. Evolution of enterprise architecture for healthcare transformation

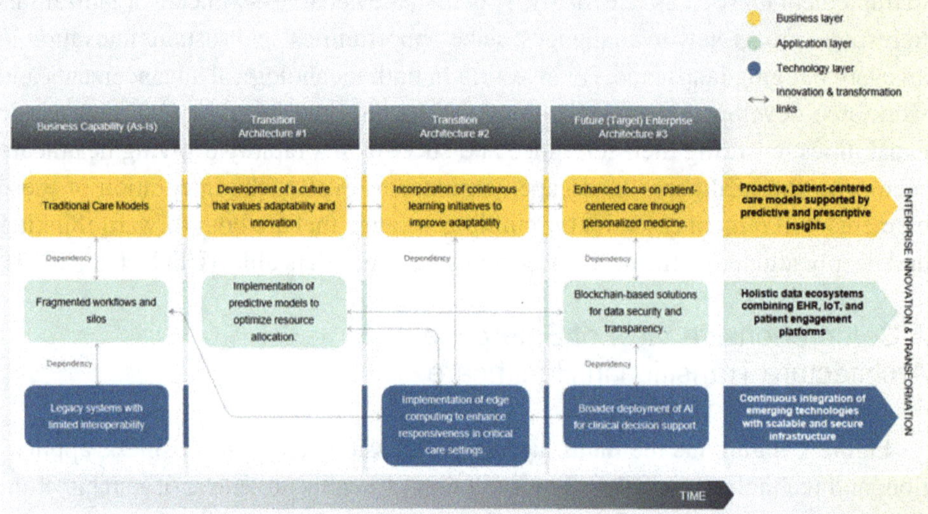

Transition Architecture #1

The first transition architecture represents the initial phase of healthcare transformation. At the business layer, this stage involves the introduction of interdisciplinary collaboration models to enhance team-based care delivery. Organizations begin to realign workflows to reduce silos, improve communication, and foster a culture that values adaptability and innovation. This cultural shift is critical to laying the groundwork for long-term transformation. Application capabilities during this phase begin to expand, with the adoption of integrated EHR systems that offer basic analytics capabilities. These systems enable providers to gain initial insights into patient data, supporting early-stage decision-making improvements. Telemedicine platforms are introduced, providing virtual consultation options that increase patient accessibility and convenience. Predictive models are implemented to optimize resource allocation, marking a significant step toward proactive healthcare management. The technology layer in Transition Architecture #1 sees the pilot implementation of advanced tools. AI is introduced for tasks such as diagnostics and predictive analytics, providing a glimpse into its transformative potential. Cloud-based solutions begin to replace legacy systems, enabling better data access and sharing across departments. IoT devices are also piloted, allowing for the monitoring of key health metrics in real time. These advancements mark the beginning of a shift toward a more technology-driven approach to healthcare delivery.

Transition Architecture #2

The second transitional phase builds upon the foundation established in the first. At the business layer, team-based care models are further refined, with clearly defined interdisciplinary roles and responsibilities. Patient-centered care becomes a focal point, supported by personalized medicine approaches that leverage data to tailor treatments to individual needs. Continuous learning initiatives are introduced to enhance adaptability, encouraging healthcare professionals to embrace innovation and change. Application capabilities at this stage become more sophisticated, with the integration of advanced analytics platforms. These platforms enable predictive and prescriptive insights, allowing providers to anticipate patient needs and optimize care delivery. Telehealth capabilities are enhanced through the integration of remote patient monitoring tools, expanding the reach and impact of virtual care. Blockchain-based solutions are also introduced to improve data security and transparency, addressing critical concerns around privacy and trust. The technology layer in Transition Architecture #2 experiences significant advancements. AI tools are deployed more broadly, providing clinical decision support and automating routine tasks. IoT devices are fully integrated into healthcare workflows, enabling the continuous monitoring and analysis of patient health metrics. Edge computing solutions are implemented to enhance responsiveness in critical care settings, ensuring that real-time data can be processed and acted upon without delays. These developments represent a maturing of the technology ecosystem, setting the stage for the target architecture.

Future (Target) Enterprise Architecture

The "Future" architecture embodies the ultimate vision for healthcare transformation. At the business layer, fully integrated systems support seamless team-based workflows, with a focus on proactive, patient-centered care. Dynamic capabilities are embedded within the organization, enabling it to sense, seize, and transform in response to emerging challenges and opportunities. This adaptability fosters a culture of continuous improvement, ensuring that the organization remains resilient and innovative in an ever-changing environment. Application capabilities in the target architecture represent the pinnacle of integration and sophistication. Holistic data ecosystems combine EHR systems, IoT platforms, and patient engagement tools, providing a comprehensive view of patient health. AI-powered tools support diagnostics, resource optimization, and real-time decision-making, ensuring that care delivery is both precise and efficient. Advanced interoperability features enable seamless data sharing across providers, enhancing collaboration and care coordination. The technology layer in the target architecture is characterized by cutting-edge advancements. AI, robotics, and digital twins are extensively used to drive precision medicine and operational efficiency. Quantum computing is introduced to address complex challenges such as drug discovery and genomic analysis, unlocking new possibilities for personalized care. Emerging technologies are continuously integrated into the system, supported by a scalable and secure infrastructure that ensures long-term sustainability. This layer exemplifies the potential of technology to transform healthcare delivery, positioning organizations at the forefront of innovation.

Interdependencies and Transformation Tracks

Changes in one layer often necessitate adjustments in others, highlighting the need for a holistic approach to transformation. For example, the adoption of AI tools in the technology layer requires corresponding changes in the application layer, such as the integration of data analytics platforms, and in the business layer, such as the development of new workflows and training programs. This interconnectedness ensures that all elements of the architecture work in harmony, driving sustainable and impactful change. Each transitional phase builds upon the previous one, creating a cohesive and incremental approach to transformation. In the current state of architecture, several challenges arise that hinder progress toward transformation. At the business layer, resistance to adopting new processes and the inefficiencies caused by outdated systems are significant barriers. Organizational culture in the current state often focuses on maintaining the status quo, making it difficult to foster the innovation and adaptability needed for future growth. Application capabilities are limited in scope, with EHRs often being underutilized and lacking interoperability. This reduces the ability of healthcare organizations to leverage data for effective decision-making. In the technology layer, reliance on legacy systems presents significant roadblocks, with minimal adoption of advanced tools such as AI or the Internet of Things. These limitations underscore the urgency for foundational changes to prepare for subsequent phases (Pesqueira, Sousa, 2022).

Transition Architecture #1 marks the initial steps toward healthcare transformation but introduces its own set of challenges. At the business layer, realigning workflows and fostering interdisciplinary collaboration requires substantial effort, particularly in overcoming entrenched silos. Building a culture that values adaptability and innovation often meets resistance, as employees and stakeholders may be hesitant to embrace change. The application layer faces challenges in implementing integrated

EHR systems and telemedicine platforms, as these require significant investments in training, infrastructure, and process redesign. Technologically, the introduction of tools such as AI for diagnostics and predictive analytics demands careful planning to ensure successful pilot implementations and scalability. Ensuring the interoperability of cloud-based solutions and IoT devices adds another layer of complexity. To overcome these challenges, strategic initiatives must focus on engaging stakeholders early in the process and fostering a sense of ownership among employees. Clear communication about the benefits of change, coupled with comprehensive training programs, helps to mitigate resistance. Pilot projects that demonstrate quick wins can build momentum and trust in the transition process. Additionally, investing in scalable infrastructure and adopting an incremental approach to technological upgrades ensures smoother integration while minimizing disruptions.

Transition Architecture #2 builds on the progress made in the first phase, but the complexity of challenges also increases. At the business layer, refining team-based care models and integrating personalized medicine approaches require significant alignment of roles, responsibilities, and resources. Creating a culture of continuous learning and innovation is essential but can be difficult to achieve consistently across all levels of the organization. In the application layer, the integration of advanced analytics platforms and blockchain-based solutions presents challenges in scaling these technologies while addressing concerns around data security and transparency. The deployment of telehealth capabilities with remote patient monitoring introduces logistical and technical barriers, including ensuring reliable connectivity and user-friendly interfaces for both providers and patients. The technology layer faces significant hurdles in scaling AI tools for clinical decision support and fully integrating IoT devices into workflows. The implementation of edge computing for real-time decision-making requires substantial investments in infrastructure and expertise.

To address these challenges, fostering collaboration across interdisciplinary teams becomes crucial. Establishing shared governance structures and promoting cross-departmental communication helps align diverse roles and responsibilities. Continuous education initiatives that emphasize adaptability and technical skills prepare the workforce for evolving demands. Leveraging partnerships with technology vendors can also facilitate the scaling of advanced solutions. Regulatory frameworks that promote data security and interoperability standards play a vital role in ensuring the seamless integration of these technologies. The future or target architecture represents the ultimate vision for healthcare transformation but is not without its challenges. At the business layer, achieving full integration of team-based workflows and embedding dynamic capabilities into the organizational culture requires sustained effort and strategic leadership. Maintaining a proactive approach to patient-centered care demands continuous evaluation and adaptation of processes and metrics. In the application layer, building holistic data ecosystems that seamlessly combine EHR systems, IoT platforms, and patient engagement tools is a highly complex undertaking. Ensuring that these systems are interoperable and secure while supporting AI-powered diagnostics and resource optimization presents a significant technical and operational challenge. At the technology layer, the adoption of cutting-edge advancements such as quantum computing and robotics must be balanced with considerations of accessibility, scalability, and cost. Ensuring that these innovations are effectively integrated into healthcare systems without creating disparities or inefficiencies is critical to the success of the target architecture (Pesqueira, Sousa, 2022).

Strategies to navigate these complexities include fostering leadership that prioritizes innovation and adaptability. Organizations can benefit from adopting flexible performance metrics that measure both short-term progress and long-term impact. Building strong partnerships with academic institutions and research centers can drive the development of cutting-edge technologies and ensure their practical application. Continuous feedback loops that involve patients, providers, and stakeholders ensure that transformations remain aligned with organizational goals and patient needs. Scaling quantum computing and robotics requires phased implementation plans and strategic investments that prioritize equitable access and sustainability. The interdependencies and transformation tracks highlighted in the figure further illuminate the challenges faced during each phase of the transition. The business changes track involves aligning organizational goals, workflows, and cultural shifts, which often requires overcoming resistance and building consensus among stakeholders. The information changes track focuses on the application layer, where integrating new data systems and analytics capabilities must be coordinated with evolving business needs and technological advancements. The technology changes track emphasizes the progression of tools and platforms, which must be implemented in a way that supports overall organizational objectives while addressing issues such as interoperability, scalability, and user adoption. These tracks underscore the interconnected nature of enterprise architecture, where changes in one layer necessitate adjustments in others, highlighting the need for a cohesive and holistic approach to transformation (Cifuentes-Faura, 2022).

The evolution of enterprise architecture for healthcare transformation is a journey fraught with challenges but also immense potential. By addressing these challenges strategically at each phase, healthcare organizations can build systems that are not only resilient and efficient but also adaptable to the needs of patients and providers. The model outlined in the figure provides a structured framework for navigating this complex process, ensuring that innovation and transformation are aligned with organizational goals and societal demands. Through a combination of strategic leadership, stakeholder engagement, and technological innovation, the vision of a fully integrated, patient-centered healthcare system can be realized.

FRAMEWORK FOR EVALUATING DYNAMIC CAPABILITIES IN HEALTHCARE

The implementation of dynamic capabilities within healthcare organizations demands not only careful integration but also an ongoing evaluation to ensure their effectiveness. This evaluation is critical for understanding how well these capabilities enable healthcare systems to adapt to change, seize opportunities, and transform processes for sustained innovation and resilience. A structured framework for assessing the presence and efficacy of dynamic capabilities provides healthcare organizations with the tools to measure progress, identify gaps, and prioritize areas for continuous improvement. By focusing on key processes—sensing, seizing, and transforming—this framework facilitates a comprehensive analysis of dynamic capabilities within complex healthcare settings. Evaluating the sensing process requires examining how well an organization identifies opportunities and threats in its external environment. Metrics for this evaluation may include the frequency and accuracy of trend analyses, the diversity and depth of data sources, and the speed of response to emerging trends. For example, a healthcare system's ability to anticipate demographic shifts or emerging diseases can be measured by the robustness of its predictive models and the timeliness of its strategic decisions. Advanced tools such as AI and big data analytics play a significant role in enhancing the sensing process, and their effectiveness can be evaluated by measuring their contribution to decision-making accuracy and strategic alignment (Pesqueira, Sousa, Pereira, 2023).

The seizing process is equally critical to the overall efficacy of dynamic capabilities. This process involves mobilizing resources and implementing strategies to capitalize on identified opportunities. Evaluating this capability often focuses on resource allocation efficiency, stakeholder engagement, and the success rate of implemented initiatives. For instance, a healthcare organization's ability to adopt telemedicine platforms or expand access to remote patient monitoring can be assessed by examining implementation timelines, utilization rates, and patient outcomes. Additionally, the organization's agility in reallocating resources during crises, such as a pandemic, serves as a strong indicator of its seizing capability. Benchmarking tools can be employed to compare these metrics against industry standards, offering insights into relative performance and areas for improvement. Transforming processes, which involve reconfiguring organizational structures and systems to sustain long-term benefits, are often the most challenging to evaluate. Metrics for assessing this capability include the rate of successful organizational restructuring, the adoption of innovative practices, and the alignment of transformation initiatives with long-term strategic goals. For example, healthcare organizations transitioning from siloed operations to integrated care models can measure success through improved care coordination, patient satisfaction, and cost efficiency. Continuous improvement frameworks, such as Lean Six Sigma, can be leveraged to monitor and enhance these transformations. Tools that track employee engagement, training completion rates, and interdepartmental collaboration provide additional layers of insight into the effectiveness of transformation efforts (Meleet al.,2023).

Benchmarking plays a pivotal role in the evaluation process, offering healthcare organizations a means to measure their dynamic capabilities against industry best practices and peers. Benchmarking tools provide quantitative and qualitative data that highlight performance gaps and guide strategic planning. For instance, healthcare organizations can benchmark their adoption of AI-driven diagnostic tools or their success in implementing precision medicine against leading institutions globally. Such comparisons not only help identify areas of underperformance but also inspire the adoption of innovative approaches and technologies. Continuous improvement is integral to the dynamic capabilities framework. The healthcare landscape is ever-changing, requiring organizations to remain agile and forward-thinking. Regular evaluations enable organizations to refine their strategies and processes, ensuring that they remain relevant and effective. Tools such as balanced scorecards and key performance indicators (KPIs) are invaluable for tracking progress and identifying areas for refinement. For example, a healthcare system might use KPIs to monitor reductions in patient wait times or improvements in diagnostic accuracy, linking these outcomes directly to the effectiveness of its dynamic capabilities. Examples of healthcare systems that have successfully implemented dynamic capabilities frameworks offer valuable insights into best practices and common challenges. One notable example is the rapid integration of telehealth services during the COVID-19 pandemic. Many healthcare organizations demonstrated exceptional sensing capabilities by recognizing the need for remote care early in the crisis. They seized the opportunity by reallocating resources to develop and deploy telehealth platforms within weeks. These organizations also showcased their transforming capabilities by embedding telehealth into their long-term care delivery models, ensuring its sustainability beyond the immediate crisis. Another example is the adoption of precision medicine in oncology, where dynamic capabilities have enabled healthcare providers to integrate genomic data into personalized treatment plans, improving patient outcomes and optimizing resource utilization.

Table 2 presents a framework for evaluating dynamic capabilities within healthcare organizations not only measures current performance but also guides future improvements. By systematically assessing sensing, seizing, and transforming processes, healthcare systems can identify strengths, address weaknesses, and capitalize on opportunities for growth and innovation. The integration of robust metrics, benchmarking tools, and continuous improvement methodologies ensures that dynamic capabilities remain a driving force for adaptability, resilience, and excellence in healthcare delivery. This framework provides a foundation for organizations to navigate the complexities of modern healthcare, fostering a culture of innovation and sustainability that ultimately benefits both providers and patients.

Table 2. Theoretical framework

Roadmap Stage	Dynamic Capability Process	Key Framework Element	Application in Enterprise Architecture
Current State	Sensing	Evaluate trends and external data sources to identify opportunities and threats.	Limited data sources and underutilized EHR systems reduce trend identification.
	Seizing	Measure resource allocation to maintain current operations.	Resource limitations hinder proactive resource deployment.
	Transforming	Assess organizational readiness for restructuring.	Siloed operations create barriers to initial transformation efforts.
Transition Architecture #1	Sensing	Implement AI and analytics to enhance trend detection and response speed.	Pilot AI tools and integrated EHR systems for predictive insights.
	Seizing	Allocate resources for initial technology adoption and team-based care models.	Begin integrating telemedicine platforms and IoT devices.
	Transforming	Redesign workflows to support interdisciplinary collaboration.	Align pilot projects with early-stage cultural shifts toward adaptability.
Transition Architecture #2	Sensing	Use advanced analytics platforms to refine understanding of patient needs.	Leverage integrated IoT systems for real-time health monitoring.
	Seizing	Scale adoption of technologies such as blockchain and precision medicine tools.	Broaden telehealth capabilities and enable secure, interoperable data sharing.
	Transforming	Develop cross-departmental governance and continuous learning initiatives.	Strengthen cultural alignment through training and shared performance metrics.
Future (Target) Architecture	Sensing	Achieve holistic integration of systems to continuously monitor environmental changes.	Establish a fully interoperable data ecosystem combining EHR, IoT, and analytics.
	Seizing	Optimize advanced resource allocation strategies using AI-powered models.	Fully embed AI in diagnostics, resource optimization, and operational workflows.
	Transforming	Sustain organizational adaptability through iterative transformation.	Implement dynamic team-based workflows for seamless patient-centered care.

continued on following page

Table 2. Continued

Roadmap Stage	Dynamic Capability Process	Key Framework Element	Application in Enterprise Architecture
Evaluation and Benchmarking	Sensing	Assess system responsiveness and data utilization efficiency.	Measure the effectiveness of AI and IoT in identifying trends and actionable insights.
	Seizing	Track project success rates and stakeholder engagement levels.	Evaluate deployment success for telehealth and other digital platforms.
	Transforming	Measure cultural alignment and innovation adoption rates.	Monitor training completion and cross-departmental collaboration.
Continuous Improvement	All	Refine metrics, methodologies, and feedback loops to sustain progress.	Ensure ongoing alignment of dynamic capabilities with enterprise transformation goals.

JUSTIFICATIONS AND VALIDATIONS FOR THE ROADMAP AND FRAMEWORK

The creation of the roadmap and framework for evaluating dynamic capabilities in healthcare is rooted in a combination of theoretical foundations, empirical evidence, and practical necessity. Healthcare organizations operate in environments characterized by high complexity, rapid technological advancements, and ever-evolving patient needs. As such, developing a structured and scientifically validated approach to assess and enhance dynamic capabilities is essential for enabling adaptability, resilience, and innovation. This section outlines the theoretical justifications and practical validations that underscore the importance of this roadmap and framework. The roadmap draws heavily on the dynamic capabilities framework, which has its theoretical foundation in the resource-based view (RBV) of organizations. The RBV posits that an organization's ability to maintain a competitive advantage lies in its internal resources and capabilities. Dynamic capabilities—defined as the organization's capacity to sense, seize, and transform—extend the RBV by emphasizing adaptability in rapidly changing environments. In the healthcare context, this theoretical underpinning is particularly relevant given the sector's dynamic nature, where external pressures such as pandemics, regulatory changes, and technological disruptions necessitate continual adaptation. The roadmap aligns with these principles by providing a structured mechanism for assessing and enhancing sensing, seizing, and transforming processes.

Empirical evidence further validates the need for such a framework. Numerous case studies demonstrate the transformative impact of dynamic capabilities in healthcare. For instance, during the COVID-19 pandemic, organizations with robust sensing capabilities were able to anticipate resource shortages and deploy telehealth solutions at scale. Similarly, seizing opportunities to implement AI-driven diagnostics and reallocate resources proved critical for many healthcare systems. These examples highlight the practical value of dynamic capabilities and the need for systematic evaluation to optimize their deployment. The roadmap, by offering measurable metrics and benchmarking tools, provides a methodical approach to replicating such successes across diverse healthcare settings. The framework's focus on measurable metrics and continuous improvement is supported by well-established methodologies in performance management and organizational theory. Tools such as balanced scorecards, key performance indicators (KPIs), and benchmarking have long been used to track progress and identify areas for improvement. Incorporating these tools into the dynamic capabilities framework ensures that the evaluation process is both rigorous and actionable. For example, KPIs measuring reductions in patient wait times or improvements in diagnostic accuracy provide tangible evidence of progress, linking dynamic capabilities directly to organizational outcomes.

Another justification for the roadmap is its alignment with systems thinking, a theoretical approach that views organizations as interconnected systems rather than isolated entities. Systems thinking emphasizes the interdependencies between different components of an organization, such as its business processes, technology, and human capital. The roadmap reflects this interconnectedness by integrating the business, application, and technology layers, demonstrating how changes in one layer necessitate adjustments in others. This holistic perspective ensures that the framework captures the complexity of healthcare organizations and provides a comprehensive approach to transformation. Validation of the framework is also achieved through its adaptability to various healthcare contexts. The roadmap's phased approach—from the current state to the target architecture—allows organizations to tailor the framework to their unique needs and constraints. For instance, a resource-limited hospital in a rural setting can focus on foundational improvements, such as adopting basic telemedicine platforms, while a technologically advanced healthcare network can concentrate on scaling AI-driven innovations. This flexibility ensures that the framework is applicable across a broad spectrum of healthcare organizations, enhancing its practical utility.

The roadmap and framework also address critical challenges in healthcare transformation, such as resistance to change and the need for stakeholder alignment. Research in organizational behavior highlights the importance of clear communication, stakeholder engagement, and demonstrating quick wins to overcome resistance. The roadmap incorporates these principles by emphasizing pilot projects and incremental implementation, allowing organizations to build momentum and trust. Additionally, the use of benchmarking tools enables organizations to compare their progress against industry standards, fostering a sense of achievement and motivation among stakeholders. Ethical considerations further validate the need for this roadmap and framework. As healthcare organizations increasingly adopt advanced technologies such as AI and IoT, concerns about data privacy, algorithmic bias, and equitable access come to the forefront. The framework addresses these issues by integrating ethical evaluation into the dynamic capabilities assessment. For instance, metrics for evaluating AI tools include not only their predictive accuracy but also their fairness and compliance with privacy regulations. By embedding ethical considerations into the framework, the roadmap ensures that healthcare transformation aligns with societal values and promotes trust among patients and providers.

Finally, the roadmap and framework are validated by their alignment with global healthcare trends and policy objectives. Initiatives such as the World Health Organization's (WHO) emphasis on universal health coverage and the United Nations Sustainable Development Goals (SDGs) highlight the need for adaptable and resilient healthcare systems. The roadmap's focus on dynamic capabilities directly supports these objectives by enabling healthcare organizations to respond proactively to global health challenges, optimize resource utilization, and improve care delivery. For example, the framework's emphasis on integrating AI and IoT aligns with global efforts to leverage technology for sustainable healthcare solutions.

The creation of the roadmap and framework for evaluating dynamic capabilities in healthcare is underpinned by robust theoretical justifications and practical validations. Drawing on the dynamic capabilities framework, systems thinking, and performance management methodologies, the roadmap provides a structured and actionable approach to assessing and enhancing organizational adaptability. Empirical evidence from healthcare transformation initiatives further underscores its practical value, while its flexibility ensures applicability across diverse contexts. By addressing ethical considerations and aligning with global health objectives, the roadmap not only facilitates innovation but also promotes trust and equity in healthcare delivery. This comprehensive framework empowers healthcare organizations to navigate complexity and drive sustainable transformation, ensuring their relevance and success in an ever-changing landscape.

CHALLENGES AND PARADOXES IN OPERATIONALIZING DYNAMIC CAPABILITIES

The operationalization of dynamic capabilities in healthcare is a complex and multifaceted endeavor, marked by inherent tensions and paradoxes. These challenges arise as organizations strive to balance competing priorities, navigate structural and cultural inertia, and align diverse stakeholder interests. Dynamic capabilities—the ability to sense opportunities and threats, seize them effectively, and transform processes for sustained advantage—offer immense potential for healthcare systems. However, implementing these capabilities in practice reveals significant obstacles that must be addressed to unlock their full value. One of the primary challenges in operationalizing dynamic capabilities is the tension between organizational inertia and the need for agility. Healthcare organizations, particularly large ones, often develop rigid structures and deeply entrenched processes over time. These characteristics, while beneficial for maintaining stability and efficiency in routine operations, can hinder adaptability in the face of change. For example, legacy systems and siloed workflows may impede the adoption of new technologies or innovative care models. Organizational inertia is further reinforced by a culture that prioritizes risk aversion and compliance with strict regulatory requirements, leaving little room for experimentation and innovation (Pesqueira & Sousa, 2022).

At the same time, healthcare organizations face increasing pressure to be agile in responding to rapid advancements in technology, shifting patient expectations, and evolving public health challenges. Agility demands the ability to pivot quickly, experiment with new approaches, and embrace uncertainty. This creates a paradox where the very structures that provide stability and reliability also act as barriers to change. Navigating this tension requires deliberate strategies, including fostering a culture of innovation, reducing bureaucratic bottlenecks, and ensuring leadership commitment to agility. Leadership plays a crucial role in setting the tone for adaptability, encouraging calculated risk-taking, and investing in initiatives that challenge the status quo. Another significant challenge lies in balancing long-term transformation goals with short-term operational demands. Dynamic capabilities emphasize the importance of forward-thinking strategies, yet healthcare organizations must also manage immediate pressures such as patient care demands, resource constraints, and financial sustainability. For example, while the integration of advanced analytics platforms or AI-driven diagnostics promises substantial long-term benefits, these initiatives often require significant upfront investments and a temporary diversion of resources from day-to-day operations. This trade-off can create resistance among stakeholders who prioritize immediate outcomes over future gains (Pesqueira, Sousa, Pereira, 2023).

Short-term operational demands often necessitate quick fixes and incremental improvements rather than transformative changes. However, focusing exclusively on short-term risks perpetuates inefficiencies and limits the potential impact of dynamic capabilities. Balancing these priorities requires a dual focus: maintaining operational excellence in the present while strategically investing in long-term transformation. Organizations can achieve this by adopting phased implementation approaches, where smaller pilot projects generate early wins that build momentum and stakeholder buy-in for larger initiatives. Additionally, aligning transformation goals with measurable short-term outcomes helps bridge the gap between immediate needs and future aspirations.

Resistance to change is a pervasive challenge in operationalizing dynamic capabilities, particularly in complex and highly regulated sectors like healthcare. Resistance may arise from various sources, including employees who fear job displacement due to automation, clinicians who are skeptical of new technologies, and administrators who are wary of disrupting established workflows. Diverse stakeholder groups within healthcare organizations often have conflicting priorities and varying levels of risk tolerance, further complicating efforts to align interests. Mitigating resistance requires a multifaceted approach that addresses both cultural and structural barriers. Open and transparent communication is essential for building trust and reducing uncertainty. Stakeholders must understand the rationale behind changes, the anticipated benefits, and the measures being taken to mitigate potential risks. Engaging stakeholders early in the process, particularly frontline employees and clinicians, fosters a sense of ownership and ensures that their insights inform decision-making. Providing adequate training and resources helps employees adapt to new systems and processes, reducing anxiety and building confidence in their ability to succeed in a transformed environment.

Structural strategies also play a critical role in overcoming resistance. For example, establishing cross-functional governance bodies can help align diverse stakeholder interests and facilitate collaboration. These bodies serve as platforms for addressing concerns, resolving conflicts, and ensuring that transformation efforts are inclusive and equitable. Incentive structures that reward innovation, collaboration, and adaptability further encourage stakeholders to embrace dynamic capabilities. For instance, performance metrics that highlight contributions to organizational transformation can shift focus from short-term productivity to long-term impact. The interplay between external pressures and internal dynamics adds another layer of complexity to operationalizing dynamic capabilities. External factors such as regulatory requirements, market competition, and public health crises create additional challenges and opportunities for healthcare organizations. For example, the COVID-19 pandemic underscored the need for dynamic capabilities as organizations rapidly adapted to deliver care through telemedicine, reallocate resources, and scale testing and vaccination efforts. However, these efforts were often constrained by regulatory uncertainties, fragmented supply chains, and workforce shortages.

Navigating external pressures requires healthcare organizations to adopt a proactive stance, leveraging dynamic capabilities to anticipate and respond to changes effectively. Collaborative partnerships with regulators, policymakers, and industry peers can help address external challenges and create an enabling environment for innovation. For example, regulatory sandboxes that allow organizations to experiment with new technologies in a controlled setting can accelerate the adoption of innovative solutions while ensuring compliance with safety and ethical standards. The operationalization of dynamic capabilities also presents ethical and equity-related challenges. Advanced technologies such as AI and machine learning, while offering significant benefits, raise concerns about data privacy, algorithmic bias, and equitable access. For instance, predictive models that rely on incomplete or biased datasets may perpetuate health disparities rather than address them. Ensuring that dynamic capabilities are implemented ethically and inclusively is critical to building trust among patients and stakeholders.

Addressing these challenges requires a commitment to ethical principles and inclusivity throughout the transformation process. This includes rigorous evaluation of technologies for fairness and transparency, as well as efforts to democratize access to innovative solutions. Healthcare organizations must actively involve diverse stakeholder groups, including underserved communities, in the design and implementation of dynamic capabilities. By prioritizing equity and ethical considerations, organizations can ensure that transformation efforts benefit all patients and contribute to broader societal goals. Despite these challenges and paradoxes, the operationalization of dynamic capabilities offers immense potential for healthcare organizations to achieve adaptability, resilience, and innovation. By addressing organizational inertia, balancing short- and long-term priorities, and aligning stakeholder interests, healthcare systems can unlock the transformative power of dynamic capabilities. A deliberate and strategic approach, supported by strong leadership, cultural alignment, and collaborative partnerships, is essential for navigating the complexities of operationalization. Through sustained efforts to overcome these challenges, healthcare organizations can position themselves to thrive in an increasingly dynamic and uncertain environment.

DYNAMIC CAPABILITIES IN GLOBAL HEALTH AND POLICY CONTEXTS

Dynamic capabilities, characterized by the ability to sense opportunities and threats, seize them strategically, and transform organizational structures, extend beyond individual healthcare systems to address global health challenges. In the interconnected world of global health, these capabilities serve as a cornerstone for resilience and adaptability, enabling organizations and governments to respond effectively to crises, drive systemic innovation, and ensure sustainable healthcare delivery. This section delves into the application of dynamic capabilities in global health contexts, focusing on their role in managing global health crises, supporting adaptive policy frameworks, and illustrating their impact through case studies of successful initiatives. The role of dynamic capabilities in responding to global health crises such as pandemics and climate-related health emergencies underscores their transformative potential. Crises of this magnitude test the agility and resilience of healthcare systems, requiring rapid adaptation to unprecedented challenges. The COVID-19 pandemic, for instance, revealed stark differences in the ability of nations and organizations to respond effectively. Countries with strong sensing capabilities—those that could identify emerging threats early through robust surveillance systems and data analytics—were better positioned to mitigate the impact of the virus. Examples include South Korea and Taiwan, where early detection measures and rapid implementation of testing and contact tracing programs were instrumental in controlling the spread of the disease.

Seizing opportunities during a global health crisis involves the rapid mobilization of resources and the implementation of innovative solutions. During COVID-19, this was exemplified by the accelerated development and deployment of vaccines. Governments and pharmaceutical companies demonstrated exceptional seizing capabilities by reallocating resources, streamlining regulatory approvals, and fostering unprecedented levels of collaboration. The establishment of public-private partnerships, such as the COVAX initiative, highlighted the importance of collaborative frameworks in ensuring equitable access to vaccines for low- and middle-income countries. The transformation process—reconfiguring systems to sustain long-term benefits—is perhaps the most challenging aspect of dynamic capabilities in the context of global health crises. Effective transformation requires institutionalizing lessons learned and integrating innovations into standard practices. For instance, the rapid expansion of telehealth services during COVID-19 demonstrated the potential for technology to enhance access to care. However, sustaining this transformation necessitates addressing structural barriers such as digital infrastructure gaps, regulatory hurdles, and workforce training. Countries that embed these changes into their healthcare systems are better equipped to handle future crises and improve overall health outcomes.

Beyond crisis management, dynamic capabilities play a pivotal role in shaping adaptive and sustainable healthcare systems through policy frameworks. Policymaking in global health must address complex and interdependent challenges, from aging populations and chronic disease burdens to health inequities and environmental sustainability. Dynamic capabilities enable policymakers to anticipate emerging trends, engage diverse stakeholders, and implement forward-looking strategies that balance immediate needs with long-term objectives. Adaptive policy frameworks that leverage dynamic capabilities are essential for building resilient healthcare systems. These frameworks prioritize flexibility and responsiveness, allowing for iterative adjustments based on real-time feedback and evolving conditions. For example, climate change poses significant health risks, including the spread of vector-borne diseases, heat-related illnesses, and the displacement of vulnerable populations. Policies that integrate dynamic capabilities into their design can enhance resilience by promoting climate-adaptive healthcare infrastructure, investing in early warning systems, and fostering cross-sector collaboration to address the social determinants of health. The implementation of universal health coverage (UHC) provides another example of how dynamic capabilities inform policy frameworks. Achieving UHC requires balancing affordability, accessibility, and quality while navigating resource constraints and diverse stakeholder interests. Countries such as Thailand and Rwanda have demonstrated strong dynamic capabilities in advancing UHC. Thailand's Universal Coverage Scheme, for instance, leveraged robust sensing capabilities through extensive data collection and analysis to identify population health needs. The program's success in seizing opportunities to expand access and transform service delivery models highlights the importance of dynamic capabilities in achieving equitable and sustainable health outcomes.

Case studies of global health initiatives illustrate the tangible impact of dynamic capabilities on systemic transformation. The Global Polio Eradication Initiative (GPEI) offers a compelling example of dynamic capabilities in action. Over several decades, this initiative has demonstrated exceptional sensing capabilities through surveillance networks that detect and monitor cases of polio worldwide. The ability to seize opportunities is evident in the rapid deployment of vaccination campaigns and innovative strategies such as the use of geographic information systems (GIS) to target underserved populations. The GPEI's transformation efforts include strengthening routine immunization systems and integrating lessons learned into broader public health programs, ensuring that progress toward eradication is sustained. Another notable example is the response to the Ebola outbreak in West Africa between 2014 and 2016. The crisis highlighted significant gaps in global health systems, including delays in recognizing the scale of the outbreak and challenges in coordinating international responses. Despite these initial setbacks, the eventual containment of Ebola demonstrated the power of dynamic capabilities. Sensing capabilities improved as governments and international organizations enhanced disease surveillance systems. Seizing capabilities were evident in the development and deployment of experimental treatments and vaccines under accelerated timelines. Transformative changes included the establishment of the Africa Centres for

Disease Control and Prevention (Africa CDC), which aims to strengthen regional preparedness and response capacities for future outbreaks.

The integration of dynamic capabilities into global health systems requires sustained investment in infrastructure, workforce development, and collaborative governance. Building sensing capabilities at the global level involves enhancing data-sharing mechanisms, standardizing reporting systems, and investing in advanced analytics platforms. For example, the World Health Organization's (WHO) Global Health Observatory provides a platform for collecting and disseminating data on global health indicators, enabling better decision-making and resource allocation. Seizing capabilities at the global level necessitates fostering partnerships that pool resources and expertise across sectors. Initiatives such as the Pandemic Fund, established to support pandemic preparedness and response, illustrate the importance of coordinated funding mechanisms in mobilizing resources effectively. Additionally, the role of technology in seizing opportunities cannot be overstated. Innovations such as mobile health applications, wearable devices, and AI-powered decision support systems offer new avenues for enhancing global health outcomes.

Transforming global health systems to ensure sustainability and resilience requires addressing structural and systemic barriers. This includes strengthening primary healthcare systems, ensuring equitable access to essential medicines and technologies, and aligning global health priorities with broader development goals such as the United Nations SDGs. The integration of dynamic capabilities into these efforts ensures that transformations are both impactful and sustainable. Dynamic capabilities serve as a critical framework for addressing the complexities of global health and policy-making. By enabling healthcare systems and policymakers to sense emerging challenges, seize opportunities for innovation, and transform processes for long-term resilience, dynamic capabilities provide a roadmap for navigating the interconnected and rapidly evolving landscape of global health. Case studies of successful initiatives, from polio eradication to pandemic response, underscore their practical value and potential for driving systemic change. As global health challenges continue to grow in scale and complexity, the integration of dynamic capabilities into policy frameworks and organizational strategies will be essential for building a healthier, more equitable, and sustainable world.

INTEGRATING DYNAMIC CAPABILITIES INTO FUTURE HEALTHCARE MODELS

As healthcare systems evolve in response to technological advancements, demographic shifts, and changing patient expectations, the integration of dynamic capabilities has become essential for ensuring adaptability and sustainability. Dynamic capabilities—the ability to sense opportunities and threats, seize them strategically, and transform organizational structures—offer a framework for navigating the complexities of future healthcare models. This section synthesizes insights from previous discussions to propose a forward-looking vision for dynamic capabilities in healthcare, focusing on future trends, integration strategies, and a roadmap for transitioning to patient-centered, sustainable healthcare systems. The future of healthcare is increasingly shaped by emerging trends such as digital twins, precision medicine, and value-based care. Digital twins—virtual replicas of physical entities—offer transformative potential for healthcare by enabling real-time monitoring, predictive modeling, and personalized interventions. For example, digital twins of individual patients can simulate treatment outcomes based on unique genetic, environmental, and lifestyle factors, empowering clinicians to make data-driven decisions. Sensing capabilities play a critical role in harnessing these innovations, as healthcare organizations must identify relevant technological advancements and their applications in clinical and operational settings. By investing in predictive analytics and advanced monitoring systems, healthcare providers can enhance their ability to detect and respond to emerging trends.

Precision medicine represents another frontier in the evolution of healthcare, emphasizing the customization of treatment based on individual patient characteristics. Dynamic capabilities enable the integration of precision medicine into healthcare systems by fostering collaboration among stakeholders, including researchers, clinicians, and policymakers. Seizing opportunities in this domain requires the development of robust data ecosystems that facilitate the collection, sharing, and analysis of genomic, clinical, and environmental data. For instance, the establishment of biobanks and data-sharing platforms accelerates research and enables the implementation of personalized treatment protocols. Transforming healthcare systems to support precision medicine necessitates the reconfiguration of workflows, training programs, and regulatory frameworks to accommodate its unique demands.

Value-based care, which prioritizes patient outcomes and cost efficiency over service volume, aligns closely with the principles of dynamic capabilities. Healthcare organizations transitioning to value-based care models must adopt strategies that balance immediate operational demands with long-term transformational goals. For example, dynamic capabilities support the shift from fee-for-service reimbursement models to outcomes-based payment structures by enabling organizations to adapt their financial, operational, and clinical processes. Sensing capabilities identify emerging opportunities for improving patient outcomes, such as the use of AI-powered tools to predict disease progression and tailor interventions. Seizing capabilities ensure the effective allocation of resources to implement these tools while transforming capabilities that embed value-based principles into organizational culture and workflows. Integrating dynamic capabilities into future healthcare models requires a holistic approach that addresses organizational, technological, and cultural dimensions. Organizationally, leadership commitment to innovation and adaptability is essential. Leaders must cultivate a culture that embraces change, encourages experimentation, and prioritizes learning from successes and failures. For instance, fostering interdisciplinary collaboration among clinicians, IT specialists, and administrators accelerates the adoption of new technologies and care models. Additionally, establishing governance structures that align transformation initiatives with strategic objectives ensures accountability and coordination across departments.

Technologically, the integration of dynamic capabilities necessitates the adoption of interoperable systems that facilitate seamless data exchange and collaboration. Advanced technologies such as blockchain can further support interoperability by providing secure and transparent mechanisms for data exchange, ensuring trust among stakeholders. By investing in scalable and flexible infrastructure, healthcare organizations can future-proof their systems and adapt to emerging innovations. Culturally, the successful integration of dynamic capabilities hinges on workforce engagement and empowerment. Training programs that enhance technical proficiency, foster interdisciplinary collaboration, and develop leadership skills prepare healthcare professionals to navigate the complexities of future healthcare models. For example, upskilling clinicians in the use of AI-driven decision support tools ensures that they can effectively leverage these technologies to improve patient care. Furthermore, engaging frontline employees in the design and implementation of transformation initiatives fosters a sense of ownership and ensures that solutions are practical and aligned with clinical realities. Recognizing and rewarding contributions to innovation and adaptability reinforces the cultural shift toward embracing dynamic capabilities.

A roadmap for transitioning to integrated, sustainable, and patient-centered healthcare systems provides a structured approach to operationalizing dynamic capabilities. The roadmap begins with an assessment of the current state, identifying gaps in sensing, seizing, and transforming processes. For example, organizations can evaluate their ability to detect emerging health trends, allocate resources effectively, and implement transformative changes. This assessment informs the development of targeted strategies to address identified gaps, such as investing in advanced analytics tools, fostering cross-functional collaboration, and aligning performance metrics with transformational goals.

The next phase of the roadmap focuses on pilot projects that demonstrate the value of dynamic capabilities in specific contexts. For instance, a pilot project may involve the integration of IoT devices into chronic disease management programs, enabling real-time monitoring and personalized interventions. By measuring the outcomes of these initiatives, organizations can generate evidence of their impact and build momentum for broader adoption. Pilot projects also provide opportunities to refine implementation strategies and address unforeseen challenges, ensuring smoother scaling in subsequent phases.

Scaling transformation efforts represents the third phase of the roadmap, emphasizing the replication and expansion of successful initiatives. For example, a healthcare network that achieves positive results with a telehealth pilot project can extend the program to additional specialties and geographic locations. Scaling efforts require robust change management strategies to address resistance and ensure alignment across diverse stakeholder groups. Additionally, continuous monitoring and evaluation ensure that scaling efforts remain aligned with organizational goals and patient needs.

The final phase of the roadmap focuses on sustaining transformation and fostering continuous improvement. Dynamic capabilities are inherently iterative, requiring organizations to adapt to evolving conditions and incorporate feedback into their strategies. For example, healthcare organizations can establish feedback loops that involve patients, providers, and administrators, ensuring that transformation efforts remain responsive to stakeholder needs. Continuous improvement frameworks such as Lean Six Sigma can support this process by identifying opportunities for optimization and fostering a culture of learning and innovation. By addressing emerging trends such as digital twins, precision medicine, and value-based care, healthcare organizations can position themselves at the forefront of innovation. A holistic approach that encompasses organizational, technological, and cultural dimensions ensures that dynamic capabilities are effectively operationalized. The proposed roadmap provides a structured framework for navigating the complexities of transformation, from assessing the current state to sustaining continuous improvement. Through strategic integration of dynamic capabilities, healthcare systems can navigate the challenges of an ever-evolving landscape and deliver meaningful improvements in patient outcomes, efficiency, and equity. The global health and policy contexts further illustrate the transformative potential of dynamic capabilities. Crises such as pandemics and climate-related health emergencies highlight the necessity for healthcare systems to sense emerging threats, seize opportunities for innovation, and transform operations for sustained resilience.

Table 3 delves into the justifications and validations for the roadmap and framework, grounding their development in robust theoretical foundations such as the RBV and systems thinking. Empirical evidence from real-world case studies, including telehealth expansion and vaccine deployment during COVID-19, underscores the practical utility and scalability of the framework. By integrating ethical considerations and inclusivity into the framework, the table reinforces the importance of equity and trust in healthcare transformation. The table underscores how this architecture guides healthcare organizations in achieving integrated, resilient systems through incremental phases of transformation. Leadership, culture, and innovation emerge as pivotal elements in sustaining dynamic transformations. The table calls for collaboration among researchers, practitioners, and policymakers to embed dynamic capabilities into healthcare strategies, ensuring that organizations remain responsive to future challenges and opportunities.

This overview serves as a foundational reference for understanding and applying dynamic capabilities in healthcare. It bridges theoretical insights with practical applications, offering a roadmap for organizations to navigate complexity, drive innovation, and achieve sustainable healthcare transformation.

Table 3. Overview and summary of dynamic capabilities in healthcare

Section	Key Insights	Applications and Implications
Challenges and Paradoxes in Operationalizing Dynamic Capabilities	Dynamic capabilities face barriers such as organizational inertia, resistance to change, and balancing short- and long-term goals.	Strategies to overcome resistance include leadership alignment, phased implementation, and stakeholder engagement.
	Trade-offs arise between stability and agility, requiring a culture that embraces calculated risks.	Operationalizing capabilities helps organizations adapt to technological advancements and public health challenges.
Dynamic Capabilities in Global Health and Policy Contexts	Dynamic capabilities enhance global health crisis management, such as during pandemics and climate-related health emergencies.	Applications include leveraging sensing, seizing, and transforming processes to manage global crises effectively.
	Adaptive policy frameworks are essential for building resilient healthcare systems.	Policies should focus on flexibility, real-time responsiveness, and sustainability goals.
	Case studies like the Global Polio Eradication Initiative and COVID-19 responses highlight the impact of collaborative frameworks.	Provides a blueprint for global and regional healthcare systems to integrate dynamic capabilities.
Integrating Dynamic Capabilities into Future Healthcare Models	Future healthcare trends, such as digital twins, precision medicine, and value-based care, align with dynamic capabilities.	These capabilities foster adaptability, patient-centered care, and technological advancements.
	Leadership, culture, and technological investments are critical for integrating dynamic capabilities into new models.	Scalable, interoperable systems enhance collaboration and data-driven decision-making.

continued on following page

Table 3. Continued

Section	Key Insights	Applications and Implications
Framework for Evaluating Dynamic Capabilities in Healthcare	Evaluation focuses on metrics for sensing, seizing, and transforming processes.	Tools like balanced scorecards and KPIs provide measurable insights into dynamic capabilities' effectiveness.
	Benchmarking enables comparisons with industry standards, identifying performance gaps.	Continuous improvement frameworks support the refinement and optimization of processes.
Justifications and Validations for the Roadmap and Framework	The roadmap is grounded in the dynamic capabilities framework and resource-based view (RBV).	Aligns with systems thinking and performance management methodologies to foster resilience.
	Empirical evidence, such as case studies of telehealth and vaccine deployment, validates its utility.	Demonstrates scalability and flexibility across diverse healthcare contexts.
Overview of Enterprise Architecture Figure	The enterprise architecture transitions through sensing, seizing, and transforming across layers.	Highlights interdependencies between business, application, and technology layers to enable systemic transformation.
	Tracks business, information, and technology changes through incremental phases.	Provides actionable steps for healthcare organizations to achieve integrated, resilient systems.
Conclusion: Rethinking Healthcare Adaptability and Sustainability	Dynamic capabilities offer a framework for driving adaptability, innovation, and resilience.	Encourages researchers, practitioners, and policymakers to embed these capabilities into strategies for modern healthcare.
	Leadership, culture, and innovation are pivotal in sustaining dynamic transformations.	Calls for collaboration among stakeholders to align dynamic capabilities with healthcare's future challenges and opportunities.

CONCLUSION

Dynamic capabilities provide a robust framework for addressing the complexities of modern healthcare, offering a pathway to enhanced adaptability, resilience, and sustainability. By synthesizing insights from organizational theory, global health contexts, and future healthcare trends, this discussion has outlined actionable strategies for integrating dynamic capabilities into healthcare organizations, fostering innovation, and driving systemic transformation. The dynamic capabilities framework, grounded in the ability to sense, seize, and transform, serves as a guiding principle for healthcare systems seeking to remain relevant and effective in a landscape characterized by rapid technological advancements, demographic shifts, and increasing patient expectations. The process of sensing enables organizations to identify emerging opportunities and threats through advanced data analytics, predictive modeling, and proactive stakeholder engagement. Seizing involves the strategic allocation of resources and the implementation of innovative solutions, ensuring that opportunities are effectively capitalized upon. Transforming, the most challenging aspect, requires organizations to reconfigure structures, processes, and cultures to sustain long-term improvements and foster continuous adaptability.

The critical role of leadership in operationalizing dynamic capabilities cannot be overstated. Leaders act as catalysts for change, setting the tone for innovation and adaptability within their organizations. By fostering a culture that values experimentation, collaboration, and continuous learning, leaders enable healthcare systems to overcome resistance, align stakeholder interests, and achieve transformational goals. Effective leadership also ensures that ethical considerations, such as equity, inclusivity, and patient trust, remain central to transformation efforts, reinforcing the social responsibility of healthcare organizations. The challenges and paradoxes associated with operationalizing dynamic capabilities, while significant, are not insurmountable. Organizational inertia, resistance to change, and the tension between short-term operational demands and long-term transformation goals require deliberate and strategic approaches. By adopting phased implementation strategies, leveraging pilot projects to build momentum, and aligning transformation initiatives with measurable outcomes, healthcare organizations can navigate these challenges effectively. The integration of benchmarking tools, continuous improvement frameworks, and collaborative governance structures further supports the successful operationalization of dynamic capabilities.

In the global health and policy context, dynamic capabilities extend beyond individual organizations to address systemic challenges and drive collective action. The ability to sense global health trends, seize opportunities for innovation, and transform policies and practices ensures that healthcare systems remain resilient in the face of crises such as pandemics and climate-related health emergencies. Case studies of global health initiatives, such as the Global Polio Eradication Initiative and the response to the Ebola outbreak, demonstrate the potential of dynamic capabilities to achieve transformative outcomes on a global scale. These examples highlight the importance of collaborative partnerships, adaptive policy frameworks, and sustained investment in infrastructure and workforce development.

Looking toward the future, the integration of dynamic capabilities into emerging healthcare models offers a vision for patient-centered, sustainable, and technologically advanced systems. Trends such as digital twins, precision medicine, and value-based care align closely with the principles of dynamic capabilities, emphasizing the importance of adaptability and innovation. By addressing organizational, technological, and cultural dimensions, healthcare systems can effectively operationalize dynamic capabilities and position themselves at the forefront of innovation. The proposed roadmap for transitioning to integrated and sustainable healthcare systems provides a structured framework for navigating this transformation, ensuring that dynamic capabilities are fully realized.

This chapter concludes with a call to action for researchers, practitioners, and policymakers to embrace dynamic capabilities as a cornerstone of healthcare adaptability and sustainability. For researchers, this involves advancing the theoretical understanding of dynamic capabilities and exploring their applications across diverse healthcare contexts. Practitioners are encouraged to integrate dynamic capabilities into their organizational strategies, leveraging them to drive innovation and improve patient outcomes. Policymakers play a critical role in creating enabling environments for dynamic capabilities, fostering collaboration, and aligning policies with the principles of adaptability and resilience. By rethinking healthcare adaptability and sustainability through the lens of dynamic capabilities, stakeholders can address the pressing challenges of modern healthcare while seizing opportunities for transformative change. The integration of dynamic capabilities into healthcare systems not only enhances their ability to navigate complexity but also ensures that they remain patient-centered, equitable, and forward-looking. In an era of rapid change and uncertainty, dynamic capabilities provide a foundation for building resilient and sustainable healthcare systems that meet the needs of present and future generations.

REFERENCES

Amini, M., & Jahanbakhsh Javid, N. (2023). A multi-perspective framework established on the diffusion of innovation (DOI) theory and technology, organization, and environment (TOE) framework toward supply chain management system based on cloud computing technology for small and medium enterprises. Organization and Environment (TOE) Framework Toward Supply Chain Management System Based on Cloud Computing Technology for Small and Medium Enterprises (January 2023). *International Journal of Information Technology and Innovation Adoption*, *11*, 1217–1234.

Ball, P. (2021). What the COVID-19 pandemic reveals about science, policy, and society. *Interface Focus*, *11*(6), 20210022. DOI: 10.1098/rsfs.2021.0022

Bhattamisra, , Banerjee, P., Gupta, P., Mayuren, J., Patra, S., & Candasamy, M. (2023). Artificial Intelligence in Pharmaceutical and Healthcare Research. *Big Data and Cognitive Computing*, *7*(1), 10. DOI: 10.3390/bdcc7010010

Bouguerra, A., Hughes, M., Cakir, M. S., & Tatoglu, E. (2022). Linking entrepreneurial orientation to environmental collaboration: A stakeholder theory and evidence from multinational companies in an emerging market. *British Journal of Management*.

Cifuentes-Faura, J. (2022). European Union policies and their role in combating climate change over the years. *Air Quality, Atmosphere & Health*, *15*(8), 1–8. DOI: 10.1007/s11869-022-01156-5

Dillard-Wright, J., & Shields-Haas, V. (2021). Nursing with the people: Reimagining futures for nursing. *Advances in Nursing Science*, *44*(3), 195–209. DOI: 10.1097/ANS.0000000000000361

Eager, B., & Brunton, R. (2023). Prompting higher education towards AI-augmented teaching and learning practice. Journal of University Teaching & Learning Practice, 20(5), 02.

Ebrahimi, S., & Bridgelall, R. (2021). A fuzzy Delphi analytic hierarchy model to rank factors influencing public transit mode choice: A case study. *Research in Transportation Business & Management*, *39*, 100496. DOI: 10.1016/j.rtbm.2020.100496

ElBaih, M. (2023). The Role of Privacy Regulations in AI Development (A Discussion of how Privacy Regulations Can Shape the Development of AI). Available at *SSRN* 4589207.

Gebhardt, M., Kopyto, M., Birkel, H., & Hartmann, E. (2022). Industry 4.0 technologies as enablers of collaboration in circular supply chains: A systematic literature review. *International Journal of Production Research*, *60*(23), 6967–6995. DOI: 10.1080/00207543.2021.1999521

Haleem, A., Javaid, M., Singh, R. P., & Suman, R. (2022). Medical 4.0 technologies for healthcare: Features, capabilities, and applications. *Internet of Things and Cyber-Physical Systems*, *2*, 12–30. DOI: 10.1016/j.iotcps.2022.04.001

Jacob, C., Bourke, S., & Heuss, S. (2022). From Testers to Cocreators—the Value of and Approaches to Successful Patient Engagement in the Development of eHealth Solutions: Qualitative Expert Interview Study. *JMIR Human Factors*, *9*(4), e41481. DOI: 10.2196/41481

Jalil, S., Rafi, S., LaToza, T. D., Moran, K., & Lam, W. (2023). Chatgpt and software testing education: Promises & perils. In *2023 IEEE International Conference on Software Testing, Verification and Validation Workshops (ICSTW)* (pp. 4130-4137). IEEE. DOI: 10.1109/ICSTW58534.2023.00078

Javaid, M., Haleem, A., & Singh, R. P. (2023). ChatGPT for healthcare services: An emerging stage for an innovative perspective. BenchCouncil Transactions on Benchmarks. *Standards and Evaluations*, *3*(1), 100105.

Junaid, M., Zhang, Q., Cao, M., & Luqman, A. (2023). Nexus between technology-enabled supply chain dynamic capabilities, integration, resilience, and sustainable performance: An empirical examination of healthcare organizations. *Technological Forecasting and Social Change*, *196*, 122828. DOI: 10.1016/j.techfore.2023.122828

Kant, N., & Anjali, K. (2021). Blockchain Technology: A Strategic Resource. In Blockchain for Healthcare Systems (pp. 1-15). CRC Press. 13

Kaplan, R. M., & Hays, R. D. (2022). Health-related quality of life measurement in public health. *Annual Review of Public Health*, *43*(1), 355–373. DOI: 10.1146/annurev-publhealth-052120-012811

Kasneci, E., Seßler, K., Küchemann, S., Bannert, M., Dementieva, D., Fischer, F., Gasser, U., Groh, G., Günnemann, S., Hüllermeier, E., Krusche, S., Kutyniok, G., Michaeli, T., Nerdel, C., Pfeffer, J., Poquet, O., Sailer, M., Schmidt, A., Seidel, T., & Kasneci, G. (2023). ChatGPT for good? On opportunities and challenges of large language models for education. *Learning and Individual Differences*, *103*, 102274. DOI: 10.1016/j.lindif.2023.102274

Kendzerska, T., Zhu, D. T., Gershon, A. S., Edwards, J. D., Peixoto, C., Robillard, R., & Kendall, C. E. (2021). The effects of the health system response to the COVID-19 pandemic on chronic disease management: A narrative review. *Risk Management and Healthcare Policy*, *14*, 575–584. DOI: 10.2147/RMHP.S293471

Kotcher, J., Maibach, E., Miller, J., Campbell, E., Alqodmani, L., Maiero, M., & Wyns, A. (2021). Views of health professionals on climate change and health: A multinational survey study. *The Lancet. Planetary Health*, *5*(5), e316–e323. DOI: 10.1016/S2542-5196(21)00053-X

Kouba, P., Kohout, P., Haddadi, F., Bushuiev, A., Samusevich, R., Sedlar, J., Damborsky, J., Pluskal, T., Sivic, J., & Mazurenko, S. (2023). Machine Learning-Guided Protein Engineering. *ACS Catalysis*, *13*(21), 13863–13895. DOI: 10.1021/acscatal.3c02743

Kwok, A. O., & Treiblmaier, H. (2023). Blockchain technology as a driver of economic development in small economies: A dynamic capabilities framework. *Journal of Decision Systems*, •••, 1–26.

Masih, E. A. (2022). Feasibility of using QR code for registration & evaluation of training and its ability to increase response rate–The learners' perception. *Nurse Education Today*, *111*, 105305. DOI: 10.1016/j.nedt.2022.105305

Mele, G., Capaldo, G., Secundo, G., & Corvello, V. (2023). Revisiting the idea of knowledge-based dynamic capabilities for digital transformation. *Journal of Knowledge Management*.

Mostafiz, M. I., Musteen, M., Saiyed, A., & Ahsan, M. (2022). COVID-19 and the global value chain: Immediate dynamics and long-term restructuring in the garment industry. *Journal of Business Research*, *139*, 1588–1603. DOI: 10.1016/j.jbusres.2021.10.078

Patil et al. (2022). "Utilization of Artificial Intelligence in Healthcare System, Pharmaceutical Industry & Education". International Journal of Advanced Research in Science, Communication and Technology.

Pereira, R., Bianchi, I. S., & Araújo, V. M. D. S. (2021). Multi-framework implementation of the problem management process. *Форсайт*, *15*(3, 3 (eng)), 94–104. DOI: 10.17323/2500-2597.2021.3.94.104

Pesqueira, A., & Sousa, M. J. (2022). *12 Social Analytics Influencing KOLs Profiling in the Dissemination of Innovations and Scientific Knowledge in the Life Sciences Industry*. Innovations and Social Media Analytics in a Digital Society.

Pesqueira, A., & Sousa, M. J. (2022). Life Sciences Industry Blockchain Value Management, Investments, and Finance Impact Assessment: Global Questionnaire Survey of 1524 Industry Professionals and Executives. In Incorporating AI Technology in the Service Sector (pp. 67-107). Apple Academic Press.

Pesqueira, A. M., Sousa, M., & Pereira, Ruben (2023). Individual dynamic capabilities are influential factors in blockchain technology innovation from hospital settings.

Secinaro, , Calandra, D., Secinaro, A., Muthurangu, V., & Biancone, P. (2021). The role of artificial intelligence in healthcare: A structured literature review. *BMC Medical Informatics and Decision Making*, *21*(1), 125. DOI: 10.1186/s12911-021-01488-9

Shiwlani, A., Khan, M., Sherani, A. M. K., & Qayyum, M. U. (2023). Synergies of AI and Smart Technology: Revolutionizing Cancer Medicine, Vaccine Development, and Patient Care. International Journal of Social. *Humanities and Life Sciences*, *1*(1), 10–18.

Tariq, , Awan, M. J., Alshudukhi, J., Alam, T. M., Alhamazani, K. T., & Meraf, Z. (2022). Software Measurement by Using Artificial Intelligence. *Journal of Nanomaterials*, *2022*(1), 7283171. DOI: 10.1155/2022/7283171

Ullah, H., Manickam, S., Obaidat, M., Laghari, S. U. A., & Uddin, M. (2023). Exploring the Potential of Metaverse Technology in Healthcare: Applications, Challenges, and Future Directions. *IEEE Access : Practical Innovations, Open Solutions*, *11*, 69686–69707. DOI: 10.1109/ACCESS.2023.3286696

Vallentin, A., Thórisson, K. R., & Latapie, H. (2023). Addressing the Unsustainability of Deep Neural Networks with Next-Gen AI. In International Conference on Artificial General Intelligence (pp. 296-306). Cham: Springer Nature Switzerland. DOI: 10.1007/978-3-031-33469-6_30

Vlasta, M. (2023). A methodological framework for European regulation of (artificial) intelligence and its limits.

Wamba, S. F., Queiroz, M. M., Jabbour, C. J. C., & Shi, C. V. (2023). Are both generative AI and ChatGPT game changers for 21st-century operations and supply chain excellence? *International Journal of Production Economics*, *265*, 109015. DOI: 10.1016/j.ijpe.2023.109015

Wani, . (2022). Utilization of Artificial Intelligence in Disease Prevention: Diagnosis, Treatment, and Implications for the Healthcare Workforce. *Health Care*.

Yulianti, T., & Sulistyawati, A. (2021). Enhancing public speaking ability through focus group discussion. [Pendidikan Dan Pengajaran]. *JURNAL PAJAR*, *5*(2), 287–295.

Chapter 12
Collaborative Leadership Effect on Implementing Team-Based Healthcare by Mediation of Inter-Professional Education in the Horn of Africa

Wako Jio
https://orcid.org/0009-0003-6192-459X
Bule Hora University, Ethiopia

Shashi Kant
https://orcid.org/0000-0003-4722-5736
Lovely Professional University, India

ABSTRACT

In this chapter, the researchers focus on the relationship between collaborative leadership and team-based healthcare implementation, while giving special attention to the role of Inter-professional education in the region of Horn of Africa. The research has a sample size of 390 respondents and employs KMO measure of sampling adequacy, confirmatory factor analysis to validate measurement model, and structural equation modeling through AMOS software to test the relationships among the variables: Inter-professional education, collaborative leadership, and team based healthcare implementation. The results demonstrate that the effectiveness of Inter-professional education is significantly improved because of working in collaboration with other professionals which helps to achieve successful implementation

DOI: 10.4018/979-8-3693-2230-7.ch012

of TBHC practices. The analysis emphasizes the role of Inter-professional education as an intermediate variable which links different kinds of leadership approaches with the healthcare results achieved.

INTRODUCTION

Over the last few years, the global perspective of the healthcare world has started to understand the importance of collaborative leadership and teamwork in achieving health goals. As health systems around the world began to integrate, the need for effective leadership that integrated different health care professionals became evident. In this chapter, the emphasis was placed on the role of collaborative leadership (CL) in the implementation of team-based healthcare practices within the African region focusing on the eastern part of Africa which had its own health inequalities and low resource availability (Moyo & Grywalski, 2024).The approach and concepts of collaborative leadership have evolved from the need to resolve complicated issues in healthcare that did not lend themselves to single discipline solutions. Emerging from participative and transformational leadership theories, the approach focused on joint decision-making, good communication, and the joint abilities of the team (Eaton *et al.*, 2024). This paradigm shift represented yet another realization that healthcare could not be delivered through vertical models alone; it required that professionals be combined in a makeup and employed in a manner designed to accomplish specific goals (Forde-Stiegler *et al.,* 2024). Evidence from past scholarship emphasized the positive relationships that exist among collaborative leadership and healthcare outcomes. Studies showed that leaders who fostered joint practices and Inter-professional relationships contributed significantly to the improvement of quality of care and satisfaction of the staff. On the other hand, a lot of the emphasis was placed on research done in the high-income countries and these largely left undeveloped important details on how such leadership models were put in practice in the context of resource poor settings particularly in the Eastern part of Africa where cultural and systemic factors affect their successful application (Stuber *et al.*, 2021).

The application of collaborative leadership practices in the Eastern part of Africa is also met with challenges such as: inadequate resources for conclusive Inter-professional education (IPE), lack of skill and cultural practices that impede healthy teamwork (Forde-Stiegler *et al.,* 2024). Most of the time, healthcare providers worked in soloed units which posed limitations on these providers with regards to inter-unit collaborations. These challenges highlighted the importance of not only the understanding of the barriers but also how leadership can assist in resolving those barriers in order to address the holistic integration of the healthcare system

(Raponi, 2024). Although the principles of CL and IPE were acknowledged, there were still knowledge disparities, in the literature and especially when these aspects interacted in limited-resource environments. To the researcher's great surprise, no previous research comprehensively explored how collaborative leadership might foster Inter-professional education, which is pivotal to improving team-based health care implementation in the Eastern part of Africa (Forde-Stiegler *et al.,* 2024). In this chapter, we have endeavored to address these above-mentioned gaps.

Given the pressing need for effective healthcare delivery in the Eastern part of Africa, this study sought to address the following question: ***"How does collaborative leadership impact the formation of team-centered healthcare delivery using Inter-professional education in this area of study?"*** Through exploring this relationship, the chapter was expected to offer policy implications for healthcare policymakers and practitioners in order to enhance cooperative approach that equally enhances health care services. Hence, this chapter aims at providing a research agenda and a guide for policymakers to understand how leadership could transfigure the delivery and implementation of healthcare in resource-scarce environments.

BACKGROUND OF STUDY

The role of team work in health care leadership has also being widely discussed as health care systems globally become more and more complex and need more interfaced care. Teamwork is as a result enhanced since the notion of collaborative leadership encourages various professionals in the healthcare system to work together. Nevertheless, the following is the overall useful concept that has faced some challenges in its practical application especially in the eastern part of Africa which is a limited resource region (Moyo & Grywalski, 2024). Regarding leadership type, one of the successful case studies published is a case of a rural health clinic in Ethiopia where collaborative leadership was attempted for improving maternal health (Forde-Stiegler *et al.,* 2024). While the initiative was meant to promote improved collaboration among the doctors, nurses and community health workers (CHWs) it was confronted with challenges as soon as it kicked off. Lack of resource as evidenced by insufficient stocks of medical equipment, inadequacy in training on team work among the healthcare providers deterred the healthcare providers from functioning optimally as a team (Moyo & Grywalski, 2024). Finally, other more profound cultural patterns in care organizations that supported bureaucratic structure inhibited the collaborative decision-making process, an aspect of collaborative leadership (Forde-Stiegler *et al.,* 2024). Consequently, the intended enhancements in maternal health were not achieved to the most extent indicating the gap among the conceptual frameworks of shared leadership and actual practice in the developing world (Mumbi & Obembe, 2022).

An example that depicts these challenges is a healthcare program in Somalia to promote collaboration of Inter-professional training of healthcare human resources. However, after completing the program with passing grades in all classes, I faced practical challenges that have no curriculum answer. A variety of healthcare employees never got an opportunity for continual learning and professional development on account of regional challenges in logistics and security risks. Thus there were no supporting structures to complement the teaching and learning of collaborative principles where even if they were taught they could not be implemented. The outcome was that working practices remained compartmentalized; professionals did not work together, doing the actual work on their own and thus negating the program objectives (Raponi, 2024; Moyo & Grywalski, 2024). These examples further bespeak the paramount of context sensitivity when engaging the collaborative leadership for dealing with matters of health care. It points out that while conceptual tools may be helpful; their implementation involves the grappling with down-to-earth local issues such as resources, culture and structures. Such context forms the basis of the current study which seeks to extend the understanding of how collaborative leadership can be realistically pursued in the Eastern part of Africa area as well as the opportunities and challenges inherent in this area of the world (Forde-Stiegler *et al.,* 2024). Consequently, the aim of the research is to identify these best practices from the discussed case studies in order to help future iterations, proposals, and policies on how to support and encourage better cooperation in the healthcare context.

STATEMENT OF PROBLEM

This chapter also identifies the importance of collaborative leadership in healthcare in an attempt to advance team work and health results in methods particularly logistics and limited equipment in the Eastern part of Africa, where this study was conducted (Forde-Stiegler *et al.,* 2024). Perfectly, covenanting leadership would enhance vertical integration of interdisciplinary healthcare workers so that, would enhance patient outcomes and satisfaction, staff satisfaction, and integrated resources utilization. Nevertheless, at the moment the process of the development of health care in this region does not always meet such an ideal (Moyo & Grywalski, 2024). Analyzing the literature, there is a lot of controversy, on the one hand, different authors state that collaborative leadership is effective; on the other hand, concrete research manifested that its implementation does not always lead to positive outcomes. For instance, a few researches manifested that CL enhances HC outcomes, while other researches finds that efforts to adopt CL models to gain these advantages did not yield the desired outcomes. This is an indication of a gap of knowledge that needs to be filled regarding the contextual factors that enhance the use of collaborative leadership (Forde-Stiegler *et al.,* 2024).

Besides, literature reviews reveal that global indexes have not been comprehensively explored, and more investigation is required (Stuber *et al.*, 2021). This lack of clarity produces theoretical deficiencies in the leadership frameworks that do not consider unique cultural, economic, and systemic context of the Eastern part of Africa Region. There continues to be question about the evidence-based ways in which collaborative leadership impacts Inter-professional education and team-based healthcare in these contexts (Raponi, 2024). Other contextual voids thus pose more challenges to the outcome of collaborative leadership. The Eastern part of Africa region is culturally, health wise and socio-economically different and these differences are likely to affect the outcomes of leadership strategies. Organizational constraints which include poor structures, few resources and low consciousness levels in collaboration impede the implementation of collaborative leadership models in healthcare facilities.

In this respect, this study will seek to offer empirical evidence to bridge these gaps with regards to the role of collaborative leadership, inter professional education and team based health care implementation in the Eastern part of Africa. In this manner, the research will present this context's individual strengths and weaknesses, as well as the applied theoretical framework. In addition, it will provide suggestions on how the effective implementation of collaborative leadership can be achieved down to practice level. Thus, this study will be useful to future researchers and policymakers to design relevant interventions to boost collaborative partnerships within the sphere of health care to ensure better health routines in the resource-scarce environments.

THEORETICAL FOUNDATION

Transformational Leadership Theory

Burns and later elaborated by Bernard Bass, the Transformational Leadership Theory pertain to the fact that leaders shall take an active part in transforming subservient followers into exceeding the normal performance threshold and become a better person. In their magnanimity, transformational leaders share common features of coming up with a vision, the provision of trust, and all-embracing cooperation amongst the working party. This theory is very applicable in health care organizations because organizational leaders are faced with multifaceted issues and have to mobilize a diverse workforce (Eaton *et al.*, 2024). Regarding the concept of the article, the transformational leadership together with the collaborative leadership give the understanding of the way that leaders can contribute into collaboration that improves the dynamics of a team and the quality of the patient services (Forde-Stiegler *et al.,* 2024).

Situational Leadership Theory

Situational Leadership Theory brought by Paul Hersey and Ken Blanchard suggests leadership depends on the environment of a business and the preparedness of the followers (Wang *et al.*, 2024). This theory postulates that one type of leadership depends on the organizational member maturity and aptitude, which may call for coaching to authoritative modes. Since some of the teams in healthcare setting may include different degrees of expertise as well as experience, the use of situational leadership come as a virtue through which leaders can effectively understand the ways through which they facilitate the working relationships. Such flexibility is important in the Eastern part of Africa which tends to have variability in the problems faced by healthcare organizations and the culture to the collaborative processes (Wang *et al.*, 2024).

Shared Leadership Theory

As is derived from its name, Shared Leadership Theory is a theory that focuses on assigning leadership roles in a team rather than being invested in a single person (Mumbi & Obembe, 2022). This kind of approach is useful in team practice health; this is because there is interaction of different persons and hence the need for cooperation. In the Eastern part of Africa where structure enhances hierarchy can create major resistance towards change while implementation of shared leadership goals can enhance collaboration among healthcare providers (Mumbi & Obembe, 2022).

Inter-professional Education (IPE) Theory

Inter-professional Education Theory embraces the aspects of sharing education or a similar course among health practitioners of distinct specialization (Kozmenko et al., 2024). Learning with others promotes effective interpersonal communication, cooperation and understanding, in broader sense leading to better patient outcomes. IPE manifested the need to provide student with the education that cannot be officially within the professional silos to work and practice together (Raponi, 2024).

Consequently, the main theoretical framework used for this research is "Transformational Leadership Theory" (Eaton *et al.*, 2024). This choice is informed by the theory postulation of how to encourage individuals within an organization, something especially important in tackling health issues. Leaders engaging in transformational leadership practices are better placed to address the peculiarities of professional practice in the Eastern part of Africa because they can also foster meaning for Inter-professional relations and harmonize a working environment that supports teamwork (Eaton *et al.*, 2024). Applying this theory therefore, the study seeks to examine how NTL can positively influence IPE and ultimately support the successful adoption of TBHC in the region (Patanian, 2024).

Definition and Origin of Terms

Collaborative Leadership

Shared empowering leadership on the other hand is the type of leadership where the leaders participate in the actual working process alongside other workers many of whom are cross disciplinary. It includes decisions with community, communication, along with respect for everyone participating in a team and manifested an environment that will help to develop innovative solutions (Forde-Stiegler *et al.*, 2024). Collaborative leadership appeared at the turn of the latest hundred years as the result of a broad realization of the shortcomings of authoritative leading styles in organizations. Born of the participative and transformational shifts in leadership, collaborative leadership emerged with a nod towards the relational processes through which such organizations might be driven toward success (Forde-Stiegler *et al.*, 2024).

Inter-professional Education (IPE)

Inter-professional Education (IPE) is understood as a process of learning within students from two or more professions under one learning event. The concept of IPE is to practice and teach healthcare professionals in teams to be able to work together successfully and efficiently in practice for the benefit of the patient (Raponi, 2024). The history of IPE can be dated as far as the 1970s when the World Health Organization called for Inter-professional practice. As the complexity of patient care needs and demands for a coordinated distributed care system continues to rise, so did the emphasis on Inter-professional learning. Since the first introduction of IPE in healthcare, it has received accreditation from several professional organizations and academies that encourage integrative learner training (Ogata *et al.*, 2021).

Team-Based Healthcare

Team-based healthcare is a concept that refers to a delivery of healthcare services by teams comprised of several individuals in a healthcare department. This model promotes the use of various skills and views in an organization with an aim of improving the patient experience, efficiency and the general quality of the health sector. Team-based care arose due to the fact that there are no simple solutions to numerous and diverse health problems that people face nowadays. The first attempts to apply the team approach to healthcare provision were made in the middle of the 20th century when it was becoming more and more apparent that different members of the healthcare team must work collaboratively. The change of focus towards the patient-orientated late in the twentieth century further boosted the use of this team-based care because it was realized by various practitioners that the use of a team would improve the health outcomes of a given patient and also would enhance the level of satisfaction of the patients (Patanian, 2024).

Collaborative Practice

Integrated practice involves the manner in which one or more healthcare workers from different disciplines come together to effectively provide care to a patient. It encompasses cooperation and collaboration of patient centered care and interdisciplinary teamwork in the management of patients' needs (Langner & Fukkink, 2023). Collaborative practice emerged as an approach to solving the problems connected with the application of the isolated models of work that dominated the health care industry. It started being developed in the several last years of the twentieth century due to the arising health care advancement projects. The Institute of Medicine (now the National Academy of Medicine) has noted that interdisciplinary practice is an essential element of health care (Langner & Fukkink, 2023).

Collaborative Leadership in Healthcare

While collaborative leadership is a general leadership approach, then collaborative leadership in healthcare means practicing this particular style of leadership solely within the realms of the healthcare industry. This can embrace managers and organizational leaders who champion teamwork in healthcare practitioners, support Inter-professional learning and improve ways of working that bring together healthcare professionals to improve client's care and efficiency of the organization (Moyo & Grywalski, 2024). With the shift in healthcare care systems to embrace team work in the late 1900s and early part of the 21st century, leadership in promoting collaboration assumed the central position towards enhancement of health outcomes. For instance, the crossing of the quality chasm report provided a heads up on the creation of environments that supported collaboration and teamwork as key to leadership (Moyo & Grywalski, 2024).

EMPIRICAL LITERATURE REVIEW

Collaborative Leadership and Team-Based Healthcare (TBHC)

This theory is known as collaborative leadership and has been introduced as an important factor for adoption of TBHC (Moyo & Grywalski, 2024). Studies have shown that shared leadership promotes the values of working in teams, facilitates the interaction among various providers and staff in the health care delivery system and also bolsters the outcomes for clients (Mumbi & Obembe, 2022). For example, a number of research findings suggest that leaders who promote Inter-professional collaboration support improvement in Inter-professional practice resources so they can address the multifaceted issues inherent to TBHC (Patanian, 2024). In addition, findings from the existing literature supporting the implementation of IPE in health care organizations shows an increases in the capacities of the members to perform their roles more effectively within a team (Raponi, 2024). This will be appropriate in areas of the globe such as the Eastern part of Africa where different groups of HLs are likely to encounter system related obstacles like inadequate equipment or restrictions arising from different cultures. A number of researchers posit that there is a positive relationship among the extent of collaborative leadership and the preparedness of the healthcare teams for adoption of TBHC given the understanding that leadership that fosters collaboration enhances voluntary commitment and satisfaction among the team members (Patanian, 2024). Collectively, the literature establishes collaborative leadership as a core component for establishing effective team work approaches in health care as a way of enhancing the delivery of health services and overall patient care (Moyo & Grywalski, 2024).

Collaborative Leadership and Inter-professional Education

Like all previous studies, this research also proves the connection among collaborative leadership and IPE in improving health outcomes (Moyo & Grywalski, 2024). It is important for IPE to thrive because collaborative leadership breeds trust and communication transparency. Leadership that encourages cooperation facilitates exchange of learning among the professions improving competence and proficiencies amongst the various branches of healthcare practice (Raponi, 2024). This result also helps improve the learning process and aligns the healthcare teams to better address associated patient needs. Additionally, IPE has been shown to improve professional attitude or team cohesiveness and enriched perspectives of interdisciplinary patient care when supported by collaborative leadership (Raponi, 2024). Whenever healthcare systems are under pressure primarily due to issues such as scarce resources and diverse cultural worlds, cooperative leadership and IPE are most effective. It has been suggested that the inclusion of collaborative leadership into IPE frameworks can further attest to augmentation of teamwork and therefore advancement of patient care and health service delivery across multiple health systems and organizations (Moyo & Grywalski, 2024).

Inter-professional Education and Implementing Team-Based Healthcare

The findings of the empirical studies reveal that IPE is crucial for effective implementation of TBHC (Patanian, 2024). Multiple studies have found that IPE improves the interaction abilities of healthcare employees and brings cohesiveness to frontline health care teams in terms of understanding role descriptions in general unique health care practicing environment. Moreover, studies reveal that IPE enables health workers to understand the characteristics of the clinical context and manifested them with appropriate skills for collaborating within the TBHC models (Raponi, 2024). More so in areas where health care systems are under stress, as is the case in a limited resource zone, IPE should be incorporated to foster strong health care teams who can optimistically provide comprehensive care. Taken collectively, it was observed from the literature that IPE is a core concept for the creation and continuation of good team-oriented models of health care (Patanian, 2024).

Collaborative Leadership, Team-Based Healthcare and Inter-professional Education

This has led to a focus on exploring and understanding the relationship among collaborative leadership, IPE, and the application of TBHC extensively in empirical work (Patanian, 2024). Research manifested that the concept of 'collaborative leadership' plays a very important role in creating a climate favorable towards the development of IPE which in turn improves cooperation and understanding among the members of the healthcare profession. This is a partnership that is important because as mentioned earlier IPE prepares learners with skills needed to practice in TBHC systems (Raponi, 2024). Published works show that only when collaborative leadership is granted for IPE initiatives do teams act even more cooperatively benefiting patient care and satisfaction. Additionally, evidence indicates that IPE mediates the relationship among collaborative leadership practices and TBHC implementation; enhancing team-based learning and promoting appreciation for each other (Moyo & Grywalski, 2024). Hence there is a synergistic benefit for collaborative leadership and IPE in situations when there is a high level of complexity and less resources; this enhances the ability of multi professional healthcare teams to meet the needs of patients from diverse backgrounds (Moyo & Grywalski, 2024). Overall, the literature underlines an incredible significance of CL and IPE for the advancement and continuity of efficient team-orientation in healthcare (Raponi, 2024).

CONCEPTUAL FRAMEWORK

Figure 1. Conceptual Framework

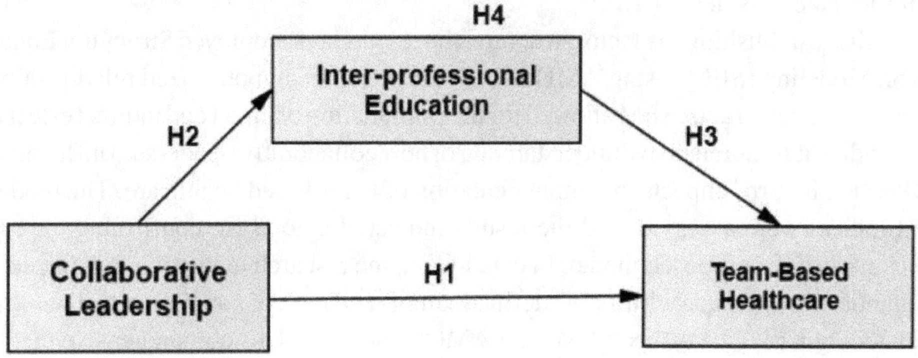

RESEARCH METHODOLOGY

The research methodology employed in this study utilized a quantitative research approach to examine the relationships among collaborative leadership, Inter-professional education (IPE), and the implementation of team-based healthcare. An aggregate of 390 respondents were surveyed for an investigation. The participants in the investigation incorporated a wide spectrum among healthcare professions: 150 health care providers including physicians, nurses, allied health professionals, and administrative staff (38.5%), 120 nursing professionals (30.8%), 80 allied health providers (20.5%), as well as 40 managerial employees (10.3%). The research study was executed across multiple states healthcare institutions in the Eastern part of Africa. The researchers aimed to gather comprehensive data on perceptions of leadership styles, Inter-professional collaboration, and the effectiveness of team-based care practices. To ensure the robustness of the data, a structured questionnaire was developed based on established scales in the literature. The scale development process involved a thorough literature review to identify relevant constructs, followed by item generation and expert validation. The initial pool of items was pre-tested with a small group of healthcare professionals to assess clarity and relevance, leading to refinements before the final administration. Prior to conducting the main analysis, the researchers performed a Kaiser-Meyer-Olkin (KMO) test to evaluate the adequacy of the sample for factor analysis. The KMO value was found to be above the recommended threshold of 0.6, indicating that the sample was suitable for further analysis. Subsequently, Exploratory Factor Analysis (EFA) was conducted to identify the underlying structure of the constructs measured in the questionnaire. The EFA revealed several distinct factors that aligned well with the theoretical constructs of collaborative leadership, IPE, and team-based healthcare, confirming the validity of the scale (Civelek, 2018).

After establishing the factor structure, the researchers employed Structural Equation Modeling (SEM) using AMOS software to test the hypothesized relationships among the constructs. SEM allowed for the examination of direct and indirect effects, providing a comprehensive understanding of how collaborative leadership influences IPE and, in turn, impacts the implementation of team-based healthcare. The model fit indices were assessed, and the results indicated a good fit, confirming the robustness of the proposed model. In conclusion, the research methodology utilized a quantitative approach with a well-defined sample and rigorous analytical techniques, including KMO, EFA, and SEM with AMOS software. This comprehensive methodology enabled the researchers to develop a reliable scale and effectively analyze the relationships among collaborative leadership, Inter-professional education, and team-based healthcare implementation, contributing valuable insights to the field. Although the principles of CL and IPE were acknowledged, there were still knowledge disparities, in the literature and especially when these aspects interacted in limited-resource environments (Civelek, 2018).

Scale Development

The development of the scale for this study was grounded in a comprehensive review of existing literature related to collaborative leadership, Inter-professional education (IPE), and team-based healthcare. The aim was to construct a reliable and valid instrument that effectively captures the key dimensions of these constructs. Initially, the researchers identified relevant theoretical frameworks and empirical studies that delineate the characteristics of collaborative leadership. Key dimensions such as communication, shared decision-making, and trust were extracted from the works of Cummings et al. (2010) and Gittell et al. (2013) cited by Luna et al., (2023), which emphasize the importance of these elements in fostering effective teamwork in healthcare settings. Based on these insights, specific items were crafted to assess each dimension, ensuring that the language used was clear and relevant to healthcare professionals. Similarly, the literature on Inter-professional education provided vital insights for developing the IPE scale. Studies by Reeves et al. (2016) and Thistlethwaite (2012) cited by Akintomide, (2023) highlighted critical components of IPE, including mutual respect, collaborative learning, and understanding of professional roles. These constructs were operationalized into scale items that reflect the attitudes and perceptions of healthcare professionals regarding their Inter-professional interactions and learning experiences. For the team-based healthcare component, the researchers drew from empirical studies that examined the effectiveness of collaborative care models. Items were developed to gauge perceptions of teamwork, communication efficacy, and patient-centered care, as discussed in the research by Patanian, (2024). Each item was designed to measure the degree to which respondents felt their team effectively collaborated in providing comprehensive patient care. To ensure content validity, the initial draft of the scale was reviewed by experts in healthcare leadership and education. Feedback from these experts led to revisions that enhanced clarity and relevance. The final scale comprised multiple items for each construct, employing a Likert-type response format to facilitate quantitative analysis. The constructed scale showed great validity as well as reliability, as proven through significant internal consistency throughout its dimensions. Cronbach's alpha values for collaborative leadership, inter-professional education, as well as team-based healthcare were 0.87, 0.85, along with 0.88, respectively. These findings suggest high internal consistency. Expert evaluations established content validity, although exploratory factor analysis proved construct validity, revealing acceptable item clusters. Furthermore, correlations with existing measures were used to establish convergent and discriminant validity, indicating that the scale accurately reflects the desired features of teamwork, IPE, along with team-based healthcare.

DATA ANALYSIS

Table 1. KMO and Bartlett's test

Kaiser-Meyer-Olkin Measure of Sampling Adequacy.		**.850**
Bartlett's Test of Sphericity	Approx. Chi-Square	1419.738
	Df	91
	Sig.	.000

Source: Authors

The findings of the Bartlett's Test of Sphericity and the Kaiser-Meyer-Olkin (KMO) Measure of Sampling Adequacy, which are crucial for determining if the data is suitable for factor analysis, are shown in Table 1. The reported KMO value of 0.850 is higher than the suggested cutoff of 0.6, indicating that the sample size is sufficient and that there is a significant amount of shared variation among the questionnaire questions. There is a good chance of finding underlying components among the variables, according to this high KMO number. A Chi-Square value of 1419.738 with 91 degrees of freedom and a significance level (Sig.) of 0.000 is also displayed by Bartlett's Test of Sphericity. This outcome supports the data's eligibility for component analysis by confirming that there are substantial correlations among the variables. All things considered, these results offer a strong basis for moving on with exploratory and confirmatory analyses, guaranteeing reliable and significant outcomes in further phases of the study.

Table 2. Total variance explained

Component	Initial Eigenvalues			Extraction Sums of Squared Loadings			Rotation Sums of Squared Loadings		
	Total	% of Variance	Cumulative %	Total	% of Variance	Cumulative %	Total	% of Variance	Cumulative %
1	4.51	32.235	32.235	4.51	32.235	32.235	3.00	21.451	21.451
2	1.37	9.787	42.022	1.37	9.787	42.022	2.16	15.491	36.942
3	1.27	9.087	51.110	1.27	9.087	51.110	1.98	14.168	51.110
4	.949	6.782	57.892						
5	.871	6.223	64.115						
6	.773	5.519	69.634						

Extraction Method: Principal Component Analysis.
Source: Authors

The findings of the Principal Component Analysis's Total Variance Explained are shown in Table 2, which sheds light on the data's underlying structure. Each component's rotation sums of squared loadings, extraction sums of squared loadings, and beginning eigenvalues are listed in the table. A substantial amount of the data in the dataset is captured by the first component, which has an eigenvalue of 4.51 and accounts for 32.235% of the total variance. This component's cumulative percentage of 32.235% indicates that it plays a significant role in explaining the variation of the data. With an eigenvalue of 1.37, the second component adds 9.787% to the overall variance, increasing the cumulative percentage to 42.022%. The eigenvalue of the third component is 1.27, contributing 9.087% to the variance and yielding a total percentage of 51.110%. Their significance in the factor structure is demonstrated by the fact that these three elements collectively account for more than half of the variation. With eigenvalues below 1.0 for the fourth, fifth, and sixth components the fourth at 0.949 the remaining components do not substantially add to the explanation of extra variance. All things considered, the study manifested that the first three factors are the most important for comprehending the data since they account for 51.110% of the variation. This finding supports the notion that a smaller number of factors can effectively represent the underlying constructs, guiding further analysis and interpretation in the research.

Confirmatory Principle Component Examination

Confirmatory principle component examination is a sort of statistics used to verify the principle component arrangement of a group of directed proxies. Research can use CFA to assess hypotheses based on the underlying frame job and correlations among observable proxies. The investigation used CFA under table 3 to assess the hypothesis that there is a relationship among the proxies being guided and the latent notions that support them.

Table 3. Covariances

Covariance			Approximation	S.E.	C.R.	P	Hy.
Inter-professional Education	**<-->**	**Collaborative Leadership**	**.242**	**.021**	**8.231**	***	**H2**
Inter-professional Education	<-->	Implementing Team-Based Healthcare	.303	.032	7.692	***	**H3**
Collaborative Leadership	<-->	Implementing Team-Based Healthcare	.254	.24	7.831	***	**H1**

Source: Authors

The correlation estimates among the dimensions examined in the study are shown in Table 3, emphasizing the connections among Collaborative Leadership, Inter-professional Education, and Implementing Team-Based Healthcare. By demonstrating how much pairs of constructs fluctuate together, the covariances shed light on how they relate to one another. At the $p < 0.001$ level, the correlation among Inter-professional Education and Collaborative Leadership is statistically significant (shown by ***), with a reported value of 0.242, a standard error (S.E.) of 0.021, and a critical ratio (C.R.) of 8.231. This large correlation supports Hypothesis 2 (H2) by indicating that greater Inter-professional education is linked to a significant collaborative leadership. The correlation among Inter-professional Education and Implementing Team-Based Healthcare is also 0.303, with a p-value of less than 0.001 and a statistical significance of 0.032 and 7.692, respectively. This result supports Hypothesis 3 (H3) by showing a strong correlation among lower Implementing Team-Based Healthcare and greater Inter-professional Education.

Last but not least, the correlation among implementing team-based healthcare and collaborative leadership is reported to be 0.254, with a C.R. of 7.831 and a S.E. of 0.24, all of which are significant at the $p < 0.001$ level. This finding supports Hypothesis 1 (H1) by indicating that higher Implementation of Team-Based Healthcare is linked to bigger Collaborative Leadership. Overall, Table 3 effectively illustrates the significant covariances among the constructs, reinforcing the theoretical framework of the study and underscoring the interconnectedness of Inter-professional Education, the Collaborative Leadership, and workplace dynamics.

Table 4. Validity concern

	CR	AVE	MSV	MaxR(H)	CL	IPE	ITBH
CL	0.732	0.643	0.219	0.852	**0.654**		
IPE	0.758	0.657	0.132	0.763	0.171	**0.665**	
ITBH	0.793	0.603	0.274	0.797	0.383	0.193	**0.684**

Note: CL= Collaborative Leadership; IPE= Inter-professional Education; ITBH= Implementing Team-Based Healthcare

Source: Authors

Table 4 shows a comprehensive assessment of the validity concerns related to three constructs: The three foci identified include Collaborative Leadership (CL), and Inter-professional Education (IPE), and Implementing Team Based Healthcare (ITBH). The following table manifested the data and analysis on CR, AVE, MSV, MaxR(H), and the construct inter-correlations. Interpreting all three constructs from the Composite Reliability analysis, they all appear to have acceptable values signifying the overall internal consistency of items in each construct is highly desirable. A result of using this method yields, CL yielded CR of 0.732, IPE registered a CR of 0.758, and ITBH had the best result of a CR of 0.793. These values mean that data measures constructs consistently, so that results of analysis can be trusted. The stability of the measure is also a expressed in AVE, for CL as 0.643, of IPE as 0.657 and of ITBH as 0.603 All the constructs carry a value more than 0.50, which validate the size of the constructs in explaining a considerable proportion of the variance in the respective SERVICEPRO quality indicators, thus justifying the convergent validity criteria.

The Maximum Shared Variance (MSV) values show the proportion of the variance shared with the constructs and is obtained with CL (.219), IPE (.132), and ITBH (.274). These values are all fair, thus lowing discriminant validity, and indicating that the constructs are not the same. Finally, the MaxR(H) for the constructs re-endorses the established reliability with CL at 0.852, IPE at 0.763 and ITBH at 0.797. The correlation coefficient among the constructs as evidenced with the correlation among ITBH and IPE of 0,684 implies a reasonable degree of integration, but with sufficiently high tolerance for independence. Thus, the results of Table 4 show a high reliability and validity of the constructs such as Collaborative Leadership,

Inter-professional Education, and Implementing Team-Based Healthcare, which will allow their further analysis in the framework of the study.

Mediating Role Examination

Figure 2. Structural Equation Model

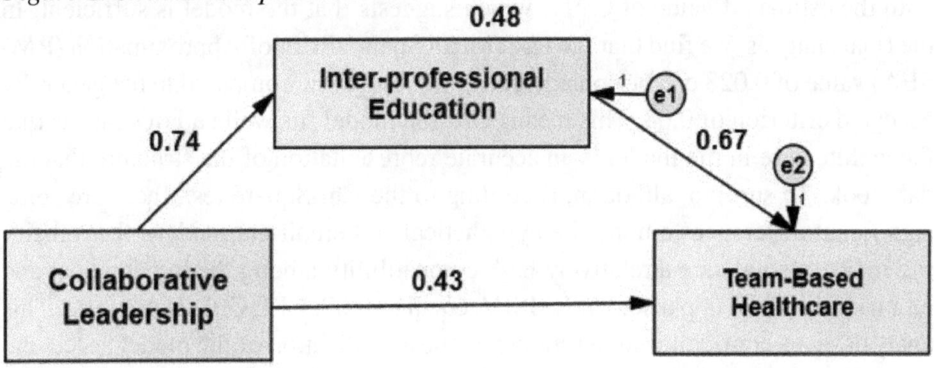

Model Fit Indices

Table 5. Indices for model fit

Sig.	Chi-Sq	RMR	Fitness Goodness	Fitness Confirmatory	TLI	RMSEA
0.004	1.954	.036	0.930	0.912	0.911	.028

Source: Authors

Table 5 manifested the indices found on the confirmatory analysis of the model providing key information to assess the proposed model. The significance value (Sig.) is reported at 0.004, which is less than the accepted level of 0.05 so the chi-square test statistic is significant, there is good evidence to believe that the model does not fit the data perfectly. But this is not to say a strange occurrence in social scientific research, as the models themselves could be developed as complicated ones. The Chi-Square has a value of 1.954, which is certainly significant although it does not paint the full picture of how well for the purpose of evaluation a given model performs. The Root Mean Square Residual (RMR) is showed 0.036, which is it is less than 0.1 so it manifested low Residual variance level which ascertains the fitness of the observed and the predicted value.

The measure of Absolute Fit is summarized by the Goodness of Fit Index (GFI) which stands a value of 0.930 and the Comparative Fit Index (CFI) reported to be 0.912. Each value is superior to 0.90 which is the standard cut off for maximized data fit in analyzing a model method. The Tucker–Lewis Index (TLI) is also high with the estimated value of 0.911, which suggests that the model is sufficient. In the final analysis, we find that the Root Mean Square Error of Approximation (RMSEA) value of 0.028 can be considered significantly low compared to the generally accepted criterion of 0.08. This means OX: the model fits well and this means that the architecture in the model is an accurate representation of the structure that the data took. To sum up, although, according to the Chi-Square test, there are some significant differences among the hypothetical and empirical models, the remaining indicators indicate a relatively high compatibility among the hypothetical and empirical models; in particular, RMSEA equal to 0.07, GFI, CFI, TLI = 0.92. This analysis gives confidence in the study and the actualization of the model tested and the ability of the model in capturing the right research relationships of the constructs.

Table 6. Regression examination

Relative			**Approx.**	**S.E.**	**C.R.**	**P**	**Ass.**
Inter-professional Education	**<---**	**Collaborative Leadership**	**.864**	**.143**	**7.583**	*******	**H2**
Implementing Team-Based Healthcare	<---	Inter-professional Education	.328	.131	2.853	***	H3
Implementing Team-Based Healthcare	<---	Collaborative Leadership	.957	.192	7.958	***	H1

Source: Authors

Table 6 shows cross tabulation, regression examination and correlation findings among the constructs of Collaborative Leadership (CL), Inter-professional Education (IPE) and Implementing Team-Based Healthcare (ITBH). The regression coefficients give the nature and the extent of these associations as well as the level of significance. The regression analysis establishes Inter-professional Education as strongly predictable by the Collaborative Leadership following coefficient = 0.864, S.E. = 0.143, C.R. = 7.583 along with $p < 0.001$ level, along with their statistical significance. The regression analysis manifested a strong relationship where Inter-professional Education is predicted by the Collaborative Leadership, with a coefficient of 0.864, a standard error (S.E.) of 0.143, and a critical ratio (C.R.) of 7.583, which is statistically significant at the $p < 0.001$ level (indicated by ***). In line with Hypothesis 2 (H2) formulated in this study, there is an increase in the value of the Inter-professional Education as the size of Collaborative Leadership is increased. The second regression path manifested that Inter-professional Education affects Implementing Team-Based Healthcare with a coefficient of 0.328, S.E. equal to 0.131 and C.R. of 2.853 which is also using the value smaller than 0.001.(ITBH). The regression coefficients indicate the strength and direction of these relationships, along with their statistical significance. The regression analysis manifested a strong relationship where Inter-professional Education is predicted by the Collaborative Leadership, with a coefficient of 0.864, a standard error (S.E.) of 0.143, and a critical ratio (C.R.) of 7.583, which is statistically significant at the $p < 0.001$ level (indicated by ***). This finding supports Hypothesis 2 (H2), suggesting that a larger Collaborative Leadership is associated with higher Inter-professional Education. In the second regression path, Implementing Team-Based Healthcare is influenced by Inter-professional Education, with a coefficient of 0.328, an S.E. of 0.131, and a C.R. of 2.853, also significant at the $p < 0.001$ level. This validates H3, which posited a negative relationship among advance in Inter-professional Education and the undertaking of Implementing Team-Based Healthcare. The third path demonstrates that Implementing Team-Based Healthcare is also significantly predicted by the Collaborative Leadership with coefficients of 0.957, S.E., 0.192, and C.R., 7.958, which is also significant on the $p < 0.001$ level. Regression coefficients indicate the strength and direction of these relationships, along with their statistical significance. The regression analysis manifested a strong relationship where Inter-professional Education is predicted by the Collaborative Leadership, with a coefficient of 0.864, a standard error (S.E.) of 0.143, and a critical ratio (C.R.) of 7.583, which is statistically significant at the $p < 0.001$ level (indicated by ***).

This finding supports Hypothesis 2 (H2), suggesting that a larger Collaborative Leadership is associated with higher Inter-professional Education. In the second regression path, Implementing Team-Based Healthcare is influenced by Inter-professional Education, with a coefficient of 0.328, an S.E. of 0.131, and a C.R. of 2.853, also significant at the $p < 0.001$ level. This result confirms Hypothesis 3 (H3), indicating that improvements in Inter-professional Education are linked to a reduction in Implementing Team-Based Healthcare. The third path manifested that Implementing Team-Based Healthcare is also significantly predicted by the Collaborative Leadership, with a coefficient of 0.957, an S.E. of 0.192, and a C.R. of 7.958, again significant at the $p < 0.001$ level. Thus, the results substantiated the first hypothesis (H1) asserting that the level of Implementing Team-Based Healthcare increases as the level of Collaborative Leadership is higher. In summary, the results presented in Table 6 demonstrate the research hypotheses and show that improvements in the Collaborative Leadership could result in positive change in Inter-professional Education, as well as a decrease in Implementing Team-Based Healthcare. The high levels of internal consistency in the stated measures and significance of the coefficients signal the interdependence of these phenomenon's in the organizational milieu.

Table 7. Mediating role effect

	Influence	Worth	Path Influence
Collaborative Leadership → Implementing Team-Based Healthcare	Direct Influence	.43	Direct influence stated
Collaborative Leadership → Inter-professional Education → Implementing Team-Based Healthcare	Indirect Influence	.74*.67=.48	Indirect Influence Ensued
	Whole influence	.91	Partial mediation

Source: Authors

Table 7 manifested how IPE is a mediator in the relationship among CL and ITBH. The table presents both straight effect and mediating effects thus giving a broad feature of how the constructs interrelate. Collaborative Leadership has a degree of 0.43 with Implementing Team-Based Healthcare which manifested the strength of positive relationship. This indicates that efficient collaborative leadership fully promotes the delivery of team-based health care practices, but highlighting leadership factors that enable healthcare convergence as key. Hence, beside the direct impact on the CL, the table also demonstrates the Indirect Effect of CL through IPL. The calculated indirect influence is derived by multiplying CL influence that is 0.74 on IPE by 0.67 influence of IPE on ITBH that gives 0.48. This finding suggests that Collaborative Leadership also has a positive impact on Implementing Team-Based Healthcare through Inter-professional Education in order to improve team implementations. The partial total effect of Collaborative Leadership through Implementing Team-Based Healthcare is 0.91. Partial mediation means that IPE still mediates among CL and ITBH at the same time CL has a direct impact. Therefore, the general message of Table 7 is to stress the complex relationship among Collaborative Leadership, Inter-professional Education and Implementing Team-Based Healthcare – Leadership plays a crucial role in supporting educational endeavors that in the long run improve the state of health care. This implies that there is potential for high return on investments in measures that could facilitate collaborative leadership.

DISCUSSION

The findings from this study unpack Collaborative Leadership (CL), Interprofessional Education (IPE), and Implementing Team-Based Healthcare (ITBH). More importantly, the causal quantitative estimate of CL on ITBH is established to be 0.43, suggesting that efficient CL is fundamental to promoting team-work oriented practices in the healthcare organization setting. This means that leaders who encourage more Inter-professional cooperation can greatly improve the effectiveness of combined health systems that are crucial for patients' quality of care and organization's organizational performance. Leadership goes beyond facilitating teamwork but also encourages teamwork and promotes the required values and beliefs in a health facility.

Also, the indirect effect of CL on the development of IPE programs as mediated by IPE is statistically significant showing a path influence of 0.48. In encouraging Inter-professional relationships, leaders foster the conditions under which members of diverse professions can learn and collaborate more efficiently. It is through such Practice Learning partnerships that competencies required for team-based health care provision are fostered and enhanced thus enhancing service delivery and patient outcomes. The total influence value of 0.91 indicates a high endogeneity suggesting that both direct and indirect effects are critical in explaining the transmission of leadership dynamics on health care practices. It is suggested that "Partial mediation" means that IPE heavily mediates the relationship among CL and ITBH but still, CL has a direct impact on ITBH. This research underscores the importance of what needs to be done to address the leadership issue to bring improvement to support collaborative leadership not only within Inter-professional education but also for the entire implementation of team-based healthcare.

CONCLUSION

Thus, the present research insists on the significance of CL for the development of efficient IPE and the implementation of ITBH. The implication of the study is that CL not only has a direct effect on the ITBH but also promotes the context for IPE and subsequent improvement in team-based practices. The overall value of the total influence score of 0.91 emphasizes the complexity of the reported constructs and points to both first order and second order effects of leadership on healthcare outcomes. Moreover, the use of the term "Partial mediation" means that, although IPE plays the role of mediator in the relationship among CL and ITBH, CL still exercise considerable direct impact. This underlines the need for healthcare organizations to consider investing in collaborative leadership competencies among their leaders because such investment will result in significantly enhanced healthcare solutions and general efficiency. Finally, the findings of this study provide notable recommendations for policymakers and healthcare managers to improve healthcare services. Socially, healthcare facilities are in a position to create conditions which promote collaboration and facilitate Inter-professional practice to generate a hard working team qualified to render patients quality care. As the healthcare environment is dynamic in the coming decade, it will be compulsory to focus on Collaborative Leadership to advance innovations and implement new team-based healthcare.

MANAGERIAL IMPLICATIONS

The implications of the finding of this study can be summarized in the following section as follows which has several implications for managers and hence superior healthcare delivery. First of all, the improvement of CL within healthcare organizations' management teams should become a major concern. Leaders should be trained in leadership practices that support IPE and ITBH as this is an indication that implementing team-based care practices will require new knowledge and different behavior from leaders who manage practice environments. Also, one of the practical steps that managers should emphasize as a strategic management activity is the support of IPE because of its positive impact on the teams. Such an approach enables training of healthcare workers from different professions to come together and be part of multispectral learning – an aspect that will enhance the workforce integration goals thus enhancing the overall patient care and organization system. This also helps to develop skills of each member of the academic medical team and fosters a culture of team-work that is central towards delivering healthcare in team-based systems. Furthermore, as mentioned earlier, more frequent self-motivation of the managers is important along with the constant assessment and review of their leadership approaches and educational processes to adjust them to the context of the developing healthcare environment. The usage of leadership performance feedback tools such as questionnaires or discussion forums can make it easier to evaluate the functionality of leadership practices and cross-disciplinary plans.

PRACTICAL IMPLICATIONS

The implications of the study are practical in that it manifested areas whereby healthcare organizations can extend improvements in their service delivery through increased focus on teamwork and leadership. To begin with, organizations ought to launch programs that facilitate acquisition of Collaborative Leadership competency by managers, leaders of teams and other upper stratified organizational members. Such programs should therefore center on ways of enhancing communication, conflict management, and collaborative decision making to enable leaders to support team-based practices. Also, healthcare institutions should consider priority promotion and development of Inter-professional Education (IPE). Through creating opportunities for collaborative learning in workshops and joint training exercises, collaborative competencies can be developed among individuals in organizations. This would also serve to demystify inter-professional barriers so that tutors and teams are better equipped to practice in these environments to the benefit of the patient. In addition, organizations should establish formal working protocols among different health disciplines on a continued basis. Maybe, the collaboration can be carried out on the basis of interdisciplinary meetings and joint projects to discuss further the existing issues and strengthen the trust among the members. The kind of actions embraced engenders culture of mutual ownership and hence problem solving, which are central tenets of well-coordinated team care. Finally, the management needs to set up indicators for evaluating the impact of leadership practices and Inter-professional work. When data on effectiveness of teams, success of particular treatments, and employee satisfaction rates are gathered and analyzed, organizations stand the chance of determining what changes may be made to the process in order to enhance its success. The use of evidence-based approach for healthcare organizations will help ensure that organizations can adapt to the dynamics of the market.

THEORETICAL IMPLICATIONS

The implication of the research findings of this study to the theoretical frameworks of leadership and healthcare management departments is crucial. To begin with, the proven link among Collaborative Leadership (CL) and the features of Implementing Team-Based Healthcare (ITBH) suggests that the primary conceptual underpinning of the presented model is the belief that leadership is a vital prerequisite for team effectiveness in the context of healthcare. This affirms existing theories, which suggest that leadership plays a critical role in creating and managing organizational cultures as well as in the synthesis of the various professional groups within an organization. Secondly, the great extent of the indirect impact of CL through Inter-professional Education (IPE) opens up a new perspective for the analysis of how educational contexts can act as mediators of leadership effects on the delivery of healthcare. This suggests that theories of Inter-professional collaboration should consider leadership dynamics as a core component when attempting to explain educational outcomes and how specific teams perform at their best. Through focusing on leadership and education as the two concepts under consideration, this study calls for the further investigation of the nature of the relationship among these variables with a view to enhancing teamwork and healthcare delivery. Further, the "Partial mediation" concluded in the study also raises conflict with the kind of models that were conventionally used for either direct or indirect effects alone.

RECOMMENDATIONS

In light of the discoveries of this research, the following suggestions can be made for healthcare organizations that want to improve their leadership and teamwork. First, in order for organizations to advance CL, leaders need to embrace the Collaborative Leadership competencies. This can be achieved by conducting training that targets developing skills in the area of communication, conflict resolution and decision making. Such training should also be fostered so that leaders can in turn create a positive organizational culture that supports teamwork and increases organizational performance. In addition, healthcare institutions should adopt Inter-professional Education (IPE). Providing occasions where interdisciplinary teams of healthcare specialists may study together allows organizations to foster improved relations in the field. This can involve collaboration of training sessions, and undertakings of cross disciplinary group projects, which provide an opportunity for the professionals to do the job in simulated environments, and this makes them update their teamwork skills as they serve the patients.

Furthermore, management should implement regular opportunities for inter-disciplinary cooperation among representatives of different healthcare specialties. Interdisciplinary conferences and jointly solved tasks should allow members of the team to discuss freely and form strong and trustful collaboration relations. It should be stated that with encouraging the concept of mutuality and shared accountability, organizations can guarantee that target teams will possess adequate tools to address multifaceted healthcare issues safely. Finally, it is the responsibility of management in organizations to provide rigorous measuring tools to evaluate the dynamics in leadership practices and Inter-professional endeavors. Through proper collection and evaluation of data regarding team performance, patients' status and other stakeholders' attitudes towards work, an organization can establish directions of further development. Assessing these utility mechanisms continuously will assist organizations to adapt to change effectively in their healthcare environment.

FUTURE DIRECTIONS

The results of this research provide direction on how future studies in leadership, Inter-professional education, and team-based health care can be conducted. One of the aforementioned directions is the identification of certain leadership approaches to improve the outcomes of CL in healthcare environments. It may be helpful for future research to explore further how teams under transformational or adaptive leaders perform, to get a deeper perception of the leadership effect in healthcare collaboration. Furthermore, it is also important that researchers assess the effects of

IPE processes that are taking a long time before we embark on more formal impacts on multi professional team efficiency and patient care effects. Future research could also establish the kind of environment that results from sustained IPE practice over time and the impact of the practices on healthcare delivery systems. It would be useful for finding out the ways of optimal integration of IPE into curriculum and studying its efficiency measures. Furthermore, the relationship among the Organizational Culture and the Collaborative Leadership needs to establish stronger ties. Organizational culture maybe another factor that determines the extent of implementation and effectiveness of collaborative processes as used in healthcare organizations; Knowledge of how a variety of organizational cultures may impact on the extent of successful implementation of collaborative practices in healthcare organizations may offer clues about how other organizations could prepare organizational culture in support of team work. It may therefore result in developmental of specific interventions suited trying to create an appropriate culture that promotes collaboration. Lastly, directional implications for future research will be based on the contribution of technology to the development of Collaborative Leadership and IPE. As technology and tele-health continues to augment the modality of healthcare delivery, it would be valuable to understand how the same technologies can be employed in the training and coordination of healthcare workers. Examining the possibility of technology in connecting the Inter-professional collaboration gaps may thus trigger enhanced team practice outcomes.

REFERENCES

Akintomide, O. (2023). *Valued Strategies in the Development and Implementation of Inter-professional Education Placements*. The University of Western Ontario.

Civelek, M. E. (2018). Essentials of Structural Equation Modeling. In *Zea Books*. Issue March., DOI: 10.13014/K2SJ1HR5

Eaton, L., Bridgman, T., & Cummings, S. (2024). Advancing the democratization of work: A new intellectual history of transformational leadership theory. *Leadership*, *20*(3), 125–143. DOI: 10.1177/17427150241232705

Forde-Stiegler, C. T., Immendorf, M. C., & Cady, S. H. (2024). Using collaborative leadership at all levels to build people-oriented organizations. In *Cases on Critical Leadership Skills* (pp. 144–152). Edward Elgar Publishing. DOI: 10.4337/9781035311866.00033

Kozmenko MD, V., Jackson MD, C., Blaseg MSIV, N., Beard MD, M., Leann, T., Kupershmidt PhD, S., Lucas Molitor, W., Taggart Pharm, D., BCCCP, K., & de la Torre-Montero, R. N. (2024). Development and implementation of an Inter-professional education (IPE) curriculum: theory and practice. *Aesculapius Journal (Health Sciences & Medicine), 5*(1), 7.

Langner, J., & Fukkink, R. G. (2023). A realist synthesis of Inter-professional collaborative practices in early intervention for children with speech, language and communication needs. *International Journal of Language & Communication Disorders*, *58*(2), 516–541. DOI: 10.1111/1460-6984.12789 PMID: 36217271

Luna, G., Kim, M., Miller, R., Parekh, P., Kim, E. S., Park, S. Y., Abdulbaseer, U., Gonzalez, C., & Stiehl, E. (2023). Inter-professional relationships and their impact on resident hospitalizations in nursing homes: A qualitative study. *Applied Nursing Research*, *74*, 151747. DOI: 10.1016/j.apnr.2023.151747 PMID: 38007247

Moyo, M., & Grywalski, M. (2024). Dynamic duo: The transformative impact of collaborative leadership on nurse turnover. *Nursing Management*, *55*(4), 40–46. DOI: 10.1097/nmg.0000000000000115 PMID: 38557750

Mumbi, H., & Obembe, D. (2022). Shared leadership in voluntary sector organisations: Exploring practice and theory development. *Voluntary Sector Review*, *13*(2), 226–242. DOI: 10.1332/204080521X16171406823270

Ogata, M. N., da Silva, J. A. M., Peduzzi, M., Costa, M. V., Fortuna, C. M., & Feliciano, A. B. (2021). Interfaces among permanent education and Inter-professional education in health. *Revista da Escola de Enfermagem da USP*, *55*, e03733. DOI: 10.1590/s1980-220x2020018903733 PMID: 34105683

Patanian, M. (2024). Sharing results from the field—implementing team-based care: Examples of practice-based evidence from recipients of CDC's heart disease and stroke prevention funding. [). LWW.]. *Journal of Public Health Management and Practice*, *30*, S101–S103. DOI: 10.1097/PHH.0000000000002015 PMID: 39041742

Raponi, J.-M. (2024). *A Multi-Method Qualitative Analysis of a Clinical Inter-professional Education Experience for Third-Year Dental Students*. University of Florida.

Stuber, F., Seifried-Dübon, T., Rieger, M. A., Gündel, H., Ruhle, S., Zipfel, S., & Junne, F. (2021). The effectiveness of health-oriented leadership interventions for the improvement of mental health of employees in the health care sector: A systematic review. *International Archives of Occupational and Environmental Health*, *94*(2), 203–220. DOI: 10.1007/s00420-020-01583-w PMID: 33011902

Wang, X., Liu, Y., Peng, Z., Li, B., Liang, Q., Liao, S., & Liu, M. (2024). Situational leadership theory in nursing management: A scoping review. *BMC Nursing*, *23*(1), 930. DOI: 10.1186/s12912-024-02582-9 PMID: 39702117

KEY TERMS AND DEFINITIONS

Collaborative Leadership (CL): The management-associated model that coordinates people in an organization by encouraging them to work together to attain set goals and improve healthcare organizational success (Moyo & Grywalski, 2024).

Communication Skills: Skills necessary to share information as well as to perceive it, non-verbal communication skills as a member of a healthcare team, listening, conflict solving in a team.

Evidence-Based Practice (EBP): An Inter-professional collaborative model to individual and team decision making in healthcare with the aim of improving client status and healthcare utility.

Inter-professional Education (IPE): An approach of integrated teaching where students of different health care field studies together presumably to enable future professionals to understand one another facilitate collaborative functioning in health care delivery system (Raponi, 2024).

Organizational Culture: System of established principles which define the behavior of people within the organization, the way work is performed and relations that concern a healthcare organization.

Team-Based Healthcare (TBH): A system where patients get cared for by a team of healthcare professionals from different fields in order to balanced combine each of their specialties (Patanian, 2024).

Transformational Leadership: A way of leading people and engaging them to the highest levels of performance and to unexpected levels by embracing creativity and positive organizational development (Eaton et al., 2024).

Chapter 13
The Future of Interprofessional Collaboration

Dawn Prentice
Brock University, Canada

ABSTRACT

In this chapter the author's vision of the future of interprofessional collaborative care is presented. The facilitators and barriers to ensuring the success of interprofessional collaborative care are discussed. Additionally, the important impact of leadership commitment of both healthcare institutions and educational institutions to the future success of interprofessional collaboration is also addressed. Finally, the influence of artificial intelligence on interprofessional care teams is also considered.

INTRODUCTION

Predicting the future is a daunting task because of all the unknown factors that could affect the expected trajectory and change the course of a direction. In this chapter I focus the discussion on what I imagine the future of interprofessional collaborative practice may look like.

Although Interprofessional Collaboration (IPC) has been mentioned in the literature for the past 20 years not all healthcare students graduate with IPC competencies nor do all healthcare settings utilize a true interprofessional collaborative approach. In my vision of the future of IPC all healthcare practitioners, will have achieved interprofessional competencies as pre-licensure students prior to starting their careers in the workplace. By having this preparation prior to starting their careers this will ensure that all healthcare practitioners will be well versed in IPC and committed

DOI: 10.4018/979-8-3693-2230-7.ch013

to achieving interprofessional collaborative care in their workplaces. Moreover, the major goals of interprofessional collaborative care will also be achieved. All team members will understand, respect and value each others' roles on the team. Additionally, all team members will be comfortable speaking out when they are not clear about a patient treatment plan or have a conflict with another team member. Healthy conflict resolution will become one of the norms for a well-functioning team.

Interprofessional Collaborative Care will be considered best practice for organizations committed to patient-centred care and demonstrate this commitment by listing interprofessional collaboration as a focus in their organization's mission and vision. To ensure this commitment to interprofessional collaborative care, healthcare organizations will provide supportive environments in their organizations to ensure sustainability of interprofessional collaborative care by providing orientation and onboarding programs to all new employees on the importance of IPC and how IPC aligns with best practice and the mission and vision of the organization. The onboarding may include didactic lectures as well as team simulations so that all new employees can understand how IPC functions in the workplace setting. Healthcare organizations will also provide resources and protected time on an ongoing basis to assist with team development and enable the teams to get to know each team member and grow as a team. Healthcare organizations will include participation in interprofessional collaboration as a key element when conducting performance reviews with all employees (Registered Nurses Association of Ontario, 2013). Achievement of these facilitators of interprofessional collaborative care will contribute to achieving an environment of patient-centred care and a focus on achieving excellent patient outcomes.

In my view of the future of IPC, educational institutions with prelicensure healthcare programs will prioritize interprofessional collaborative care competencies in their curricula. Educational institutions will provide sufficient resources to ensure all students are well-grounded in IPC. Additionally, schools that educate interprofessional healthcare students will provide different modalities of teaching and learning of IPC across the curriculum such as lectures, simulations and opportunities in clinical practicums for students to learn, understand and practice IPC in a safe setting, to ensure that students will be competent when they graduate and transition to the clinical setting.

INTERPROFESSIONAL CARE OUTCOMES

In the future, research findings will clearly show the impact of interprofessional collaboration. The positive outcomes of IPC will be demonstrated by a significant decrease in errors, and harm reduction that is attributable to IPC. Staff satisfaction surveys and retention data reports will be favourable due to the impact of working on effective interprofessional teams. Finally, and most importantly, patient satisfaction scores will increase and will demonstrate a direct correlation to the interprofessional collaboration among team members.

THE REALITIES OF INTERPROFESSIONAL COLLABORATIVE CARE

Despite my utopian view of the future of interprofessional collaborative care I must present the realities and challenges to making IPC a global reality in all healthcare settings. Presently we do not know how artificial intelligence (AI) will impact on teams and decision-making in the hospital setting. With the fast-paced changes in technology and acceptance of AI use in the clinical setting, it is not clear if algorithms for care will replace or alter team decision-making as we currently know it. The use of AI may influence a team's decision-making and the overall team process. Currently AI is used in predicting outcomes in radiology (Bera et al., 2002), used to examine the effectiveness in finding clinical deterioration (Gallo et al., 2024) and to benefit care in older adults (Shiwani et al., 2023). Furthermore, there is a possibility that robots may be used more in the healthcare setting in the future and the impact on teams, team culture and communication in care will also need to be considered (Sangseok & Robert, 2023).

The global healthcare workforce shortage (Boniol et al., 2022; World Health Organization, 2024) is already affecting healthcare resources, but with the turnover in healthcare staff we do not know the impact on team formation and team members having the time to become acquainted, learn about each other's roles and develop trust in their colleagues. Furthermore, with the shortage of healthcare workers and the emphasis on maximizing time with patients, there may be a shift to having more team meetings conducted virtually, and we do not know how this will affect team development and in turn, interprofessional collaborative care.

COST CONSTRAINTS

Another reality in the practice setting that must be considered is cost constraints. Sustaining IPC in the practice setting and providing resources and time for team development is a concern. Providing IPC training for onboarding/orientation for all new employees comes at a cost especially if using intensive educational methods such as simulation. In their overall budget strategy, leaders of healthcare organizations must be committed to IPC and allocate funds to financially support IPC initiatives in the workplace.

REALTIES IN THE EDUCATION SECTOR

The curriculum in pre-licensure healthcare professional programs is rife with competing elements that need to be included, and as patient care continues to evolve, and new technology and treatments are developed there will be a need to include this information in the curriculum. I am not convinced that IPC competencies are prioritized in all pre-licensure healthcare professional program curricula, nor is the amount of IPC content being measured. There needs to be consistency in IPC curriculum across academic programs. The content provided to medical students on IPC should be the same as is provided to nursing students. However, it is not, and a major challenge will be having all pre-licensure healthcare professional programs in agreement on the amount and type of IPC content in their respective curriculums and approach to teaching IPC.

Research outcomes that clearly demonstrate the effectiveness of interprofessional care and interprofessional education is it at best mixed. There has been some criticism of the types of studies conducted and published about the benefits of interprofessional collaboration and interprofessional education (Reeves et al., 2018a; Reeves et al., 2018b). In order to ensure adoption of IPC globally the research needs to be clear and fulsome to show the links between IPC and patient outcomes and interprofessional education and learners.

CONCLUSION

In order for IPC to flourish in both academic and healthcare organizations the leaders of these organizations will need to continue to believe in the value of IPC and interprofessional education and provide strategic direction. Furthermore, these leaders must model interprofessional collaboration for their employees and their students. Financial resources must be designated to support IPC initiatives and there will need to be faculty to teach IPC in pre-licensure programs. Ideally there will be agreement of all professions in what IPC content is taught across the curriculum.

When all the barriers have been addressed and the facilitators to IPC are in place, then we will truly see the implementation of interprofessional education in all health care professional schools and interprofessional collaborative care in all healthcare organizations.

REFERENCES

Bera, L., Braman, N., Gupta, A., Velcheti, V., & Madabhushi, A. (2002). Predicting cancer outcomes with radiomics and artificial intelligence in radiology. *Nature Reviews. Clinical Oncology*, *19*(2), 132–146. DOI: 10.1038/s41571-021-00560-7 PMID: 34663898

Boniol, M., Kunjumen, T., Nair, T. S., Siyam, A., Campbell, J., & Diallo, K. (2022). The global health workforce stock and distribution in 2020 and 2030:A threat to equity and 'universal' health coverage? *BMJ Global Health*, *7*(6), 009316. https://gh.bmj.com/content/bmjgh/7/6/e009316.full.pdf. DOI: 10.1136/bmjgh-2022-009316 PMID: 35760437

Gallo, R. J., Shieh, L., Smith, M., Marafino, B. J., Geldsetzer, P., Asch, S. M., Shum, K., Lin, S., Westphal, J., Hong, G., & Li, R. C. (2024). Effectiveness of an artificial intelligence-enabled intervention for detecting clinical deterioration. *JAMA Internal Medicine*, *184*(5), 557–563. DOI: 10.1001/jamainternmed.2024.0084 PMID: 38526472

Reeves, S., Pelone, F., Harrison, R., Goldman, J., & Zwarenstein, M. (2018a). Interprofessional collaboration to improve professional practice and healthcare outcomes. *Cochrane Database of Systematic Reviews*, (8). Retrieved from https://ovidsp.ovid.com/ovidweb.cgi?T=JS&PAGE=reference&D=coch&NEWS=N&AN=00075320-100000000-00589

Reeves, S., Perrier, L., Goldman, J., Freeth, D., & Zwarenstein, M. (2018b). Interprofessional education: effects on professional practice and healthcare outcomes. *Cochrane Database of Systematic Reviews*, (8). Retrieved from https://ovidsp.ovid.com/ovidweb.cgi?T=JS&PAGE=reference&D=coch&NEWS=N&AN=00075320-100000000-01679

Registered Nurses Association of Ontario. (2013). *Best practice guideline. Developing and sustaining interprofessional health care: Optimizing patient, organizational and system outcomes*. Retrieved July 25, 2024 https://rnao.ca/bpg/guidelines/interprofessional-team-work-healthcare

Reilly, S., Hobson-Merrett, C., Gibbons, B., Jones, B., Richards, D., Plappert, H., & Planner, C. L. (2024). Collaborative care approaches for people with severe mental illness. *Cochrane Database of Systematic Reviews*, (5). Retrieved from https://ovidsp.ovid.com/ovidweb.cgi?T=JS&PAGE=reference&D=coch&NEWS=N&AN=00075320-100000000-07931

Sangseok, Y., & Robert, L. P. (2023). Subgroup formation in human-robot teams: A multi-study mixed methods approach with implications for theory and practice. *Journal of the Association for Information Science and Technology*, *74*(3), 323–338. DOI: 10.1002/asi.24626

Shiwani, T., Relton, S., Evans, R., Kale, A., Heaven, A., Clegg, A., Abuzour, A., Alderman, J., Anand, A., Bhanu, C., Bunn, J., Collins, J., Cutillo, L., Hall, M., Keevil, V., Mitchell, L., Ogliari, G., Penfold, R., van Oppen, J., & Todd, O.Ageing Data Research Collaborative. (2023). New horizons in artificial intelligence in the healthcare of older people. *Age and Ageing*, *52*(12), afad219. Advance online publication. DOI: 10.1093/ageing/afad219 PMID: 38124256

World Health Organization. 2024. *Health workforce.* Retrieved June 26, 2024, https://www.who.int/health-topics/health-workforce#tab=tab_1

Compilation of References

Aakhus, M. (2007). Communication as design. *Communication Monographs, 74*(1), 112–117. DOI: 10.1080/03637750701196383

Aakhus, M., & Bzdak, M. (2015). Stakeholder engagement as communication design practice. *Journal of Public Affairs, 15*(2), 188–200. DOI: 10.1002/pa.1569

Agbejule, A., Rapo, J., & Saarikoski, L. (2021). Vertical and horizontal trust and team learning: The role of organizational climate. *International Journal of Managing Projects in Business, 14*(8), 1425–1443. DOI: 10.1108/IJMPB-05-2020-0155

Agurs-Collins, T., Persky, S., Paskett, E. D., Barkin, S. L., Meissner, H. I., Nansel, T. R., Arteaga, S. S., Zhang, X., Das, R., & Farhat, T. (2019). Designing and assessing multilevel interventions to improve minority health and reduce health disparities. *American Journal of Public Health, 109*(S1), S86–S93. DOI: 10.2105/AJPH.2018.304730 PMID: 30699029

Ahlquist, J. S., & Levi, M. (2011). Leadership: What it means, what it does, and what we want to know about it. *Annual Review. Annual Review of Political Science, 14*(1), 1–24. DOI: 10.1146/annurev-polisci-042409-152654

Akintomide, O. (2023). *Valued Strategies in the Development and Implementation of Inter-professional Education Placements*. The University of Western Ontario.

Amini, M., & Jahanbakhsh Javid, N. (2023). A multi-perspective framework established on the diffusion of innovation (DOI) theory and technology, organization, and environment (TOE) framework toward supply chain management system based on cloud computing technology for small and medium enterprises. Organization and Environment (TOE) Framework Toward Supply Chain Management System Based on Cloud Computing Technology for Small and Medium Enterprises (January 2023). *International Journal of Information Technology and Innovation Adoption, 11*, 1217–1234.

Ang'ana, G., & Kilika, J. M. (2022). Collaborative leadership in an organizational context: A research agenda. *Journal of Human Resource & Leadership*, *6*(1), 48–71. DOI: 10.53819/81018102t2050

Archer, D., & Cameron, A. (2009). *Collaborative leadership: How to succeed in an interconnected world*. Elsevier. DOI: 10.4324/9780080943008

Argyris, C., & Schön, D. A. (1978). *Organizational learning: A theory of action perspective*. Addison Wesley.

Arnst, J. (2018, February 1). Addressing the tangled roots of health disparities. *ASBMB Today*. https://www.asbmb.org/asbmb-today/science/020118/addressing-the-tangled-roots-of-health-disparities

Aveyard, H., Edwards, S., & West, S. (2005). Core topics of health care ethics: The identification for interprofessional education. *Journal of Interprofessional Care*, *19*(1), 63–69. DOI: 10.1080/13561820400021692 PMID: 15842081

Aveyard, H., Kolawole, A., Gurung, P., Cridlund, E., & Kozlowska, O. (2022). Informed consent prior to nursing care: Nurses' use of information. *Nursing Ethics*, *29*(5), 1244–1252. DOI: 10.1177/09697330221095148 PMID: 35724324

Azzam, M. B., Girard, M. A., Andrews, C., Bilinski, H., Connelly, D. M., Gilbert, J. H. V., Newton, C., & Grymonpre, R. E. (2022). RE. Correction: Accreditation as a driver of interprofessional education: the Canadian experience. *Human Resources for Health*, *20*(1), 77. DOI: 10.1186/s12960-022-00775-4 PMID: 36333726

Babnik, K., Sirca, N. T., & Dermol, V. (2014). Individuals learning in work teams: Support of knowledge management initiatives and an important source of organizational learning. *Procedia: Social and Behavioral Sciences*, *124*, 178–185. DOI: 10.1016/j.sbspro.2014.02.475

Baik, D. (2016). Team-based care: A concept analysis. *Nursing Forum*, *52*(4), 313–322. DOI: 10.1111/nuf.12194 PMID: 27935047

Ballini, L. (2014). *Governance in health systems innovation*. Il Pensiero Scientifico Editore.

Ball, P. (2021). What the COVID-19 pandemic reveals about science, policy, and society. *Interface Focus*, *11*(6), 20210022. DOI: 10.1098/rsfs.2021.0022

Bard, S. K., Rench, T. A., & Kozlowski, S. W. J. (2014). Performance adaptation: A theoretical integration and review. *Journal of Management*, *40*(1), 48–99. DOI: 10.1177/0149206313488210

Barge, J. K. (2002). Enlarging the meaning of group deliberation: From discussion to dialogue. (2002). In *New Directions in Group Communication* (p. 159). SAGE Publications, Inc., DOI: 10.4135/9781412990042.n9

Barnato, A. E., Moore, R., Moore, C. G., Kohatsu, N. D., & Sudore, R. L. (2017). Financial incentives to increase advance care planning among medicaid beneficiaries: Lessons learned from two pragmatic randomized trials. *Journal of Pain and Symptom Management*, *54*(1), 85–95. DOI: 10.1016/j.jpainsymman.2017.02.016 PMID: 28450218

Barr, H., Koppel, I., Reeves, S., Hammick, M., & Freeth, D. (2005). *Effective interprofessional education: Argument, assumption, and evidence*. Blackwell. DOI: 10.1002/9780470776445

Bauwens, R., Audenaert, M., & Decramer, A. (2024). Performance management systems, innovative work behavior and the role of transformational leadership: An experimental approach. *Journal of Organizational Effectiveness: People and Performance*, *11*(1), 178–195. DOI: 10.1108/JOEPP-03-2022-0066

Beauchamp, T., & Childress, J. (1994). *Principles of biomedical ethics*. Oxford University Press.

Benoliel, P., & Somech, A. (2014). The role of leader boundary activities in enhancing interdisciplinary team effectiveness. *Small Group Research*, *46*(1), 83–124. DOI: 10.1177/1046496414560028

Bera, L., Braman, N., Gupta, A., Velcheti, V., & Madabhushi, A. (2002). Predicting cancer outcomes with radiomics and artificial intelligence in radiology. *Nature Reviews. Clinical Oncology*, *19*(2), 132–146. DOI: 10.1038/s41571-021-00560-7 PMID: 34663898

Bhattamisra, , Banerjee, P., Gupta, P., Mayuren, J., Patra, S., & Candasamy, M. (2023). Artificial Intelligence in Pharmaceutical and Healthcare Research. *Big Data and Cognitive Computing*, *7*(1), 10. DOI: 10.3390/bdcc7010010

Bianchi Martini, B. (2013). Corporate development strategies, corporate governance processes and value creation. In *Theories, empirical analyses and experiences in comparison*. Franco Angeli Editore.

Bland, J. M., & Altman, D. G. (1997). Cronbach's Alpha. *British Medical Journal*, *314*(7080), 572. DOI: 10.1136/bmj.314.7080.572 PMID: 9055718

Boix Mansilla, V., Lamont, M., & Sato, K. (2015). Shared cognitive–emotional–interactional platforms. *Science, Technology & Human Values*, *41*(4), 571–612. DOI: 10.1177/0162243915614103

Boniol, M., Kunjumen, T., Nair, T. S., Siyam, A., Campbell, J., & Diallo, K. (2022). The global health workforce stock and distribution in 2020 and 2030:A threat to equity and 'universal' health coverage? *BMJ Global Health*, *7*(6), 009316. https://gh.bmj.com/content/bmjgh/7/6/e009316.full.pdf. DOI: 10.1136/bmjgh-2022-009316 PMID: 35760437

Borgonovi, E. (2004). Corporateisation and clinical governance. In *MECOSAN, 49*, 2-6.

Borgonovi, E. (2021). *Gestione per la salute. Scienza, diritti, responsabilità sociale, efficienza*. Franco Angeli.

Borgonovi, E., Fattore, G., & Longo, F. (2013). *Management of public institutions*. Egea.

Bosquillon, C., Cujko, L., Gautel, G., Di Pippo, S., & Vittori, E. (2024). Is the lunar economy solely for the space industry? Opportunities for nonspace companies in lunar infrastructure leveraging technological synergies. *New Space*, *12*(3), 174–187. DOI: 10.1089/space.2023.0057

Bouguerra, A., Hughes, M., Cakir, M. S., & Tatoglu, E. (2022). Linking entrepreneurial orientation to environmental collaboration: A stakeholder theory and evidence from multinational companies in an emerging market. *British Journal of Management*.

Boyle, D. K., & Kochinda, C. (2004). Enhancing collaborative communication of nurses and physician leadership in two intensive care units. *The Journal of Nursing Administration*, *34*(2), 60–70. DOI: 10.1097/00005110-200402000-00003 PMID: 14770064

Braveman, P. (2006). Health disparities and health equity: Concepts and measurement. *Annual Review of Public Health*, *27*(1), 167–194. DOI: 10.1146/annurev.publhealth.27.021405.102103 PMID: 16533114

Brennan, N. M., & Flynn, M. A. (2013). Differentiating clinical governance, clinical management and clinical practice. *Clinical Governance*, *18*(2), 114–131. DOI: 10.1108/14777271311317909

Brown Whitehead, P., Swope, M. G., & Ferren Carter, K. (2020, Spring-Fall). Impact of a team-based, interprofessional, clinical ethics immersion on moral resilience. *Teaching Ethics*, *20*(1-2), 65–74. Advance online publication. DOI: 10.5840/tej202132585

Brown, A. F., Ma, G. X., Miranda, J., Eng, E., Castille, D., Brockie, T., Jones, P., Airhihenbuwa, C. O., Farhat, T., Zhu, L., & Trinh-Shevrin, C. (2019). Structural Interventions to Reduce and Eliminate Health Disparities. *American Journal of Public Health (1971), 109*(S1), S72–S78. https://doi.org/DOI: 10.2105/AJPH.2018.304844

Brush, B. L., Mentz, G., Jensen, M., Jacobs, B., Saylor, K. M., Rowe, Z., Israel, B. A., & Lachance, L. (2020). Success in long-standing community-based participatory research (CBPR) partnerships: A scoping literature review. *Health Education & Behavior*, *47*(4), 556–568. DOI: 10.1177/1090198119882989 PMID: 31619072

Bulduk, S., Özel, İ., & Dinçer, Y. (2016). Informal communication in healthcare (gossip and rumour): Nurses' attitudes. *Athens Journal of Health*, *3*(4), 23–29. DOI: 10.30958/ajh.3-4-3

Burkhardt, M., & Nathaniel, A. (2013). *Ethics and issues in contemporary nursing*. Delmar Cengage Learning.

Burm, S., Boese, K., Faden, L., DeLuca, S., Huda, N., Hibbert, K., & Goldszmidt, M. (2019). Recognizing the importance of informal communication events in improving collaborative care. *BMJ Quality & Safety*, *28*(4), 289–295. DOI: 10.1136/bmjqs-2017-007441 PMID: 30121585

Burns, L. R., Bradley, E. H., Weiner, B. J., & Shortell, S. (2012). *Shortell and Kaluzny health management: organisation, design and behaviour*. Delmar Cengage Learning.

Butcher, L., & Mackie, E. (2021). *Ethics frameworks: an annotated bibliography*. Retrieved from https://healthethics.ca

Cameron, K. A. (2013). Advancing equity in clinical preventive services: The role of health communication. *Journal of Communication*, *63*(1), 31–50. DOI: 10.1111/jcom.12005

Campbell, A. R., Layne, D., Scott, E., & Wei, H. (2020). Interventions to promote teamwork, delegation and communication among registered nurses and nursing assistants: An integrative review. *Journal of Nursing Management*, *28*(7), 1465–1472. DOI: 10.1111/jonm.13083 PMID: 32621342

Canadian Interprofessional Health Collaborative (CIHC). (2024) CIHC Competency Framework for Advancing Collaboration. Retrieved from: https://cihc-cpis.com/wp-content/uploads/2024/06/CIHC-Competency-Framework.pdf

Canadian Interprofessional Health Collaborative. (2010). *A national interprofessional competency framework*. Retrieved from https://health.ubc.ca/sites/health. ubc.ca/files/documents/CIHC_IPCompetencies_Feb1210.pdf

Canadian Interprofessional Health Collaborative. (April 2024). CIHC competency framework for advancing collaboration. Retrieved June 20, 2024. https://cihc-cpis.com/wp-content/uploads/2024/06/CIHC-Competency-Framework.pdf

Canadian Interprofessional Health Collaborative. *Glossary*. Retrieved June 25, 2024. lhttps://cihc-cpis.com/resources/glossary/

Carlton, E. L., Whiting, J. B., Bradford, K., Dyk, P. H., & Vail, A. (2009). Defining factors of successful university-community collaborations: An exploration of one healthy marriage project. *Family Relations*, *58*(1), 28–40. DOI: 10.1111/j.1741-3729.2008.00532.x

Cassano, R. (2013). *Accountability and stakeholder relations in public enterprises*. Franco Angeli Editore.

Castriota, S., Delmastro, M., & Tonin, M. (2023). National or local infodemic? The demand for news during the COVID-19 pandemic. *International Journal of Health Economics and Management*, *23*(4), 507–536. DOI: 10.1007/s10754-023-09350-3 PMID: 37069418

Centers for Disease Control and Prevention (CDC). (2020, December 10). Risk of severe illness or death from COVID-19. https://www.cdc.gov/coronavirus/2019-ncov/community/health-equity/racial-ethnic-disparities/disparities-illness.html

Centers for Disease Control and Prevention (CDC). (2021, January 28). The Social-Ecological Model: A framework for prevention. https://www.cdc.gov/violenceprevention/about/social-ecologicalmodel.html

Chen HW, O'Donnell JM, Chiu YJ, Chen YC, Kang YN, Tuan YT, Kuo SY, Wu JC. (2022). Comparison of learning outcomes of interprofessional education simulation with traditional single-profession education simulation: A mixed-methods study. *BMC Med Educ 30*, 22(1):651. . PMID: 36042449; PMCID: PMC9429663.DOI: 10.1186/s12909-022-03640-z

Chrislip, D. D. (2002). *The collaborative leadership fieldbook: A guide for citizens and civic leaders*. Jossey-Bass.

Ciambotti, M. (2015). *Topics and research in business economics: firms, entrepreneurship, human capital*. Franco Angeli publisher.

Cifuentes-Faura, J. (2022). European Union policies and their role in combating climate change over the years. *Air Quality, Atmosphere & Health*, *15*(8), 1–8. DOI: 10.1007/s11869-022-01156-5

Civelek, M. E. (2018). Essentials of Structural Equation Modeling. In *Zea Books*. DOI: 10.13014/K2SJ1HR5

Coda, V., Invernizzi, G., & Russo, P. (2017). *Business strategy*. McGraw Hill Education.

Comite, U. (2022). The hospital company in the perspective of process reengineering: between health services and care profiles. In Teliti, E., & Laghi, P. (Eds.), *Process, processes and the technological revolution*. Cedam.

Cook, C., & Brunton, M. (2018). The importance of moral emotions for effective collaboration in culturally diverse healthcare teams. *Nursing Inquiry*, *25*(2), e12214. Advance online publication. DOI: 10.1111/nin.12214 PMID: 28730736

Cooperrider, D. L., & Srivastva, S. (1987). Appreciative inquiry in organizational life. In Woodman, R. W., & Pasmore, W. A. (Eds.), *Research in organizational change and development* (Vol. 1, pp. 129–169). JAI Press., DOI: 10.1108/S1475-9152(2013)0000004001

Coronella, S., Risaliti, G., & Verona, R. (2016). Fiscal policy in the doctrine of business economics: critical reflections. In Il governo tra tradizione e innovazione, edited by M. Luciano, R. Lombardi, L. Anselmi. Milan: Franco Angeli editore.

Crevani, L., Lindgfren, M., & Packendorff, J. (2009). Leadership, not leaders: On the study of leadership as practices and interactions. *Scandinavian Journal of Management*, *26*(1), 77–86. DOI: 10.1016/j.scaman.2009.12.003

Criado-Perez, C., Jackson, C., Minbashian, A., & Collins, C. G. (2024). Cognitive reflection and decision-making accuracy: Examining their relation and boundary conditions in the context of evidence-based management. *Journal of Business and Psychology*, *39*(1), 249–273. DOI: 10.1007/s10869-023-09883-x

Cyna, A. M., & Simmons, S. W. (2017). Guidelines on informed consent in anaesthesia: Unrealistic, unethical, untenable…. *British Journal of Anaesthesia*, *119*(6), 1086–1089. DOI: 10.1093/bja/aex347 PMID: 29028983

D'Amico, E. (2009). *Evolution of planning and managerial controls in central state administrations*. Wolters Kluwer.

D'Amour, D., Ferrada-Videla, M, San Martin Rodriguez, L., & Beaulieu, M.D. (2005). The conceptual basis for interprofessional collaboration: Core concepts and theoretical frameworks. *Journal of Interprofessional Care*, Supplement 1: 116 – 131DOI: DOI: 10.1080/13561820500082529

Dankwa-Mullan, I., Rhee, K. B., Williams, K., Sanchez, I., Sy, F. S., Stinson, N.Jr, & Ruffin, J. (2010). The science of eliminating health disparities: Summary and analysis of the NIH summit recommendations. *American Journal of Public Health, 100*(S1), S12–S18. DOI: 10.2105/AJPH.2010.191619 PMID: 20147660

Dean, M., Gill, R., & Barbour, J. B. (2016). "Let's sit forward": Investigating interprofessional communication, collaboration, professional roles, and physical space at EmergiCare. *Health Communication, 31*(12), 1506–1516. DOI: 10.1080/10410236.2015.1089457 PMID: 27093130

Decuyper, S., Dochy, F., & Van den Bossche, P. (2010). Grasping the dynamic - complexity of team learning: An integrative model for effective team learning in organizations. *Educational Research Review, 5*(2), 111–133. DOI: 10.1016/j.edurev.2010.02.002

Defila, R., & di Giulio, A. (2017). Managing Consensus in Inter- and Transdisciplinary Teams: Tasks and Expertise. In *The Oxford Handbook of Interdisciplinarity* (2nd ed.). Oxford University Press. https://doi.org/DOI: 10.1093/oxfordhb/9780198733522.013.27

Del Gesso, C. (2014). The systemic view of the public health enterprise. Evolutionary trends of organisation, management and detection in the health protection system. Milan: Franco Angeli editore.

Del Grosso, P., & Van Roey, K. (2024). Diversifying evidence in evidence-based management. *Philosophy of Management, 23*(4), 439–460. DOI: 10.1007/s40926-024-00318-y

DeVellis, R. F. (2003). *Scale Development: Theory and Applications* (2nd ed.). Sage.

Di Cagno, N., Adamo, S., & Giaccari, F. (2019). The company. Purpose-structure-administration. In *Collana di Studi Aziendali, Serie Studi Istituzionali*. Cacucci publisher.

DiBello, K. (2019). Collaborative leadership. *AAACN Viewpoint: Pitman, 41*(4), 15–16.

Dillard-Wright, J., & Shields-Haas, V. (2021). Nursing with the people: Reimagining futures for nursing. *Advances in Nursing Science, 44*(3), 195–209. DOI: 10.1097/ANS.0000000000000361

Donabedian, A. (1985). *The Methods and Findings of Quality Assessment and Monitoring: An Illustrated Analysis*. Health Administration Press.

Dyer, S. M., Perracini, M. R., Smith, T., Fairhall, N. J., Cameron, I. D., Sherrington, C., & Crotty, M. (2020). Rehabilitation Following Hip Fracture. 2020 Aug 21. In: Falaschi P, Marsh D, editors. Orthogeriatrics: The Management of Older Patients with Fragility Fractures [Internet]. 2nd edition. Cham (CH): Springer; 2021. Chapter 12. Available from: https://www.ncbi.nlm.nih.gov/books/NBK565580/pdf/Bookshelf_NBK565580.pdf

Eager, B., & Brunton, R. (2023). Prompting higher education towards AI-augmented teaching and learning practice. Journal of University Teaching & Learning Practice, 20(5), 02.

Eaton, L., Bridgman, T., & Cummings, S. (2024). Advancing the democratization of work: A new intellectual history of transformational leadership theory. *Leadership*, *20*(3), 125–143. DOI: 10.1177/17427150241232705

Ebrahimi, S., & Bridgelall, R. (2021). A fuzzy Delphi analytic hierarchy model to rank factors influencing public transit mode choice: A case study. *Research in Transportation Business & Management*, *39*, 100496. DOI: 10.1016/j.rtbm.2020.100496

Edmondson, A. (1999). Psychological safety and learning behavior in work teams. *Administrative Science Quarterly*, *44*(2), 350–383. DOI: 10.2307/2666999

Edmonstone, J. (2009). Clinical leadership: The elephant in the room. *The International Journal of Health Planning and Management*, *24*(4), 290–305. DOI: 10.1002/hpm.959 PMID: 18770874

ElBaih, M. (2023). The Role of Privacy Regulations in AI Development (A Discussion of how Privacy Regulations Can Shape the Development of AI). Available at *SSRN* 4589207.

Ellinor, L., & Gerard, G. (1998). *Dialogue: Rediscover the transforming power of conversation*. John Wiley.

Engel, J., & Prentice, D. (2013). The ethics of interprofessional collaboration. *Nursing Ethics*, *20*(4), 426–435. DOI: 10.1177/0969733012468466 PMID: 23329780

Engel, J., Prentice, D., & Hicks, R. (2019). Where does the patient fit? An analysis of word use within the context of interprofessional collaborative care. *Global Qualitative Nursing Research*, *6*, 2333393619889353. Advance online publication. DOI: 10.1177/2333393619889353 PMID: 31840037

Esperat, M. C., Hust, C., Song, H., Garcia, M., & McMurry, L. J. (2023). Interprofessional collaborative practice: Management of chronic disease and mental health issues in primary care. *Public Health Reports*, *138*(1, suppl), 29S–35S. DOI: 10.1177/00333549231155469 PMID: 37226954

Espinoza, P., Peduzzi, M., Agreli, H. F., & Sutherland, M. A. (2018). Interprofessional team member's satisfaction: A mixed methods study of a Chilean hospital. *Human Resources for Health, 16*(30), 30. Advance online publication. DOI: 10.1186/s12960-018-0290-z PMID: 29996936

Essex, R., Kennedy, J., Miller, D., & Jameson, J. (2023). A scoping review exploring the impact and negotiation of hierarchy in healthcare organisations. *Nursing Inquiry, 30*(4), e12571. DOI: 10.1111/nin.12571 PMID: 37338510

Ezra, W., & Charles, M. (2023). Organizational Culture Among Religious Founded Schools in Enhancing Teachers' Performance: A Case Study of Bishop Willigers Secondary School in Bugweri District, Eastern Uganda. *Research and Advances in Education, 2*(9), 61–73. DOI: 10.56397/RAE.2023.09.06

Farrell, C. (2016). The ethics and value of true interprofessionalism. *AMA Journal of Ethics, 18*(9), 887–890. DOI: 10.1001/journalofethics.2016.18.9.fred1-1609

Febrian, W. D., & Solihin, A. (2024). Analysis of Improving Organizational Culture Through Employee Engagement, Talent Management, Training and Development Human Resources. *Siber Journal of Advanced Multidisciplinary, 1*(4), 185–195. DOI: 10.38035/sjam.v1i4.86

Feller, I. (2002). New organizations, old cultures: Strategy and implementation of interdisciplinary programs. *Research Evaluation, 11*(2), 109–116. DOI: 10.3152/147154402781776862

Fernandes, A. Palombella, J. Salfi, & B. Wainman. (2015). Dissecting through barriers: A mixed-methods study on the effect of interprofessional education in a dissection course with health care professional students. *Anatomic Science Education (ASE). Journal, 8*, 305–316. PMID: 25641912

Ferrari, F. (2014). Evidence-based management. In *Rivista di Management per le professioni sanitarie*. Maggioli Editore.

Forde-Stiegler, C. T., Immendorf, M. C., & Cady, S. H. (2024). Using collaborative leadership at all levels to build people-oriented organizations. In *Cases on Critical Leadership Skills* (pp. 144–152). Edward Elgar Publishing. DOI: 10.4337/9781035311866.00033

Francesconi, A. (2007). *Organisational and technological innovation in health care. The role of health technology assessment*. FrancoAngeli Editore.

Freedman, D. B. (2002). Clinical governance: Bringing together management and clinical approaches to quality in the UK. *Clinica Chimica Acta, 319*(2), 133–141. DOI: 10.1016/S0009-8981(02)00034-7 PMID: 11955490

Frydman, B., Wilson, I., & Wyer, J. A. (2000). *The power of collaborative leadership: Lessons for the learning organization*. Butterworth-Heinemann. HD58.82. F79 2000 658.4'063-dc21

Fukui, M., & Abe, H. (2013). The Graphic interpretation of the Co-occurrence Network Diagram in a different writing style. *Journal of Graphic Science of Japan, 47* (4), 3-9.

Funari, A., Lecci, F., & Ricci, A. (2019). Middle management in public health companies: national census and analysis of empowerment and empowerment mechanisms. In Report, O. A. S. I. (Ed.). EGEA.

Furukawa, H. (1990). Indispensable theoretical place to practice organizational transformation, a critical challenge for corporate organizations. "Ko-zo kowashi – soshiki henkaku no shinrigaku". In *Japapanese*. Seisin-Shobo.

Gachira, J. N., & Ntara, C. (2024). Effect of Transformational Leadership on Organisational Performance of Top 100 SMEs in Nairobi, Kenya. *Journal of Human Resource & Leadership*, *8*(2), 82–99.

Gallo, R. J., Shieh, L., Smith, M., Marafino, B. J., Geldsetzer, P., Asch, S. M., Shum, K., Lin, S., Westphal, J., Hong, G., & Li, R. C. (2024). Effectiveness of an artificial intelligence-enabled intervention for detecting clinical deterioration. *JAMA Internal Medicine*, *184*(5), 557–563. DOI: 10.1001/jamainternmed.2024.0084 PMID: 38526472

Ganz, S. C. (2020). Hyperopic search: Organisations learning about managers learning about strategies. *Organization Science*, *31*(4), 821–838. DOI: 10.1287/orsc.2019.1330

Garmston, R. J., & Wellman, B. M. (1999). *The adaptive school: A sourcebook for developing collaborative groups*. Christopher-Gordon.

Gebhardt, M., Kopyto, M., Birkel, H., & Hartmann, E. (2022). Industry 4.0 technologies as enablers of collaboration in circular supply chains: A systematic literature review. *International Journal of Production Research*, *60*(23), 6967–6995. DOI: 10.1080/00207543.2021.1999521

Gehlert, S., Murray, A., Sohmer, D., McClintock, M., Conzen, S., & Olopade, O. (2010). The importance of transdisciplinary collaborations for understanding and resolving health disparities. *Social Work in Public Health*, *25*(3-4), 408–422. DOI: 10.1080/19371910903241124 PMID: 20446184

Gehlert, S., Sohmer, D., Sacks, T., Mininger, C., McClintock, M., & Olopade, O. (2008). Targeting health disparities: A model linking upstream determinants to downstream interventions. *Health Affairs*, *27*(2), 339–349. DOI: 10.1377/hlthaff.27.2.339 PMID: 18332488

Gergerich, E., Boland, D., & Scott, M. A. (2019). Hierarchies in interprofessional training. *Journal of Interprofessional Care*, *33*(5), 528–535. DOI: 10.1080/13561820.2018.1538110 PMID: 30383437

Gibson, C. B., & Gibbs, J. (2006). Unpacking the concept of virtuality: The effects of geographic dispersion, electronic dependence, dynamic structure, and national diversity on team innovation. *Administrative Science Quarterly*, *51*(3), 451–495. DOI: 10.2189/asqu.51.3.451

Gigliotti, R. A., & Goldthwaite, C. (2021). *Leadership in academic health centers: Core concepts and critical cases*. Kendall Hunt.

Gigliotti, R. A., Weidner, M., Jansen, M., Greenberg, P., Bachmann, G., Dominguez-Bello, M. G., Parmar, V., Panettieri, R. A., Reilly, N., Ayers, C. A., Cohen, B., Denzin, L. K., Feldman-Zohn, C., Fiedler, N., Jimenez, M. E., Laumbach, R. J., Malin, S. K., Mazzaferro, N., Pai, S., & Horton, D. B. (2024). Assessments of working group effectiveness in the planning of the New Jersey Kids Study: An applied mixed-methods study on the science of team science. *Journal of Clinical and Translational Science*, *8*(1), e163.

Gilliland, C. T., White, J., Gee, B., Kreeftmeijer-Vegter, R., Bietrix, F., Ussi, A. E., Hajduch, M., Kocis, P., Chiba, N., Hirasawa, R., Suematsu, M., Bryans, J., Newman, S., Hall, M. D., & Austin, C. P. (2019). The fundamental characteristics of a translational scientist. *ACS Pharmacology & Translational Science*, *2*(3), 213–216. DOI: 10.1021/acsptsci.9b00022 PMID: 32259057

Gitell, J. H., Godfrey, M., & Thistlethwaite, J. (2013). Interprofessional collaborative practice and relational coordination: Improving healthcare through relationships. *Journal of Interprofessional Care*, *27*(3), 210–213. DOI: 10.3109/13561820.2012.730564 PMID: 23082769

Gittell, J. H. (2011). *Relational Coordination: Guidelines for Theory, Measurement and Analysis*. Relational Coordination Research Collaborative.

Gleeson, L. A., O'Brien, G. L., O'Mahony, D., & Byre, S. (2023). Interprofessional communication in the hospital setting: A systematic review of the qualitative literature. *Journal of Interprofessional Care*, *37*(2), 203–213. DOI: 10.1080/13561820.2022.2028746 PMID: 35109753

Gold, M. (2014). Reducing health care disparities: Where are we now? *Mathematica Policy Research.* Robert Wood Johnson Foundation. https://www.mathematica.org/our-publications-and-findings/publications/reducing-health-care-disparities-where-are-we-now

Greenfield, B. (2007). The role of emotions in ethical decision making: Implications for physical therapist education. *Journal, Physical Therapy Education, 21*(1), 14–21. DOI: 10.1097/00001416-200701000-00003

Greenleaf, R. K. (1977). *Servant Leadership: A Journey into the Nature of Legitimate Power and Greatness.* Paulist Press.

Grice, G., Thomason, A., Meny, L., Pinelli, N., Martello, J., & Zorek, J. (2018). Intentional interprofessional experiential education. *American Journal of Pharmaceutical Education, 82*(3), 6502. https://www.ncbi.nlm.nih.gov/pmc/articles/PMC5909877/pdf/ajpe6502.pdf. DOI: 10.5688/ajpe6502 PMID: 29692445

Grymonpre, R. E., Bainbridge, L., Nasmith, L., & Baker, C. (2021). Development of accreditation standards for interprofessional education: A Canadian Case Study. *Human Resources for Health, 19*(1), 12. DOI: 10.1186/s12960-020-00551-2 PMID: 33472633

Haleem, A., Javaid, M., Singh, R. P., & Suman, R. (2022). Medical 4.0 technologies for healthcare: Features, capabilities, and applications. *Internet of Things and Cyber-Physical Systems, 2*, 12–30. DOI: 10.1016/j.iotcps.2022.04.001

Hall, P. (2005). Interprofessional teamwork: Professional cultures as barriers. *Journal of Interprofessional Care, 19*(sup1), 188-196. https://doi.org/DOI: 10.1080/13561820500081745

Hammick, M., Freeth, D., Koppel, I., Reeves, S., & Barr, H. (2007). A best evidence systematic review of inter-professional education: BEME Guide no.9. *Medical Teacher, 29*(8), 735–751. DOI: 10.1080/01421590701682576 PMID: 18236271

Harrington, N. G. (2013). Introduction to the special issue: Communication strategies to reduce health disparities. *Journal of Communication, 63*(1), 1–7. DOI: 10.1111/jcom.12004

Harrison, J. S., & Thompson, S. (2014). *Strategic management of healthcare organisations: A stakeholder management approach.* Business Expert Press.

Haruta, J., Breugelmans, R., & Nishigori, H. (2018). Translation and cultural adaptation of the Japanese version of the interprofessional facilitation scale. *Journal of Interprofessional Care, 32*(3), 321–328. DOI: 10.1080/13561820.2017.1398720 PMID: 29161176

Haruta, J., Yoshida, K., Goto, M., Yoshimoto, H., Ichikawa, S., Mori, Y., Yoshimi, K., & Otsuka, M. (2018). Development of an interprofessional competency framework for collaborative practice in Japan. *Journal of Interprofessional Care*, *32*(4), 436–443. https://doi-org.proxy.library.brocku.ca/10.1080/13561820.2018.1426559. DOI: 10.1080/13561820.2018.1426559 PMID: 29381091

Helmstadter, C. (2002). Early nursing reform in nineteenth-century London: A doctor-driven phenomenon. *Medical History*, *46*(3), 325–350. https://www.cambridge.org/core/journals/medical-history/article/early-nursing-reform-in-nineteenthcentury-london-a-doctordriven-phenomenon/B78A155787D8643EFB9296ECC561B845. DOI: 10.1017/S0025727300069386 PMID: 12194424

Higuchi, K. (2017). A two-step approach to quantitative content analysis: KH coder tutorial using Anne of Green Gables (part II). *Ritsumeikan Social Sciences Review*, *53*(1), 137. https://www.ritsumei.ac.jp/file.jsp?id=346128

Hirokawa, R. Y. (1988). Group communication and decision-making performance: A continued test of the functional perspective. *Human Communication Research*, *14*(4), 487–515. DOI: 10.1111/j.1468-2958.1988.tb00165.x

Hogan, R., & Kariser, R. B. (2005). What we know about leadership. *Review of General Psychology*, *9*(2), 169–180. DOI: 10.1037/1089-2680.9.2.169

Hood, C. (1991). A public management for all seasons? *Public Administration*, *69*(1), 3–19. DOI: 10.1111/j.1467-9299.1991.tb00779.x

Hosoda, M. (2021). *"Team-iryo" towa nani-ka 2nd edi. Toward Patient/service user-centered approach*. Japanese Nursing Association Publishing Company. (in Japanese)

Hsieh, J. Y., & Liou, K. T. (2018). Collaborative leadership and organizational performance: Assessing the structural relation in a public service agency. *Review of Public Personnel Administration*, *38*(1), 83–109. DOI: 10.1177/0734371X15623619

Hu, L. T., & Bentler, P. M. (1999). Cutoff Criteria for Fit Indexes in Covariance Structure Analysis: Conventional Criteria versus New Alternatives. *Structural Equation Modeling*, *6*(1), 1–55. DOI: 10.1080/10705519909540118

Hwang, K. (2015). Morality 'East' and 'West': cultural concerns. In Wright, J. (Ed.), *International Encyclopedia of the Social and Behavioral Sciences* (pp. 806–810). Elsevier. DOI: 10.1016/B978-0-08-097086-8.64005-9

Institute of Medicine. (2015). *Measuring the impact of interprofessional practice on collaborative practice and patient outcomes*. National Academies Press.

Interprofessional Education Collaborative (IPEC). (2023). *IPEC Core Competencies Revision: Version 3 (2021-2023)*. Retrieved from: https://www.ipecollaborative.org/assets/core-competencies/IPEC_Core_Competencies_Version_3_2023.pdf

Jacob, C., Bourke, S., & Heuss, S. (2022). From Testers to Cocreators—the Value of and Approaches to Successful Patient Engagement in the Development of eHealth Solutions: Qualitative Expert Interview Study. *JMIR Human Factors*, *9*(4), e41481. DOI: 10.2196/41481

Jagosh, J., Bush, P. L., Salsberg, J., Macaulay, A. C., Greenhalgh, T., Wong, G., Cargo, M., Green, L. W., Herbert, C. P., & Pluye, P. (2015). A realist evaluation of community-based participatory research: Partnership synergy, trust building and related ripple effects. *BMC Public Health*, *15*(725), 1–11. DOI: 10.1186/s12889-015-1949-1 PMID: 26223523

Jalil, S., Rafi, S., LaToza, T. D., Moran, K., & Lam, W. (2023). Chatgpt and software testing education: Promises & perils. In *2023 IEEE International Conference on Software Testing, Verification and Validation Workshops (ICSTW)* (pp. 4130-4137). IEEE. DOI: 10.1109/ICSTW58534.2023.00078

Jarvis, P. (2010). *Adult education & lifelong learning: Theory and practice* (4th ed.). Routledge.

Javaid, M., Haleem, A., & Singh, R. P. (2023). ChatGPT for healthcare services: An emerging stage for an innovative perspective. BenchCouncil Transactions on Benchmarks. *Standards and Evaluations*, *3*(1), 100105.

Jehn, K. A. (1997). A qualitative analysis of conflict types and dimensions in organizational groups. *Administrative Science Quarterly*, *42*(3), 530–557. DOI: 10.2307/2393737

Jensen, R., & Lund, A. (2014). Horizontal dynamics in an inter-professional school improvement team. *International Journal of Leadership in Education*, *17*(3), 286–303. DOI: 10.1080/13603124.2013.794302

Jiang, G. (2023). Collaborative leadership in team science: dynamics of sense making, decision making, and action taking. *Frontiers in Research Metrics and Analytics*, 01-06. DOI: 10.3389/frma.2023.1211407

Johnstone, M., Hutchinson, A., & Peter, E. (2015). Moral distress' – time to abandon a flawed nursing construct? *Nursing Ethics*, *22*(1), 5–14. DOI: 10.1177/0969733013505312 PMID: 24311238

Jones, L. R., & Mussari, R. (2000). Public management reform in the United States and Italy: Accounting, measurement and finance. *International. Public Management Review*, *1*(1), 56–83.

Junaid, M., Zhang, Q., Cao, M., & Luqman, A. (2023). Nexus between technology-enabled supply chain dynamic capabilities, integration, resilience, and sustainable performance: An empirical examination of healthcare organizations. *Technological Forecasting and Social Change*, *196*, 122828. DOI: 10.1016/j.techfore.2023.122828

Kaiser, S., Patras, J., & Martinussen, M. (2018). Linking interprofessional work to outcomes for employees. *Research in Nursing & Health*, *41*(3), 265–280. DOI: 10.1002/nur.21858 PMID: 29906320

Kant, N., & Anjali, K. (2021). Blockchain Technology: A Strategic Resource. In Blockchain for Healthcare Systems (pp. 1-15). CRC Press. 13

Kaplan, R. M., & Hays, R. D. (2022). Health-related quality of life measurement in public health. *Annual Review of Public Health*, *43*(1), 355–373. DOI: 10.1146/annurev-publhealth-052120-012811

Kariuki, B. W., Gichuhi, D., & Mwaura, P. (2024). Influence of Corporate Culture on the Implementation of Change Initiatives in Kirinyaga County Government, Kenya. *African Journal of Empirical Research*, *5*(4), 957–965. DOI: 10.51867/ajernet.5.4.78

Karpf, M. (2019). The role of academic health centers in addressing health equity and social determinants of health. *Academic Medicine*, *94*(9), 1273–1275. DOI: 10.1097/ACM.0000000000002834 PMID: 31460914

Kasneci, E., Seßler, K., Küchemann, S., Bannert, M., Dementieva, D., Fischer, F., Gasser, U., Groh, G., Günnemann, S., Hüllermeier, E., Krusche, S., Kutyniok, G., Michaeli, T., Nerdel, C., Pfeffer, J., Poquet, O., Sailer, M., Schmidt, A., Seidel, T., & Kasneci, G. (2023). ChatGPT for good? On opportunities and challenges of large language models for education. *Learning and Individual Differences*, *103*, 102274. DOI: 10.1016/j.lindif.2023.102274

Katz, D. (1982). The effects of group longevity on project communication and performance. *Administrative Science Quarterly*, *27*(1), 81–104. DOI: 10.2307/2392547

Keddy, B., Gillis Jones, M., Jacobs, P., Burton, H., & Rogers, M. (1986). The doctor-nurse relationship: An historical perspective. *Journal of Advanced Nursing*, *11*(6), 745–753. DOI: 10.1111/j.1365-2648.1986.tb03393.x PMID: 3540064

Kelstrup, J. D. (2024). Understanding the role of practical knowledge in evidence-based welfare reform-a three-stage model. *Humanities & Social Sciences Communications*, *11*(1), 1438. DOI: 10.1057/s41599-024-03937-y

Kendzerska, T., Zhu, D. T., Gershon, A. S., Edwards, J. D., Peixoto, C., Robillard, R., & Kendall, C. E. (2021). The effects of the health system response to the COVID-19 pandemic on chronic disease management: A narrative review. *Risk Management and Healthcare Policy*, *14*, 575–584. DOI: 10.2147/RMHP.S293471

Keyton, J., Ford, D. J., & Smith, F. I. (2008). A mesolevel communicative model of collaboration. *Communication Theory*, *18*(3), 376–406. DOI: 10.1111/j.1468-2885.2008.00327.x

Khalili, H., Lackie, K., Langlois, S., Wetzlmair, L. C., & the Working Group. (2022). Global IPE Situational Analysis Result Final Report. InterprofessionalResearch. Global Publication (ISBN: 978-1-7366963-2-3). Available at: https://interprofessionalresearch.global/wp-content/uploads/2022/10/Global-IPE-Situational-Analysis-Final-Report-October-2022-1.pdf

Khalili, H., & Orchard, C. (2020). The effects of an IPS-based IPE program on interprofessional socialization and dual identity development. *Journal of Interprofessional Care*, •••, 1–11. DOI: 10.1080/13561820.2019.1709427 PMID: 32019374

Kivits, J., Ricci, L., & Minary, L. (2019). Interdisciplinary research in public health: the "why" and the "how." *Journal of Epidemiology and Community Health (1979)*, *73*(12), 1061–1062. https://doi.org/DOI: 10.1136/jech-2019-212511

Klein, J. T. (2017). Typologies of interdisciplinarity: The boundary work of definition. In *The Oxford Handbook of Interdisciplinarity* (2nd ed.). Oxford University Press., DOI: 10.1093/oxfordhb/9780198733522.013.3

Klein, J. T., & Porter, A. L. (1990). Preconditions for interdisciplinary research. In *International Research Management*. Oxford University Press., DOI: 10.1093/acprof:oso/9780195062526.003.0002

Klein, K. J., Knight, A. P., Ziegert, J. C., Lim, B. C., & Slatz, J. L. (2010). When team members' values differ: The moderating role of team leadership. *Organizational Behavior and Human Decision Processes*, *114*(1), 25–36. DOI: 10.1016/j.obhdp.2010.08.004

Koh, H. K., Oppenheimer, S. C., Massin-Short, S. B., Emmons, K. M., Geller, A. C., & Viswanath, K. (2010). Translating research evidence into practice to reduce health disparities: A social determinants approach. *American Journal of Public Health*, *10*(1), S72–S80. DOI: 10.2105/AJPH.2009.167353 PMID: 20147686

König, B., Diehl, K., Tscherning, K., & Helming, K. (2013). A framework for structuring interdisciplinary research management. *Research Policy*, *42*(1), 261–272. DOI: 10.1016/j.respol.2012.05.006

Körner, M. (2010). Interprofessional teamwork in medical rehabilitation: A comparison of multidisciplinary and interdisciplinary team approach. *Clinical Rehabilitation*, *24*(8), 745–755. DOI: 10.1177/0269215510367538 PMID: 20530646

Kotcher, J., Maibach, E., Miller, J., Campbell, E., Alqodmani, L., Maiero, M., & Wyns, A. (2021). Views of health professionals on climate change and health: A multinational survey study. *The Lancet. Planetary Health*, *5*(5), e316–e323. DOI: 10.1016/S2542-5196(21)00053-X

Kouba, P., Kohout, P., Haddadi, F., Bushuiev, A., Samusevich, R., Sedlar, J., Damborsky, J., Pluskal, T., Sivic, J., & Mazurenko, S. (2023). Machine Learning-Guided Protein Engineering. *ACS Catalysis*, *13*(21), 13863–13895. DOI: 10.1021/acscatal.3c02743

Kouzes, J., & Posner, B. (2012). *The leadership challenge: How to make extraordinary things happen in organizations* (5th ed.). Jossey-Bass.

Kovner, A. R., Elton, J. J., & Billings, J. (2000). Evidence-based management. *Frontiers of Health Services Management*, *16*(4), 3–24. DOI: 10.1097/01974520-200004000-00002 PMID: 11183283

Kozlowski, S. W. J. (2018). Enhancing the effectiveness of work groups and teams: A reflection. *Perspectives on Psychological Science*, *13*(2), 205–212. DOI: 10.1177/1745691617697078 PMID: 29232536

Kozlowski, S. W., & Bell, B. S. (2007). Team learning, development, and adaptation. In *Work group learning* (pp. 39–68). Psychology Press.

Kozmenko MD, V., Jackson MD, C., Blaseg MSIV, N., Beard MD, M., Leann, T., Kupershmidt PhD, S., Lucas Molitor, W., Taggart Pharm, D., BCCCP, K., & de la Torre-Montero, R. N. (2024). Development and implementation of an Interprofessional education (IPE) curriculum: theory and practice. *Aesculapius Journal (Health Sciences & Medicine)*, *5*(1), 7.

Kruse, K. (2013). *What is leadership?* Forbes.com, April 9, 2013. 1-3

Kuzemski, D., Thirlwall, A., Brunton, M., & Brownie, S. (2022). I speak a little Arabic: Nursing communication in a cross-cultural context. *Journal of Clinical Nursing*, *31*(1-2), 145–157. DOI: 10.1111/jocn.15891 PMID: 34263493

Kwok, A. O., & Treiblmaier, H. (2023). Blockchain technology as a driver of economic development in small economies: A dynamic capabilities framework. *Journal of Decision Systems*, •••, 1–26.

Labrague, L. J., Al Subei, S., Al Rawajfah, O., AbuAlrub, R., & Burney, I. (2022). Interprofessional collaboration as a mediator in the relationship between nurse work environment, patient safety outcomes and job satisfaction among nurses. *Journal of Nursing Management*, *30*(1), 268–278. DOI: 10.1111/jonm.13491 PMID: 34601772

Lai, A., & Gomes, D. (2018). Accounting in different cultures and from different perspectives. In *Accounting and business culture*. Franco Angeli publisher.

Lai, A., Lionzo, A., Stacchezzini, F., & Rossignoli, F. (2015). *From enterprise to network. Governance profiles and business models*. FrancoAngeli Editore.

Langner, J., & Fukkink, R. G. (2023). A realist synthesis of Inter-professional collaborative practices in early intervention for children with speech, language and communication needs. *International Journal of Language & Communication Disorders*, *58*(2), 516–541. DOI: 10.1111/1460-6984.12789 PMID: 36217271

Lathabhavan, R. (2024). Mental well-being through HR analytics: Investigating an employee supportive framework. *Personnel Review*, *53*(5), 1110–1128. DOI: 10.1108/PR-11-2022-0836

League, F. (2013). *Healthcare management: Essential frameworks and recent developments in healthcare and business*. EGEA.

Lechasseur, K., Caux, C., Dolle, S., & Legault, A. (2018). Nursing ethics: An integrative review. *Nursing Ethics*, *26*(6), 694–706. DOI: 10.1177/0969733016667773 PMID: 27694548

Lega, F. (2023). *Economia e management sanitario. Settore, sistema, aziende, protagonisti* (3rd ed.). EGEA.

Lega, F., & Vendramini, E. (2008). Budgeting and performance management in the Italian National Health Service (NHS): Assessment and constructive criticism. *Journal of Health Organization and Management*, *22*(1), 11–22. DOI: 10.1108/14777260810862371 PMID: 18488516

Lengwiler, M. (2006). Between charisma and heuristics: Four styles of interdisciplinarity. *Science & Public Policy*, *33*(6), 423–434. DOI: 10.3152/147154306781778821

Liang, Z., Zhao, Y., Yu, H., Habibi, M., & Mahmoudi, T. (2024). Artificial neural networks coupled with numerical approach for the stability prediction of non-uniform functionally graded microscale cylindrical structures. *Structures (Oxford)*, *60*, 105826. DOI: 10.1016/j.istruc.2023.105826

Lindqvist, S., Duncan, A., Shepstone, L., Watts, F., & Pearce, S. (2005). Development of the 'Attitudes to Health Professionals Questionnaire' (AHPQ): A measure to assess interprofessional attitudes. *Journal of Interprofessional Care, 19*(3), 269–279. DOI: 10.1080/13561820400026071 PMID: 16029980

Long, S., Irving, K., & Murphy, C. (2023). Is therapeutic lying contradictory to person-centred care? Toward understanding the connection. *Aging & Mental Health, 28*(3), 520–530. DOI: 10.1080/13607863.2023.2202632 PMID: 37139937

Luna, G., Kim, M., Miller, R., Parekh, P., Kim, E. S., Park, S. Y., Abdulbaseer, U., Gonzalez, C., & Stiehl, E. (2023). Inter-professional relationships and their impact on resident hospitalizations in nursing homes: A qualitative study. *Applied Nursing Research, 74*, 151747. DOI: 10.1016/j.apnr.2023.151747 PMID: 38007247

Mabry, P. L., Olster, D. H., Morgan, G. D., & Abrams, D. B. (2008). Interdisciplinarity and systems science to improve population health. *American Journal of Preventive Medicine, 35*(2), S211–S224. DOI: 10.1016/j.amepre.2008.05.018 PMID: 18619402

Ma, C., Park, S. H., & Shang, J. (2018). Inter- and intra-disciplinary collaboration and patient safety outcomes in U.S. acute care hospitals: A cross sectional study. *International Journal of Nursing Studies, 85*, 1–6. DOI: 10.1016/j.ijnurstu.2018.05.001 PMID: 29783090

Marks, L. (2020). From crisis to sustainable development: The role of measurement and control systems. *Management Control, 3*, 5–16.

Martin, A. K., Green, T. L., McCarthy, A. L., Marcin Sowa, P., & Laakso, E. L. (2022). Healthcare teams: Terminology, confusion, and ramifications. *Journal of Multidisciplinary Healthcare, 15*, 765–772. DOI: 10.2147/JMDH.S342197 PMID: 35422626

Masih, E. A. (2022). Feasibility of using QR code for registration & evaluation of training and its ability to increase response rate–The learners' perception. *Nurse Education Today, 111*, 105305. DOI: 10.1016/j.nedt.2022.105305

Matsushita, H. (2010). *Creative Leadership and Team Medical Care*. Japan Medical Planning.

McAuliffe, D. (2022). *Interprofessional ethics: collaboration in the social, health and human sciences*. Cambridge University Press.

McCartney, S., & Fu, N. (2021). Bridging the gap: Why, how and when human resource analysis can impact organisational performance. *Management Decision, 60*(13), 25–47. DOI: 10.1108/MD-12-2020-1581

Mele, G., Capaldo, G., Secundo, G., & Corvello, V. (2023). Revisiting the idea of knowledge-based dynamic capabilities for digital transformation. *Journal of Knowledge Management*.

Miranda, D., & Watts, R. (2022). What is a RACI chart? How this project management tool can boost your productivity. www.forbes.com

Mitchell, P., Wynia, M., Golden, R., McNellis, B., Okun, S., Webb, C. E., Rohrbach, V., & Kohorn, I. V. (2012) Discussion Paper: Core Principles & Values of Effective Team-Based Health Care - National Academy of Medicine (IOM).

Miyoshi, Y., Yoshioka, S. I., & Yamamoto, M. (2024). Transferability of Effective Consultation Skills for Decision-Making Support in the Voluntary Surrender of Older Adult Drivers' Licences in Super-Aged Japan. *International Journal of Older People Nursing*, *19*(4), e12630. DOI: 10.1111/opn.12630 PMID: 38990513

Monteiro, M., & Keating, E. (2009). Managing misunderstandings: The role of language in interdisciplinary scientific collaboration. *Science Communication*, *31*(1), 6–28. DOI: 10.1177/1075547008330922

Montgomery, A., Lainidi, O., & Georganta, K. (2024). Why talking is not cheap: Adverse events and informal communication. *Healthcare (Basel)*, *12*(6), 635. Advance online publication. DOI: 10.3390/healthcare12060635 PMID: 38540601

Moore, J., Engel, J., & Prentice, D. (2014). Relational ethics in everyday practice. *Canadian Oncology Nursing Journal = Revue Canadienne de Nursing Oncologique*, *24*(1), 31–34. DOI: 10.5737/1181912x2413134 PMID: 24707705

Morgan, K. H., Barroso, C. S., Bateman, S., Dixson, M., & Conroy Brown, J. (2020). Patients' experiences of interprofessional collaborative practice in primary care: A scoping review of the literature. *Journal of Patient Experience*, *7*(6), 1466–1475. DOI: 10.1177/2374373520925725 PMID: 33457603

Morita, T., Irisawa,S., Nagashio, A., Nomura, K.,Tsukada, T.,Otsuka, H., & Sugita, H.(2012). An analysis on the image of the city by text mining using free answer data. *Japanese Journal of Japan Society of Civil Engineers*, 68(5), I_315-I_323. DOI: 10.2208/jscejipm.68.I_315

Mostafiz, M. I., Musteen, M., Saiyed, A., & Ahsan, M. (2022). COVID-19 and the global value chain: Immediate dynamics and long-term restructuring in the garment industry. *Journal of Business Research*, *139*, 1588–1603. DOI: 10.1016/j.jbusres.2021.10.078

Moyo, M., & Grywalski, M. (2024). Dynamic duo: The transformative impact of collaborative leadership on nurse turnover. *Nursing Management*, *55*(4), 40–46. DOI: 10.1097/nmg.0000000000000115 PMID: 38557750

Mumbi, H., & Obembe, D. (2022). Shared leadership in voluntary sector organisations: Exploring practice and theory development. *Voluntary Sector Review*, *13*(2), 226–242. DOI: 10.1332/204080521X16171406823270

Musgrove, H., Ruby, A., Chami, E., Pollak, E., Suleyman, G., & Gupta, A. (2024). Using interprofessional collaboration to reduce reported rates of central-line-associated bloodstream infection in an intensive care setting. *Infection Control and Hospital Epidemiology*, *1-3*(5), 674–676. Advance online publication. DOI: 10.1017/ice.2023.279 PMID: 38163995

Musto, L., Starzomski, R., Rodney, P., & Dodek, P. (2023). Nurses and health care providers as moral agents: from moral distress to moral action. In (R. Starzomski, J. Storch, & P. Rodney, Eds.) *Towards a moral horizon: nursing ethics for leadership and practice* (pp. 225-266), University of Victoria Libraries ePublishing Services.

National Institute on Minority Health and Health Disparities (NIMHD). (2017). *NIMHD research framework*. https://www.nimhd.nih.gov/about/overview/research-framework.html

National Institutes of Health (NIH). (2020, December 4). *The NIH almanac: National Institute on Minority Health and Health Disparities (NIMHD)*. https://www.nih.gov/about-nih/what-we-do/nih-almanac/national-institute-minority-health-health-disparities-nimhd

Nilushi Holmes, S., & Illing, J. (2021). Breaking bad news: Tackling cultural dilemmas. *BMJ Supportive & Palliative Care*, *11*(2), 128–132. DOI: 10.1136/bmjspcare-2020-002700 PMID: 33762267

Nortje, N., Jones-Bonofiglio, K., & Sotomayor, C. (2021). Exploring values among three cultures from a global bioethics perspective. *Global Bioethics = Problemi di Bioetica*, *32*(1), 1–14. DOI: 10.1080/11287462.2021.1879462 PMID: 33658749

O'Rourke, B., Widenhoefer, T., Reimer, N., Vazquez, E., & Wolpert, C. (2018). Roles, Responsibilities, and implications of health care practitioners providing interprofessional collaborative practice to the geriatric population. *Topics in Geriatric Rehabilitation*, *34*(3), 165–170. DOI: 10.1097/TGR.0000000000000189

Oberle, K., & Raffin-Bouchal, S. (2009). *Ethics in Canadian nursing practice: navigating the journey*. Pearson Prentice Hall.

Ogata, M. N., da Silva, J. A. M., Peduzzi, M., Costa, M. V., Fortuna, C. M., & Feliciano, A. B. (2021). Interfaces among permanent education and Inter-professional education in health. *Revista da Escola de Enfermagem da USP*, *55*, e03733. DOI: 10.1590/s1980-220x2020018903733 PMID: 34105683

Onesti, T., & Angiola, N. (2009). *Il controllo strategico nelle amministrazioni pubbliche*. Franco Angeli.

Ong, A. K. S., German, J. D., Dangaran, P. C., Paz, J. J. B., & Macatangay, R. R. G. (2024). Service quality and customer satisfaction analysis among motorcycle taxi transportation in the Philippines through SERVQUAL dimensions and social exchange theory. *Case Studies on Transport Policy*, *15*, 101139. DOI: 10.1016/j.cstp.2023.101139

Orchard, C. (2020). The advanced practice nurse and interprofessional collaborative practice. In E. Staples, R. Pilon, & R.A. Hannon (Eds) *Canadian perspectives on advanced practice nursing (2nd. Ed.)* (pp. 406-432). Canadian Scholars. ISBN: 9781773382173

Orchard, C. (2022). *A further update of the Assessment of Interprofessional Collaborative Leadership Scale (AICLS)*. Unpublished.

Orchard, C., (2024). (in review). Health Care Transitions: A critical literature review. *The Journal of Continuing Education in the Health Professions*.

Orchard, C., & Rykhoff, M. (2015). Collaborative leadership within interprofessional practice. In *Leadership and collaboration: Further developments for interprofessional education* (pp. 71-94). Palgrave Macmillan UK.

Orchard, C. A., King, G. A., Khalili, H. L., & Bezzina, M. B. (2012). Assessment of inter-professional team collaboration scale (AITCS): Development and testing of the instrument. *The Journal of Continuing Education in the Health Professions*, *32*(1), 58–67. DOI: 10.1002/chp.21123 PMID: 22447712

Orchard, C., King, G., Tryphonopoulos, P., Gorman, E., Ugirase, S., Lising, D., & Fung, K. (2023). Interprofessional team conflict resolution: A critical literature review. *The Journal of Continuing Education in the Health Professions*, *44*(3), 203–2010. DOI: 10.1097/CEH.0000000000000524 PMID: 37458607

Orchard, C., & Rykhoff, M. (2015). Collaborative leadership within inter-professional practice. In Forman, D., Jones, M., & Thistlethwaite, J. (Eds.), *Leadership and collaboration: Further developments for inter-professional education* (pp. 71–94). Palgrave Macmillan. DOI: 10.1057/9781137432094_5

Orchard, C., Sinclair, E., & Rykhoff, M. (2019). The new leadership in health care teams: Progress report of development on a promising measure. *Archives of Healthcare*, *1*(1), 20–26.

Orchard, C., Sonibare, O., Morse, A., Collins, J., & Al-Hamad, A. (2017). Collaborative leadership, part 1: The nurse leader's role within inter-professional teams. *Nursing Leadership*, *30*(2), 14–25. DOI: 10.12927/cjnl.2017.25258 PMID: 29083290

Pakkanen, P., Haggman-Laitila, A., & Kangasniemi, M. (2022). Ethical issues identified in nurses' interprofessional collaboration in clinical practice: a meta-synthesis. *Journal of Interprofessional Care, 36*(5), 725-734. Doi: . 1892612epub. DOI: 10.1080/13561820.2021

Papsiene, P. (2024). Theoretical modeling of organizational reflex in human resource management from the perspective of organizational biological approach. *Humanities & Social Sciences Communications*, *11*(1), 1–13. DOI: 10.1057/s41599-024-02644-y

Patanian, M. (2024). Sharing results from the field—implementing team-based care: Examples of practice-based evidence from recipients of CDC's heart disease and stroke prevention funding. []. LWW.]. *Journal of Public Health Management and Practice*, *30*, S101–S103. DOI: 10.1097/PHH.0000000000002015 PMID: 39041742

Patil et al. (2022). "Utilization of Artificial Intelligence in Healthcare System, Pharmaceutical Industry & Education". International Journal of Advanced Research in Science, Communication and Technology.

Paxson, T. D.Jr. (1996). Modes of interaction between disciplines. *The Journal of General Education*, *45*(2), 79–94.

Payscale (2016). *2016 Workforce-Skills Preparedness Report.* Retrieved June 28, 2024 from https://www.payscale.com/data-packages/job-skills

Pearce, C. L. (2004). The future of leadership: Combining vertical and shared leadership to transform knowledge work. *The Academy of Management Perspectives*, *18*(1), 47–57. DOI: 10.5465/ame.2004.12690298

Pearce, C. L., & Sims, H. P.Jr. (2002). Vertical versus shared leadership as predictors of the effectiveness of change management teams: An examination of aversive, directive, transactional, transformational, and empowering leader behaviours. *Group Dynamics*, *6*(2), 172–197. DOI: 10.1037/1089-2699.6.2.172

Pereira, R., Bianchi, I. S., & Araújo, V. M. D. S. (2021). Multi-framework implementation of the problem management process. *Форсайт*, *15*(3, 3 (eng)), 94–104. DOI: 10.17323/2500-2597.2021.3.94.104

Pesqueira, A. M., Sousa, M., & Pereira, Ruben (2023). Individual dynamic capabilities are influential factors in blockchain technology innovation from hospital settings.

Pesqueira, A., & Sousa, M. J. (2022). Life Sciences Industry Blockchain Value Management, Investments, and Finance Impact Assessment: Global Questionnaire Survey of 1524 Industry Professionals and Executives. In Incorporating AI Technology in the Service Sector (pp. 67-107). Apple Academic Press.

Pesqueira, A., & Sousa, M. J. (2022). *12 Social Analytics Influencing KOLs Profiling in the Dissemination of Innovations and Scientific Knowledge in the Life Sciences Industry*. Innovations and Social Media Analytics in a Digital Society.

Pettigrew, T. F. (1998). Intergroup contact theory. *Annual Review of Psychology, 49*(1), 65–85. DOI: 10.1146/annurev.psych.49.1.65 PMID: 15012467

Pettigrew, T. F., & Tropp, L. R. (2008). How does intergroup contact reduce prejudice? Meta-analytic tests of three mediators. *European Journal of Social Psychology, 38*(6), 122–134. DOI: 10.1002/ejsp.504

Pfeffer, J., & Sutton, R. (2006). *Hard facts, dangerous half-truths and total nonsense: Making money from evidence-based management.* Harvard Business Press.

Pollard, K., Sellman, D., & Senior, B. (2005). The need for interprofessional working. In Barret, G., Sellman, D., & Thomas, J. (Eds.), *Interprofessional Working in Health and Social Care: Professional Perspectives*. Palgrave Macmillan.

Pomare, C., Long, J. C., Churruca, K., Ellis, L. A., & Braithwaite, J. (2020). Interprofessional collaboration in hospitals: A critical, broad-based review of the literature. *Journal of Interprofessional Care, 34*(4), 509–519. DOI: 10.1080/13561820.2019.1702515 PMID: 31928245

Porter, A. L., Roessner, J. D., Cohen, A. S., & Perreault, M. (2006). Interdisciplinary research: Meaning, metrics and nurture. *Research Evaluation, 15*(3), 187–195. DOI: 10.3152/147154406781775841

Prenestini, A. (2012). The formation of strategies in public health companies. In *Strategia e performance management nelle Aziende pubbliche, 19.33*. EGEA.

Prentice, D., & Salfi, J. (2021). Translating evidence into practice: An experience with interprofessional education (IPE). In Matsushita, H. (Ed.), *Health Informatics. Translational Systems Sciences, 24*. Springer., DOI: 10.1007/978-981-15-3781-3_7

Raelin, J. A. (Ed.). (2016*). Leadership-as-practice: Theory and application.* Routledge Studies in Leadership Research, ISBN: 978-138-92485-7

Raelin, J. A. (2016). Imagine there are no leaders: Reframing leadership as collaborative agency. *Leadership*, *12*(2), 131–158. DOI: 10.1177/1742715014558076

Rangachari, P. (2020). Understanding the implementation of evidence-based practice (EBP) in HCOS through the lens of organisational theory. *Health Leadership Journal*, *12*, 35–48. PMID: 32607042

Raponi, J.-M. (2024). *A Multi-Method Qualitative Analysis of a Clinical Interprofessional Education Experience for Third-Year Dental Students*. University of Florida.

Rashid, A. M., Ling, K., Tassone, R. D., Resnick, P., Kraut, R., & Riedl, J. (2006). Motivating participation by displaying the value of contribution. *Proceedings of the SIGCHI Conference on Human Factors in Computing Systems, 2*, 955–958. DOI: 10.1145/1124772.1124915

Reeves S, Perrier L, Goldman J et al (2007). Inter-professional education: effects on professional practice and healthcare outcomes, Cochrane Database of systematic reviews 3,h t t p s: / / w w w. c o c h r a n e l i b r a r y. c o m / c d s r / d o i /, accessed on Jul 3, 2021DOI: 10.1002/14651858.CD002213.pub3/full

Reeves, S., Pelone, F., Harrison, R., Goldman, J., & Zwarenstein, M. (2018a). Interprofessional collaboration to improve professional practice and healthcare outcomes. *Cochrane Database of Systematic Reviews*, (8). Retrieved from https://ovidsp.ovid.com/ovidweb.cgi?T=JS&PAGE=reference&D=coch&NEWS=N&AN=00075320-100000000-00589

Reeves, S., Perrier, L., Goldman, J., Freeth, D., & Zwarenstein, M. (2018b). Interprofessional education: effects on professional practice and healthcare outcomes. *Cochrane Database of Systematic Reviews*, (8). Retrieved from https://ovidsp.ovid.com/ovidweb.cgi?T=JS&PAGE=reference&D=coch&NEWS=N&AN=00075320-100000000-01679

Reeves, S., & Hean, S. (2013). EDITORIAL Why we need theory to help us better understand the nature of interprofessional education, practice and care. *Journal of Interprofessional Care*, *27*(1), 1–3. DOI: 10.3109/13561820.2013.751293 PMID: 23256880

Reeves, S., Lewin, S., Espin, S., & Zwarenstein, M. (2010). *Interprofessional teamwork for health and social care*. Blackwell- Wiley. DOI: 10.1002/9781444325027

Reeves, S., Zwarenstein, M., Goldman, J., Barr, H., Freeth, D., Hammick, M., & Koppel, I. (2008). Interprofessional education: Effects on professional practice and health care outcomes. *Cochrane Database of Systematic Reviews*, (1). Advance online publication. DOI: 10.1002/14651858.CD002213.pub2 PMID: 18254002

Registered Nurses Association of Ontario. (2013). *Best practice guideline. Developing and sustaining interprofessional health care: Optimizing patient, organizational and system outcomes*. Retrieved July 25, 2024 https://rnao.ca/bpg/guidelines/interprofessional-team-work-healthcare

Reichers, A. E., Wanous, J. P., & Austin, J. T. (1997). Understanding and managing cynicism about organizational change. *The Academy of Management Perspectives*, *11*(1), 48–59. DOI: 10.5465/ame.1997.9707100659

Reilly, S., Hobson-Merrett, C., Gibbons, B., Jones, B., Richards, D., Plappert, H., & Planner, C. L. (2024). Collaborative care approaches for people with severe mental illness. *Cochrane Database of Systematic Reviews*, (5). Retrieved from https://ovidsp.ovid.com/ovidweb.cgi?T=JS&PAGE=reference&D=coch&NEWS=N&AN=00075320-100000000-07931

Rhoten, D. (2004). Interdisciplinary research: Trend or transition. *Items & Issues*, *5*(1-2), 6–11. https://items.ssrc.org/from-our-archives/interdisciplinary-research-trend-or-transition/

Riani, D. (2024). Reimagining Human Resource: Redefine Human Resource Management Practices for the Future. *Jurnal Riset Bisnis Dan Manajemen*, *17*(1), 149–157. DOI: 10.23969/jrbm.v17i1.12997

Rojak, J. A., Sanaji, S., Witjaksono, A. D., & Kistyanto, A. (2024). The influence of transformational leadership and organizational culture on employee performance. *EDUKASIA: Jurnal Pendidikan Dan Pembelajaran*, *5*(1), 977–990. DOI: 10.62775/edukasia.v5i1.926

Rosenman, E. D., Ilgen, J. S., Shandro, J. R., Harper, A. L., & Fernandez, R. (2015). A systematic review of tools used to assess team leadership in health care action teams. *Academic Medicine*, *90*(10), 1408–1422. DOI: 10.1097/ACM.0000000000000848 PMID: 26200585

Roussos, S. T., & Fawcett, S. B. (2000). A review of collaborative partnerships as a strategy for improving community health. *Annual Review of Public Health*, *21*(1), 369–402. DOI: 10.1146/annurev.publhealth.21.1.369 PMID: 10884958

Ruben, B. D., De Lisi, R., & Gigliotti, R. A. (2021). *A guide for leaders in higher education: Core concepts, competencies, and tools* (2nd ed.). Stylus.

Rundall, T. G. (2007). Evidence-based management. *Hospitals & Health Networks*, *81*(11), 72. PMID: 18175596

Rykhoff, M., Orchard, C., & Wong, C. (2015). *Interprofessional Collaborative Leadership: a concept analysis*. Unpublished PhD work. University of Western Ontario.

Sá, C. M. (2007). 'Interdisciplinary strategies' in U.S. research universities. *Higher Education*, *55*(5), 537–552. DOI: 10.1007/s10734-007-9073-5

Salfi, J., Prentice, D., Podwinski, K., Triemstra, C., & Hildebrand, L. (2019). The Impact of an Interprofessional Education (IPE) Clinical Teaching Unit on Developing Collaborative Skills and Behaviors: A Pilot Case Study. Unpublished manuscript.

Salfi, J., Solomon, P., Allen, D., Mohaupt, J., & Patterson, C. (2012). Overcoming all obstacles: A framework for embedding interprofessional education (IPE) into a large, multi-site BScN program. *The Journal of Nursing Education*, *51*, 106–110. DOI: 10.3928/01484834-20111230-05 PMID: 22201276

Salvatore, F. P. (2022). *Management and performance in healthcare: economic and business aspects of healthcare companies*. Giuffrè Francesco Lefebvre.

Salvioni, D. (2007). Corporate governance, control and transparency. Milan: Franco Angeli editore.

Sangseok, Y., & Robert, L. P. (2023). Subgroup formation in human-robot teams: A multi-study mixed methods approach with implications for theory and practice. *Journal of the Association for Information Science and Technology*, *74*(3), 323–338. DOI: 10.1002/asi.24626

Schein, E. H., & Schein, P. A. (2018). *Humble Leadership: The Power of Relationships, Openness and Trust*. Berrett-Koehler Publishers.

Schot, E., Tummers, L., & Noordegraaf, M. (2020). Working on working together. A systematic review on how healthcare professionals contribute to interprofessional collaboration. *Journal of Interprofessional Care*, *34*(3), 332–342. DOI: 10.1080/13561820.2019.1636007 PMID: 31329469

Secinaro, , Calandra, D., Secinaro, A., Muthurangu, V., & Biancone, P. (2021). The role of artificial intelligence in healthcare: A structured literature review. *BMC Medical Informatics and Decision Making*, *21*(1), 125. DOI: 10.1186/s12911-021-01488-9

Senge, P. M. (2006) *The fifth discipline: The art and practice of the learning organization*. Broadway.

Senge, P. M. (2006). *The fifth discipline: The art and practice of the learning organization*. Doubleday Publishing Group, Inc.

Shiwani, T., Relton, S., Evans, R., Kale, A., Heaven, A., Clegg, A., Abuzour, A., Alderman, J., Anand, A., Bhanu, C., Bunn, J., Collins, J., Cutillo, L., Hall, M., Keevil, V., Mitchell, L., Ogliari, G., Penfold, R., van Oppen, J., & Todd, O.Ageing Data Research Collaborative. (2023). New horizons in artificial intelligence in the healthcare of older people. *Age and Ageing*, *52*(12), afad219. Advance online publication. DOI: 10.1093/ageing/afad219 PMID: 38124256

Shiwlani, A., Khan, M., Sherani, A. M. K., & Qayyum, M. U. (2023). Synergies of AI and Smart Technology: Revolutionizing Cancer Medicine, Vaccine Development, and Patient Care. International Journal of Social. *Humanities and Life Sciences*, *1*(1), 10–18.

Shulman, L. S. (2005). Signature pedagogies in the professions. *Daedalus*, *134*(3), 52–59. DOI: 10.1162/0011526054622015

Siedlok, F., & Hibbert, P. (2014). The organization of interdisciplinary research: Modes, drivers and barriers. *International Journal of Management Reviews*, *16*(2), 194–210. DOI: 10.1111/ijmr.12016

Siedlok, F., Hibbert, P., & Sillince, J. (2015). From practice to collaborative community in interdisciplinary research contexts. *Research Policy*, *44*(1), 96–107. DOI: 10.1016/j.respol.2014.07.018

Simms, L. W., Dalston, J. W., & Roberts, P. W. (1984). Collaborative practice: Myth or reality? *Hospital & Health Services Administration*, *29*(6), 36–48. PMID: 10268659

Slawomirski, L., & Klazinga, N. (2020). *The economics of patient safety: from analysis to action*. Organisation for Economic Co-operation and Development., https://www.oecd.org/health/health-systems/Economics-of-Patient-Safety-October-2020.pdf

Smedley, B. D., Stith, A. Y., & Nelson, A. R. (Eds.). (2003). Unequal treatment: Confronting racial and ethnics disparities in health care. In *Journal of the National Medical Association*: Vol. 94. *Issue 8* (pp. 666–668). National Academies Press., DOI: 10.17226/12875

Smith, C., Baveja, R., Grieb, T., & Mashour, G. A. (2017). Toward a science of translational science. *Journal of Clinical and Translational Science*, *1*(4), 253–255. DOI: 10.1017/cts.2017.14 PMID: 29657860

Stuber, F., Seifried-Dübon, T., Rieger, M. A., Gündel, H., Ruhle, S., Zipfel, S., & Junne, F. (2021). The effectiveness of health-oriented leadership interventions for the improvement of mental health of employees in the health care sector: A systematic review. *International Archives of Occupational and Environmental Health*, *94*(2), 203–220. DOI: 10.1007/s00420-020-01583-w PMID: 33011902

Sturm, A., Ager, A., & Roth, R. (2022). Western ideals and global realities – physiotherapists' views on factors that play a role in ethical decision-making: an international qualitative analysis. *European Journal of Physiotherapy, 26* (1), 12-24. Doi: . 2022.2155.240.DOI: 10.1080/21679169

Sumeth, T., & Li, X. (2013). Is there a relationship between individual learning, team learning, and organizational learning? *The Alberta Journal of Educational Research, 59*(1), 1–16. DOI: 10.55016/ojs/ajer.v59i1.55542

Sun, T., Wang, J., Zhang, S., Shi, Y., Liu, B., & Wang, X. (2021). Status, causes and consequences of physicians' self-perceived reputation damage in China: A cross-sectional survey. *BMC Health Services Research, 21*(1), 344. DOI: 10.1186/s12913-021-06306-6 PMID: 33853589

Tannenbaum, S. I., & Cerasoli, C. P. (2013) Do Team and Individual Debriefs Enhance Performance? A Meta-Analysis._https://journals.sagepub.com/doi/epub/10.1177/0018720812448394

Tannenbaum, S.I., Beard,R.L., & Cerasoli, C.P.(2013) Conducting team debriefings the work.

Tariq, , Awan, M. J., Alshudukhi, J., Alam, T. M., Alhamazani, K. T., & Meraf, Z. (2022). Software Measurement by Using Artificial Intelligence. *Journal of Nanomaterials, 2022*(1), 7283171. DOI: 10.1155/2022/7283171

Tavakol, M., & Dennick, R. (2011). Making sense of Cronbach's alpha. *International Journal of Medical Education, 2*, 53–55. DOI: 10.5116/ijme.4dfb.8dfd PMID: 28029643

Thistlethwaite, J., & Xyrichis, A. (2022). Forecasting interprofessional education and collaborative practice: Towards a dystopian or utopian future? *Journal of Interprofessional Care, 36*(2), 165–167. DOI: 10.1080/13561820.2022.2056696 PMID: 35484900

Thompson, J. L. (2009). Building collective communication competence in interdisciplinary research teams. *Journal of Applied Communication Research, 37*(3), 278–297. DOI: 10.1080/00909880903025911

Thorpe, H., Clark, M., Brice, J., & Sims, S. (2020). The transdisciplinary health research apparatus: A Baradian account of knowledge boundaries and beyond. *Health*. Advance online publication. DOI: 10.1177/1363459320961429 PMID: 33012195

Touati, N., Rodríguez, C., Paquette, M.-A., & Denis, J.-L. (2018). Understanding the emergence and development of medical collaboration across organizational boundaries: A longitudinal case study. *Health*, *22*(6), 580–602. DOI: 10.1177/1363459317724852 PMID: 28795577

Tsakitzidis, G., Timmermans, O., Callewaert, N., Verhoeven, V., Lopez-Hartmann, M., Truijen, S., Meulemans, H., & Van Royen, P. (2016). Outcome indicators on interprofessional collaboration interventions for elderly. *International Journal of Integrated Care*, *16*(2), 5. Advance online publication. DOI: 10.5334/ijic.2017 PMID: 27616961

Tuckman, B. W. (1965). Developmental sequence in small groups. *Psychological Bulletin*, *63*(6), 384–399. DOI: 10.1037/h0022100 PMID: 14314073

Tuckman, B. W., & Jensen, M. A. (1977). Stages of Small-Group Development Revisited. *Group & Organization Studies*, *2*(4), 419–427. Advance online publication. DOI: 10.1177/105960117700200404

U.S. Department of Health & Human Services (HHS). (n.d.). Healthy people 2030. https://health.gov/healthypeople/objectives-and-data/social-determinants-health

Ullah, H., Manickam, S., Obaidat, M., Laghari, S. U. A., & Uddin, M. (2023). Exploring the Potential of Metaverse Technology in Healthcare: Applications, Challenges, and Future Directions. *IEEE Access : Practical Innovations, Open Solutions*, *11*, 69686–69707. DOI: 10.1109/ACCESS.2023.3286696

Vallentin, A., Thórisson, K. R., & Latapie, H. (2023). Addressing the Unsustainability of Deep Neural Networks with Next-Gen AI. In International Conference on Artificial General Intelligence (pp. 296-306). Cham: Springer Nature Switzerland. DOI: 10.1007/978-3-031-33469-6_30

Van Klaveren, L., Geukers, V., & de Vos, R. (2024). Care complexity, perceptions of complexity and preferences for interprofessional collaboration: An analysis of relationships and social networks in paediatrics. *BMC Medical Education*, *24*(1), 334. DOI: 10.1186/s12909-024-05304-6 PMID: 38528513

VanVactor, J. D. (2012). Collaborative leadership model in the management of health care. *Journal of Business Research*, *65*(4), 555–561. DOI: 10.1016/j.jbusres.2011.02.021

Varkey, B. (2021). Principles of clinical ethics and their application to practice. *Medical Principles and Practice : International Journal of the Kuwait University, Health Science Centre*, *30*(1), 17–28. DOI: 10.1159/000509119 PMID: 32498071

Vaughn, L. M., Jacquez, F., & Zhen-Duan, J. (2018). Perspectives of community co-researchers about group dynamics and equitable partnership within a community-academic research team. *Health Education & Behavior*, *45*(5), 682–689. DOI: 10.1177/1090198118769374 PMID: 29618239

Vicarelli, G. (2004). Corporateisation and management in the evolution of the Italian health system. In Health and society. Milan: Franco Angeli editore.

Vlasta, M. (2023). A methodological framework for European regulation of (artificial) intelligence and its limits.

Voyer, B. (2013). Changes in the relations and roles of doctors and nurses. *British Journal of Health Care Management*, *19*(1), 16–21. DOI: 10.12968/bjhc.2013.19.1.16

Wagter, J. M., van de Bunt, G., Honing, M., Eckenhausen, M., & Scherpbier, A. (2012). Informal interprofessional learning: Visualizing the clinical workplace. *Journal of Interprofessional Care*, *26*(3), 173–182. DOI: 10.3109/13561820.2012.656773 PMID: 22332642

Walker, L., & Avant, K. C. (2005). *Strategies for theory construction in nursing* (4th ed.). Pearson Prentice Hall.

Walter, C., Soni, T., Gavin, M. A., Kubes, J., & Paciullo, K. (2022). An interprofessional approach to reducing hospital-onset *Clostridioides difficile* infections. *American Journal of Infection Control*, *50*(12), 1346–1351. DOI: 10.1016/j.ajic.2022.02.017 PMID: 35569613

Wamba, S. F., Queiroz, M. M., Jabbour, C. J. C., & Shi, C. V. (2023). Are both generative AI and ChatGPT game changers for 21st-century operations and supply chain excellence? *International Journal of Production Economics*, *265*, 109015. DOI: 10.1016/j.ijpe.2023.109015

Wang, X., Liu, Y., Peng, Z., Li, B., Liang, Q., Liao, S., & Liu, M. (2024). Situational leadership theory in nursing management: A scoping review. *BMC Nursing*, *23*(1), 930. DOI: 10.1186/s12912-024-02582-9 PMID: 39702117

Wani, . (2022). Utilization of Artificial Intelligence in Disease Prevention: Diagnosis, Treatment, and Implications for the Healthcare Workforce. *Health Care*.

Weber, E., Wyverkens, A., & Leuridan, B. (2024). Rethinking evidence-based management. *Philosophy of Management*, *23*(1), 59–84. DOI: 10.1007/s40926-023-00236-5

Webster, L., & Shirley, J. (2016). No need to object: Ethical obligations for interprofessional collaboration in emergency department discharge planning. *Annual Review of Nursing Research, 34*(1), 183–XI. DOI: 10.1891/0739-6686.34.183 PMID: 26673382

Wei, H., Horns, P., Sears, S. F., Huang, K., Smith, C. M., & Wei, T. H. (2022). A systematic meta-review of systematic reviews about interprofessional collaboration: Facilitators, barriers, and outcomes. *Journal of Interprofessional Care, 36*(5), 735–749. DOI: 10.1080/13561820.2021.1973975 PMID: 35129041

Weinstein, J. N., Geller, A., Negussie, Y., & Baciu, A. (Eds.). (2017). *Communities in action: Pathways to health equity*. The National Academies Press. DOI: 10.17226/24624

Whitmer, A., Ogden, L., Lawton, J., Sturner, P., Groffman, P. M., Schneider, L., Hart, D., Halpern, B., Schlesinger, W., Raciti, S., Bettez, N., Ortega, S., Rustad, L., Pickett, S. T., & Killilea, M. (2010). The engaged university: Providing a platform for research that transforms society. *Frontiers in Ecology and the Environment, 8*(6), 314–321. DOI: 10.1890/090241

Will, K. K., Johnson, M. L., & Lamb, G. (2019). Team-based care and patient satisfaction in the hospital setting: A systematic review. *Journal of Patient-Centered Research and Reviews, 6*(2), 158–171. DOI: 10.17294/2330-0698.1695 PMID: 31414027

World Health Organization (WHO). (2010) *Framework for action on IPE & collaborative practice.* WHO, Geneva, Switzerland. Retrieved from: https://iris.who.int/bitstream/handle/10665/70185/WHO_HRH_HPN_10.3_eng.pdf

World Health Organization (WHO). (2010). *Framework for action on interprofessional education and collaborative practice. (WHO/HRH/HPN/10.3)*. WHO.

World Health Organization. (2010). Framework for action on interprofessional education and collaborative practice. Geneva, Switzerland: WHO https://www.who.int/publications/i/item/framework-for-action-on-interprofessional-education-collaborative-practice

World Health Organization. (2018). Health professions networks: nursing and midwifery human resources: Framework for action on interprofessional education and collaborative practice. *https://interprofessional.global/wp-content/uploads/2018/11/WHO-2010-WHO-framework-for-action-on-interprofessional-education-collaborative-practice.pdf*

World Health Organization. (September 11, 2023). *Patient safety*. Retrieved January 4, 2024. https://www.who.int/news-room/fact-sheets/detail/patient-safety

World Health Organization. 2024. *Health workforce*. Retrieved June 26, 2024, https://www.who.int/health-topics/health-workforce#tab=tab_1

World Health Organization. Health Professions Network Nursing and Midwifery Office within the Department of Human Resources for Health (2010) Framework for action on interprofessional education and collaborative practice. Geneva Switzerland: World Health Organization. https://www.who.int/hrh/nursing-midwifery/en/

Wright, D., & Brajtman, S. (2011). Relational and embodied knowing: Nursing ethics within the interprofessional team. *Nursing Ethics*, *18*(1), 20–30. DOI: 10.1177/0969733010386165 PMID: 21285194

Wright, K. N., Williams, P., Wright, S., Lieber, E., Carrasco, S. R., & Gedjeyan, H. (2011). Ties that bind: Creating and sustaining community-academic partnerships. *Gateways : International Journal of Community Research & Engagement*, *4*, 83–99. DOI: 10.5130/ijcre.v4i0.1784

Yamaguchi, E. (2017). Cultivating a learning hospital organization: striving for better quality and safety in medical care (Japanese) *System/Control/Information*, Vol. 61, No. 6, pp. 233–239.

Yamamoto, T. (2014). Empirical research on organizational change in hospitals through team medical care (Japanese). *Kawasaki Medical Welfare Journal*, *23*(2), 255–267.

Yasuda, H., Kawamukai, H., & Nishimura, H. (2021). Relationship analysis of failure risk factors in small and medium-sized company projects focusing on co-occurrence. *Journal of Japan Society of Information and Knowledge*, *31*(2), 181–185. DOI: 10.2964/jsik_2021_024

Yoon, S. W., Song, J. H., Lim, D. H., & Joo, B.-K. (2010). Structural determinants of team performance: The mutual influences of learning culture, creativity, and knowledge. *Human Resource Development International*, *13*(3), 249–264. DOI: 10.1080/13678868.2010.483815

Young, G. (2019). Personhood across disciplines: Application to ethical theory and mental health ethics. *Ethics, Medicine, and Public Health*, *10*, 93–101. DOI: 10.1016/j.jemep.2019.100407

Yulianti, T., & Sulistyawati, A. (2021). Enhancing public speaking ability through focus group discussion. [Pendidikan Dan Pengajaran]. *JURNAL PAJAR*, *5*(2), 287–295.

Zheng, Y., Palombella, A., Salfi, J., & Wainman, B. (2018). Dissecting through barriers: A follow-up study on the long-term effects of interprofessional education in a dissection course with healthcare professional students. *Anatomic Science Education (ASE). Anatomical Sciences Education, 12*(1), 52–60. DOI: 10.1002/ase.1791 PMID: 29659188

Zwarenstein, M., Goldman, J., & Reeves, S. (2009). Interprofessional collaboration: Effects of practice-based interventions on professional practice and healthcare outcomes. *Cochrane Database of Systematic Reviews*, (3). Advance online publication. DOI: 10.1002/14651858.CD000072.pub2 PMID: 19588316

About the Contributors

Dawn Prentice is a Professor and Concurrent BNMN Graduate Program Director in the Department of Nursing, Brock University. Dr. Prentice has worked in a variety of nursing roles including staff nurse, researcher, educator and leadership positions. Her research interests include intraprofessional and interprofessional collaboration.

***

Dora Almeida is a University Professor and a research fellow at Universidade Europeia. Her research interests currently are public policies and political science, innovation and business management issues. She is also External Expert of Dynamic Capabilities Operational Progressive Institute, Switzerland.

Noah Mike Barr is an accomplished professional with a dynamic career in technology and healthcare management. He holds advanced degrees that blend his expertise in computer science and health administration, which underpin his innovative approaches to solving industry challenges. Barr's career spans significant achievements across healthcare technology, financial systems, and administrative strategy. With a unique combination of technical expertise and management acumen, he has contributed to transformative projects, advancing innovation in critical sectors. Barr's dedication to improving systems through integrated methodologies has made him a respected voice in his fields of study and practice.

Ubaldo Comite was born in Cosenza, Italy, June 14 1971. He has a degree in Law (1994) and Economics (1996) at the University of Messina (Italy), and earned his Ph.D. in Public Administration at the University of Calabria, Rende (Cs) Italy, in 2005. Currently he is a professor of Budget and Business Organization at the Faculty of Economy, Department of Business Sciences, University of Calabria. Furthermore he is a professor of Business Administration and Health Management at the Faculty of Economy, University Giustino Fortunato (Benevento – Italy). His Research interests are: Private and Public Management, Non profit Organizations and Accounting, Health Management. E-mail, u.comite@unifortunato.eu Key words areas specialization: management, public administration, accountancy, health management

Joyce Engel has a PhD (U of Alberta) in nursing, as well as a MEd (U of Calgary), BEd (U of Calgary), and a RN Diploma (Lethbridge). As a staff nurse in mental health and community settings, educator, researcher, leader, and administrator, interprofessional practice and programming have been significant components of her practice and as an educator, author, and researcher, ethics has been of particular interest. Currently, Dr. Engel is a project consultant in curriculum and evaluation and is also an adjunct professor at Brock University, where she was an assistant and then associate professor in nursing.

Ralph A Gigliotti, Rutgers University (ralph.gigliotti@rutgers.edu) Ralph serves as Assistant Vice President for Organizational Leadership in University Academic Affairs at Rutgers University. In this role, he directs the Rutgers Office of Organizational Leadership and provides executive leadership for a portfolio of signature leadership development programs, consultation services, and applied research initiatives. Ralph serves as a trusted advisor for senior leaders across Rutgers in the areas of change leadership, crisis leadership, organizational strategy, and continuous improvement. He is responsible for the advancement of academic change and transformation projects of strategic importance to the university. Ralph holds part-time faculty appointments in the Department of Communication (School of Communication and Information), Ph.D. Program in Higher Education (Graduate School of Education), Department of Family Medicine and Community Health (Robert Wood Johnson Medical School), and Rutgers Business School. He teaches courses in undergraduate, master's, doctoral, and executive education programs. His research and consulting interests explore topics related to leadership, crisis, strategy, team dynamics, organizational communication, and training and development within the context of higher education. He is author and editor of 10 books and over 50 peer-reviewed journal articles and book chapters. Ralph is president of the Network for Change and Continuous Innovation (NCCI)—an organization of nearly 100 colleges and universities from across North America who seek to advance sustainable excellence in higher education by promoting successful practices and approaches used to drive change, innovation, and continuous improvement across academic and administrative functions. Additionally, he serves as a member of the Malcolm Baldrige National Quality Award Board of Examiners (National Institute of Standards and Technology, United States Department of Commerce), co-lead for the New Jersey Alliance for Clinical and Translational Science (NJ ACTS) Team Science Core, and co-lead of the Distinction in Leadership in Academic Healthcare Program at Rutgers University. Ralph is the recipient of numerous national and local teaching, research, and service awards.

Christine Goldthwaite (cgoldthwaite@me.com) Christine Goldthwaite, Ph.D., is an organizational development consultant, leadership coach, and educator with over 15 years of experience in higher education. She currently serves as a Senior Organizational Development Consultant at Yale University, where she partners with units across the institution to develop comprehensive strategies for staff learning and development. She is an Associate Certified Coach (ACC) through the International Coaching Federation (ICF), holds a certification in coaching for Emotional and Social Competency through Korn Ferry International, and a certification in Leadership Coaching for Organizational Performance through Rutgers University. She is a co-author of Leadership in Digital Contexts (Kendall Hunt, 2023); Leadership in Academic Health Centers: Core Concepts and Critical Cases (Kendall Hunt, 2021); and Leadership: Social Influence in Personal and Professional Settings (Kendall Hunt, 2017). As an organizational communication scholar, her research and consulting interests explore the intersection of organization design and communication design in relation to interdisciplinary and interprofessional collaboration. She is also a part-time lecturer at the Rutgers School of Communication and Information, where she teaches Organizational Leadership. Education Rutgers University Ph.D., Organizational Communication Rutgers University M.C.I.S., Organizational Communication Montclair State University B.A., Communication Studies

Wako Jio, PhD Research Scholar, Department of Management, Bule Hora University, Ethiopia

Shashi Kant, Associate Professor, Mittal School of Business, Lovely Professional University, India

Yuka Murata, Educational Background 1983 Graduated from Yamaguchi Red Cross College of Nursing 2005 Graduated from Tamagawa University, Department of Education, Faculty of Literature, Correspondence Course 2008 Completed Master's Degree in Nursing Administration, Japanese Red Cross Hiroshima College of Nursing Master's degree in nursing 9. 2019 Withdrawal with Completion of Course Credits from Hiroshima University Graduate School of Integrated Arts and Sciences, Second Semester Doctoral Course 3. 2020 Completed Doctoral program, Graduate School of Integrated Arts and Sciences, Hiroshima University Career 1983- Japanese Red Cross Yamaguchi Hospital 2004- Lecturer at Japanese Red

Cross Hiroshima College of Nursing 2022- Vice President at Japanese Red Cross Hiroshima College of Nursing

Carole Orchard is currently Professor Emerita and Adjunct Research Professor in the Arthur Labatt Family School of Nursing and the former Coordinator of Interprofessional Health Education & Research at the University of Western Ontario. Her research focuses on interprofessional client-centred collaborative practice. Dr. Orchard and her colleagues have developed several measurement instruments: Interprofessional Socialization & Valuing Scale (ISVS) and the Assessment of Interprofessional Team Collaboration Scale-II (AITCS-II for practitioners), AITCS-II for students, and Interprofessional Collaborative Leadership Scale (AICLS). Dr. Orchard co-chaired the Canadian Interprofessional Health Collaborative's IP Competency Working Group who developed the 2010 CIHC National IP Competency Framework and has been involved in its 2024 revision. In 2015 she published a book with colleagues on Interprofessional Client-Centered Collaborative Practice: What does it look like? How can it be achieved? Her research currently focuses on the role of patients both in their own self-care and in collaborative teams. Currently she and colleagues are testing an online training program in Interprofessional Team Conflict Resolution. Her work is frequently cited in the field of IPC.

Antonio Pesqueira is a healthcare and pharmaceutical commercial and supply chain management leader, with an emphasis on technological advancements and process improvement. Concurrently, he holds esteemed academic positions as a professor and research fellow at ISCTE/IUL. Within the Technology and Architecture Research Department, he contributes to the Ph.D. program, focusing his research on digital technologies, healthcare data management, blockchain, and the nexus of innovation and business management. He has notably chaired the Pharmaceutical Supply Chain & Security World Forum and is often invited as a keynote speaker at events such as the Pharma Track & Trace, and Serialization & Labeling Summit. Co-authored more than 20 scholarly articles and book chapters that have been featured in prestigious scientific journals. These include the Journal of Business Research, Future Generations Computer Systems, Journal of Medical Systems, Knowledge Management, WSEAS Transactions on Business and Economics, and Information Systems Frontiers, to name a few. Moreover, his outstanding contributions have been acknowledged at various peer-reviewed international conferences.

Jenn Salfi worked at McMaster University as Faculty Lead for Interprofessional Education (IPE) for 14 years before coming to Brock University in September 2013. She is currently Assistant Chair and Associate Professor with the Department of Nursing and continues to be involved in a variety of nursing and interprofessional education initiatives. Jenn is also a core faculty member with the Master of Applied Gerontology (MAG) program where she teaches a course on interprofessional collaboration.

Sara E Spear, Yale University (sara.spear@yale.edu) Sara is Director of Academic Affairs and Director of the First-Year Scholars at Yale (FSY) Program at Yale University. In this role, Sara provides strategic leadership to Yale Summer Session, overseeing curricular and course development of 150+ summer courses, faculty recruitment and appointments, and student academic advising. Sara is also responsible for executing the vision and strategy of the FSY Program, a residential summer bridge program for 96 first-generation, low-income (FGLI) incoming first-year students at Yale. Prior to Yale, Sara worked at Rutgers University as Assistant Director at the Center for Organizational Leadership and Assistant Dean at the Office of Advising & Academic Services for the School of Arts and Sciences. Sara completed her B.A. in History at Mount Holyoke College followed by a Master's and Ph.D. in Higher Education at Rutgers University.

Risa Suzuki is an Associate Professor at Faculty of Human Sciences at Waseda University, physiotherapist. She holds a Doctor of Human Sciences from the Graduate School of Human Sciences, Waseda University, and a master's degree from the Graduate School of Media and Governance, Keio University. Her research interests include biofeedback, health management, bio instrumentation, ICT application, and neurorehabilitation. She has significantly contributed to physiotherapist education at Japanese physiotherapist training institutions such as Bunkyo Gakuin University and Tokoha University. Her recent research interests reflect her commitment to advancing the field of rehabilitation. Her focus has expanded to include therapist education, inter-professional collaboration, and the organizational climate in the medical field. She is also involved in the development of innovative movement analysis systems and biofeedback devices for rehabilitation.

Yumi Tamura, March 1977: Graduated from Matsuyama Red Cross Nursing College April 1977: Matsuyama Red Cross Hospital (Neurosurgery Ward) May 1979: Osaka Red Cross Hospital (Surgery, Urology, Dermatology Mixed Ward) September 1981: Matsuyama Red Cross Hospital (Surgery, Intensive Care Unit, Urology Ward, Head Nurse of Urology Ward since April 1990) July 1990: ICRC International Relief Dispatch (Quetta, Islamic Republic of Pakistan) July 1991: IFRC International Relief Dispatch (Yerevan, Republic of Armenia) September 1993: Graduated from Bukkyo University, Faculty of Sociology, Department of Social Welfare March 1996: London South Bank University (LSBU), Graduate School of Health and Social Care, Inter-professional Education Graduated from London

South Bank University Graduate School of Health and Social Welfare Studies (MSc. Interprofessional Education and Research Course) April 1996: Assistant, Nursing Department, Faculty of Medicine, Kagawa Medical University (now Kagawa University) April 1997: Lecturer, Nursing Department, Faculty of Medicine, Kagawa Medical University (now Kagawa University) April 2001: Associate Professor, Department of Health Sciences, Kobe University Faculty of Medicine, Kobe University Graduate School of Medicine April 2005: Professor, Department of Health Sciences, Kobe University Faculty of Medicine, Kobe University Graduate School of Medicine April 2011: Professor, Shigeki University Graduate School of Medical Sciences September 2012: Waseda University Faculty of Human Sciences (PhD, Human Sciences) April 2014: Professor, Japanese Red Cross College of Nursing (Disaster Nursing Global Leader Program: DNGL) April 2020: President, Japanese Red Cross Hiroshima College of Nursing (current position)

Index

L

M

P

R

S

T

V

Z

www.ingramcontent.com/pod-product-compliance
Lightning Source LLC
LaVergne TN
LVHW080643011026
849160LV00014B/1309
* 9 7 9 8 3 3 7 3 3 6 3 1 2 *